CANCER ETIOLOGY, DIAGNOSIS AND TREATMENTS

MULTIPLE MYELOMA

RISK FACTORS, DIAGNOSIS AND TREATMENTS

CANCER ETIOLOGY, DIAGNOSIS AND TREATMENTS

Additional books in this series can be found on Nova's website under the Series tab.

Additional e-books in this series can be found on Nova's website under the e-book tab.

CANCER ETIOLOGY, DIAGNOSIS AND TREATMENTS

MULTIPLE MYELOMA

RISK FACTORS, DIAGNOSIS AND TREATMENTS

STEVE HOLT
EDITOR

NOVA BIOMEDICAL

New York

For permission to use material from this book please contact us:
Telephone 631-231-7269; Fax 631-231-8175
Web Site: http://www.novapublishers.com

Library of Congress Cataloging-in-Publication Data

ISBN: 978-1-63321-514-6
Library of Congress Control Number: 2014944852

Published by Nova Science Publishers, Inc. † New York

Contents

Preface

Multiple myeloma (MM) is a hematological malignancy characterized by the clonal expansion of monoclonal immunoglobulin-secreting plasma cells in the bone marrow (BM). MM is associated with lytic bone lesions, anemia, immunodeficiency, and renal impairment. Multiple myeloma accounts for more than 10% of all hematologic malignancies and about 1% of all cancers. Multiple myeloma remains mostly incurable despite conventional intensive high dose chemotherapy followed by hematopoietic stem cell transplant. The costs associated with multiple myeloma are among the highest. This book discusses the diagnosis of multiple myeloma along with the risk factors involved and the treatments that are available.

Chapter 1 - Multiple myeloma (MM) is a stem cell malignancy arising from a single plasma cell clone that secretes a monoclonal immunoglobulin. Clinical outcome depend on multiple risk factors which include performance status, age, international stage and cytogenetics including mutated and translocated oncogenes. The Mayo clinic's risk-stratification tool (mSMART) based on cytogenetic markers categorizes patients into low, intermediate, and high risk that guides initial therapy. Despite the addition of newer and more effective therapeutic options for MM, the disease remains incurable. The goal of therapy is focused on improving overall survival, progression free survival, duration of complete response, and quality of life. This is largely due to novel agents, combination therapies, better targeting of the tumor microenvironment and autologous stem cell transplantation. Currently FDA approved therapeutic options include immunomodulatory (iMiDs) drugs, proteaosome inhibitors, alkylators, anthracycline, vinca alkaloid, and steroids. Bortezomib and lenalidomide have become the backbone for transplant eligible patients with induction therapy in combination with other agents. Various combinations exist; bortezomib and dexamethasone with lenalidomide, thalidomide, cyclophosphamide, or liposomal doxorubicin. In transplant ineligible patients induction therapies overlap but include mephalan plus dexamethasone with bortezomib, lenalidomide, or thalidomide. As knowledge of the molecular pathways in combination of whole exome sequencing continues to expand, novel therapies will be matched to underlying biology. The authors discuss these exciting drugs, their mechanism of action, pathways, and their incorporation into ongoing clinical trials to improve overall syrvival. Examples of cell surface and extracellular targets include EGFR, CS-1, IGF-1R, CD40, CD38, CD138, PD-1 and PD-L1 respectively. Of the novel agents, a humanized IgG1 monoclonal antibody to CD38 SAR650984 (SAR) showed a favorable toxicity profile and encouraging single agent activity in an early phase clinical trial. OSI-906 an oral IGF-1R kinase inhibitor in combination with bortezomib was cytotoxic to

MM cell lines in a dose-dependent manner suggesting a high degree of synergy for combination therapy. A phase I trial evaluating OSI-906 in combination with bortezomib plus dexamethasone is underway. Of the intracellular targeted agents novel proteosome inhibitors, Bcl2 inhibitors, HSP90 inhibitors, AKT inhibitors, mTOR inhibitors, p38 MAPK inhibitors, autophagy inducers, HDAC inhibitors, aurora kinase and CDK inhibitors have shown promising in vivo activity. TGO2 a multi-kinase inhibitor of CDK 1, 2, 9, JAK2, FLT3, in addition to MAPK, ERK5 in MM cell lines resulted in arrest and rapid apoptosis. TGO2 is under evaluation in phase I clinical trials alone or in combination with carfilzomib. Finally, chimeric antigen receptors (CARs) which are synthetic trans-membrane proteins are being utilized to redirect autologous T-cells with specificity for surface antigens on MM cells. Current targets are the Kappa light chain, CD138, and Lewis Y antigen. CARs targeting BCMA, CS1, and CD38 are in pre-clinical investigation. Initial CARs therapy would focus on R/R MM, while consolidation strategies after first-line therapy or in conjunction with autologous stem cell transplantation are promising.

Chapter 2 - Multiple myeloma (MM) is the most common primary bone malignancy, characterized by accumulation of terminally differentiated B-lymphocytes, malignant plasma cells, within bone marrow.

MM remains mostly an incurable disease with high morbidity in the most cases. The introduction of novel agents has improved outcomes for patients with MM during the last years. The ubiquitin-proteasome path-way (UPP) is responsible for degradation of numerous proteins involved in MM cell proliferation, survival, and drug resistance. UPP is a major proteolytic system for proteins mediating the cell cycle and controlling apoptosis including cyclin-dependent kinase inhibitors (p21/CIP1, WAF1 and p27/KIP1), cyclin D, cyclin E, the dual-specificity phosphatase cdc 25, the protein kinase Wee1, p53, inhibitors of apoptosis proteins /IAPs/, caspases, NF-κB inhibitor IκB and others).

Bortezomib (Velcade^{TM}, PS-341) is boronate-based dipeptide proteasome inhibitor (PI) that primarily targets the chymotrypsin-like activities of the intracellular proteasome enzyme complex. Bortezomib was approved by the US Food and Drug Administration in 2003 and fully in 2005 in MM patients who have received at least one prior therapy. For optimization of clinical response and disease control bortezomib-based combination strategies (with alkylating agents: melphalan, cyclophospha-mide, bendamustine; glucocoticoids: prednisone, dexamethasone; and immunomodulatory drugs) have been effectively used, particularly in relapsed or refractory MM patients who have exhausted the standard therapies or those who are not eligible for autologous stem cell trans-plantation. Bortezomib directly induces apoptosis of tumor cells and reverses drug resistance of MM cells by affecting cytosine circuits, cell adhesion and angiogenesis in bone marrow microenvironment.

However, a considerable proportion of MM patients fail to respond to bortezomib and many MM patients relapse from this drug, either when it is used alone or as bortezomib-based combinations.

Therefore the new PI generation with the higher efficacy of proteasome inhibition, the enhanced antitumor activity and the decreased toxicity was developed.

Chapter 3 - Cereblon (CRBN) was named according to its putative role in cerebral development, especially in memory and learning. A nonsense mutation in CRBN causes autosomal recessive nonsyndromic mental retardation. CRBN is a member and substrate receptor of the cullin 4 ring E3 ubiquitin ligase complex (CRL4). CRL4 consists of Cullin 4,

RING finger protein (Roc1), and DNA damage binding protein 1 (DDB1). CRBN binds to its substrate proteins and it leads to ubiquitination of these substrates by the CRL4.

CRBN is a primary target of thalidomide teratogenicity. The binding of immunomodulatory drugs (IMiDs) to CRBN is associated with cytotoxicity of IMiDs and is used to treat multiple myeloma (MM), myelo-dysplastic syndromes (MDS) and lymphomas. The *CRBN* gene consists of 1329 base pairs, 11 exons, and encodes a protein of 443 amino acids. Exons 10-11 code for the binding site of IMiDs and exons 5-7 for the binding site of DDB1. CRBN plays a key role in mediating the antiproliferative and immunomodulatory activities of IMiDs in MM cells and T cells, respectively. Two target proteins, the zinc finger containing transcription factors Ikaros (IKZF1) and Aiolos (IKZF3) have been recently revealed by analysis of MM cell lines treated with lenalidomide. IMiDs induce the CRBN-dependent proteasomal degradation of IKZF1 and IKZF3. Both these factors are required for the viability of MM cell lines. IKZF1 bind and activate interferon regulatory factor 4 gene (*IRF4*) promoters and *MYC* expression in B cells. IKZF1/3 are known repressors of the interleukin 2 gene (*IL-2*) promoter in T cells. CRBN directly interacts with the α-subunit of 5´-adenosine monophosphate-activated protein kinase (AMPK) and reduces the enzymatic activity of AMPK by suppressing phosphorylation of its catalytic subunit. This AMPK inhibition activates MdmX (murine double minute X, also known as MDM4) and the mammalian target of rapamycin (mTOR) pathway.

Chapter 4 – *Introduction:* Multiple myeloma (MM) is a malignant disease characterized by uncontrolled plasma tumor cell proliferation, produced by extrinsic stromal cell support and intrinsic chromosomal abnormalities together with the presence of monoclonal protein in blood or urine or both. Typical clinical presentation at diagnosis includes anemia, skeletal lesions, renal impairment, and hypercalcemia. In recent years, the introduction of novel agents such as proteasome inhibitor bortezomib, thalidomide, lenalidomide, which are associated with high dose therapy and autologous stem cell transplantation in young patients and standard chemotherapy in elderly patients, has changed the management of myeloma and extended overall survival (OS) times. In this chapter, the authors will review the risks factors, diagnosis and treatment of Multiple myeloma.

Risk Factors: There are few risk factors that may affect someone's chance of getting multiple myeloma, for example age, other plasma cell diseases, sex, race, radiation, family history or obesity. A causal relationship between MGUS and MM and chronic antigenic stimulation has been suggested by the results of several studies. Hyperphosphorylated paratarg-7 carrier state was shown to be the first molecularly defined autosomal dominantly inherited risk factor for MGUS and MM.

Multiple myeloma diagnosis is based on a step by step diagnosis approach. Screening test: Full Blood Counts, Urea, creatinine, calcium, albumin, electrophoresis of serum and urine, quantification of non-isotypic immunoglobulins, X-ray of symptomatic areas. Test to establish diagnostic: Bone marrow aspirates and trephine biopsy with plasma cell phenotyping, skeletal survey, immunofixation of serum and urine. Tests to estimate tumour burden and prognosis: FISH analysis, quantification of Monoclonal protein in serum and urine, Albumin, b2-microglobulin. Tests to assess myeloma related organ impairment (ROTI): Full blood count, Serum urea and creatinine, creatinine clearance (measured or calculated), Calcium, Albumin, Plasma viscosity, Tissue biopsy (or fat pad aspirate) for amyloid (if suspected) Quantification of non-isotypic immunoglobulins, Skeletal survery. The diagnosis criteria proposed by International Multiple myeloma working Group, in 2003, distinguish between myeloma and MGUS principally. Other differential diagnoses in patient with Multiple myeloma are solitary plasmacytoma and other B-cell lymphoproliferative disorders.

Treatment: Therapy for multiple myeloma has advanced over the past 5 to 7 years, but with this progress, be uncertainty which is the optimal therapy, particularly in the newly diagnosed patient. A reasonable aim of Multiple myeloma treatment in younger “transplant eligible” patients is to initiate therapy with a target of durable complete remission, and the anticipated consequence of long-term disease control. To achieve this situation, recommended induction therapy with multiagent combination chemotherapies (usually selected from bortezomib, lenalidomide, thalidomide, cyclophosphamide, and corticosteriods) which when employed together elicit frequent, rapid, and good responses. The earliest reports say that there are a very good partial response rates combining various drugs in triplets or even using 4 drugs together. After that, consolidation with high-dose melphalan and autologous stem cell transplantation in the majority of patients, especially in those failing to achieve a complete response or at high risk for early relapse based on prognostic, genetically defined risk factors.

Chapter 5 - The oral manifestations arising from Multiple myeloma (MM) are resultant effects of the moclonal proliferation of atypical plasmocytes derived from bone marrow, kappa and lambda light chains and osteoclast activating factors. The initial manifestation of the MM in maxillofacial complex involves 12-15% of cases, mainly the posterior region of the jaw, justified by the intense hematopoietic activity. The main signs and symptoms include facial pain, gingival bleeding, paresthesias, tooth mobility, ulceration, soft tissue edema, pathological fractures and deposition of amyloidosis in the tongue. The radiographic aspects vary from discreet localized bone resorption until generalized bone rarefaction, may present osteolytic areas in “punched-out”. Other osteolytic lesions as osteoporosis, chronic osteomyelitis, bone metastasis, osteoradionecrosis, arteriovenous malformations, osteonecrosis associated with bisphosphonates should be included in the differential diagnosis due to clinical and radiographic similarity. For elucidation of the diagnosis, laboratory exams and biopsy are indicated. Atypical plasmocytes with hyperchromatic core in histopathological analysis and kappa and lambda chains in immunohistochemistry analysis lead to the diagnosis of multiple myeloma.

From the established diagnosis, treatment is given in conjunction with the oncohematologist. Oral care include: oral preparation prior to chemotherapy, with the removal of focus of infection, such as caries, periodontal disease and residual roots; prevention of osteonecrosis associated with bisphosphonates and prevention and treatment of oral complications resulting from chemotherapy, such as oral mucositis, xerostomia, and opportunistic infections. The knowledge of the oral manifestations of the MM can lead to early diagnosis and optimal management of patients during the various stages of treatment.

Chapter 6 - Multiple myeloma still remains an incurable disease with a high incidence rate in the elderly. Near the old active classes of drugs: alkylators (e.g., melphalan and cyclophosphamide), corticosteroids (e.g., prednisone and dexamethasone), and anthracyclines (e.g., doxorubicin), new drug formulations (e.g., liposomal doxorubicin) and new active classes of drugs such as proteasome inhibitors (e.g., bortezomib) and immunomodulatory drugs (e.g., thalidomide and lenalidomide) have been introduced in myeloma therapy. The high heterogeneity of this disease leads to large differences in clinical responses to treatments. High response rates and good quality responses with a long-term disease control can be observed with the introduction of new drugs. Changes in treatment strategies due to the introduction of novel drugs have been able to improve significantly the quality of responses. In fact, if in the past, Complete Remission (CR) in MM was rare to achieve, while the introduction of new treatments have increased the rate in younger patients as well as in non-transplant setting. CR represents a surrogated marker of long survival. It correlates with the long-term Progression-Free Survival (PFS) and Overall Survival (OS). Achieving CR and sustaining CR within a 3-year landmark from the treatment initiation is associated with highly superior survival. Actually, the authors agree that "The more profound the remission, the longer the duration of response".

Moreover, the interactions between tumor cells and their bone marrow microenvironment play a pivotal role in myeloma progression, inducing also drug resistance. This knowledge has improved treatment options leading to the approval of new drugs which target the malignant cell itself and also its microenvironment. These agents are in preclinical/early clinical evaluation and they appear to further improve disease control but their use is still not approved outside of clinical trials.

Chapter 7 - Multiple myeloma (MM) arises through an accumulation of multiple genetic and epigenetic changes, which play a significant role in tumorigenesis and tumor development. DNA methylation is often found in cancers including MM at the 5-carbon on cytosine residues within CpG islands of genes whose products are associated with the promoter regions of protein-coding genes. This methylation is an epigenetic alteration that leads to heritable changes in gene expression through the recruitment of histone deacetylases and histone methyltransferases. The authors and other researchers have reported the association of global and regional DNA methylation status with MM. Global DNA hypomethylation is the predominant early change during plasma cell oncogenesis from monoclonal gammopathy of undetermined significance to MM, while regional DNA hypermethylation occurs in tumor relapse and during disease progression. Thus, DNA methylation could be a useful biomarker of MM tumorigenesis and progression. In the current review, the authors discuss the role of DNA methylation changes; their potential application as epigenetic biomarkers to facilitate risk assessment, diagnosis, prediction of prognosis, and sensitivity to treatment; and epigenetic therapy in MM.

Chapter 8 - Intravenous bisphosphonates are used in multiple myeloma to reduce pathologic bone fracture, bone pain and to correct hypercalcemia. However, bisphosphonates related necrosis of the jaw (BRONJ) has been reported frequently in those who received intravenous bisphosphonates since 2003. Bisphosphonate related osteonecrosis of the jaw is initiated with dental extraction, dental implant surgery, denture wearing, and periodontal surgery or disease, however, it occurs spontaneously. The purpose of this study was to report 15 cases of BRONJ in multiple myeloma. The male to female ratio was 8:7. Six maxilla and nine mandibles were involved. The etiology of the BRONJ was dental extraction (6 cases), dental implant (2 cases), denture wearing (1 case), untreated vertical tooth fracture (1 case), however, five patients did not have any etiology to cause BRONJ. Conservative medical treatment to reduce pain, discomfort and infection is recommended for the initial therapy. However, if there is a sequestrum, which is separated from the basal bone of the jaw, surgical debridement and primary closure is the key to treat the BRONJ. In this study, surgical debridement was performed in 11 patients with success in 9 patients. Six patients died of multiple myeloma during follow-up periods.

Chapter 9 - Several decades of "stagnation" in the introduction of new antimyeloma agents beyond the traditional corticosteroids and alkylating agents have been occupied from the late nineties by an exciting new era characterized by rapid or even 'explosive' development of a variety of new agents starting from the dramatic comeback of thalidomide, this time as a novel agent against multiple myeloma (MM) followed by the appearance of completely new classes of agents directed against specific molecular targets. The revolution in drug development since then has been manifested by the growing number of clinical trials assessing numerous combinations of older and new first and second generation agents and more recently also by modified routs of drug administrations. Despite this, the progress in elucidation of the basic mechanism of action of many of the novel agents in use has been lagging behind the clinical data acquired and this knowledge gap is becoming an obstacle for the ability to improve the available treatments against resistant disease or to design newer molecules which target the desired pathways more directly. This chapter will summarize the current knowledge on the mechanism of action of some of the mostly used classes of novel agents and those under advanced stage of evaluation. It is noteworthy that in many instances modern research failed to support the general idea standing behind the mechanism offered originally and new theories came instead. Thalidomide is one of the most fascinating examples in all times, for which the obscure binding site and the unknown molecular pathway mediating its diversified physiological effects turned much of the attention towards the clinical manifestations seen and the biological changes observed under experimental conditions, whether of clinical relevance or just another speculation as also happened with the second generation IMiDs. The proteasome inhibitors in contrast have their binding site recognized already from the first introduction to clinic but even there the means by which the proteasome blockade translates into tumor cell killing remains largely unknown considering the failure to confirm the historical attribution of the cytotoxicity to NFkB inhibition. Another therapeutic modality that has gained a lot of success in the treatment of cancer but in myeloma is still seeking for its place is targeted therapy using monoclonal antibodies directed against specific tumor associated antigens or extracellular factors. The limited benefit of the antibodies studied so far in myeloma is an indication that our targets are not optimally selected and we have to improve our knowledge on myeloma initiating cells and their unique immunophenotype. All these issues will be addressed comprehensively and new insights will be introduced, which will be many times inconsistent with the established literature dogmas.

In: Multiple Myeloma: Risk Factors, Diagnosis and Treatments ISBN: 978-1-63321-514-6
Editor: Steve Holt

Chapter 1

Recent Advances in Diagnosis and Treatment of Multiple Myeloma

Drew Dill, M.D., Mansoor Ul Haq, M.D. and Daruka Mahadevan, M.D., Ph.D.
The West Cancer Center/University of Tennessee Health Sciences Center, Memphis, Tennessee, US

Abstract

Multiple myeloma (MM) is a stem cell malignancy arising from a single plasma cell clone that secretes a monoclonal immunoglobulin. Clinical outcome depend on multiple risk factors which include performance status, age, international stage and cytogenetics including mutated and translocated oncogenes. The Mayo clinic's risk-stratification tool (mSMART) based on cytogenetic markers categorizes patients into low, intermediate, and high risk that guides initial therapy. Despite the addition of newer and more effective therapeutic options for MM, the disease remains incurable. The goal of therapy is focused on improving overall survival, progression free survival, duration of complete response, and quality of life. This is largely due to novel agents, combination therapies, better targeting of the tumor microenvironment and autologous stem cell transplantation. Currently FDA approved therapeutic options include immunomodulatory (iMiDs) drugs, proteaosome inhibitors, alkylators, anthracycline, vinca alkaloid, and steroids. Bortezomib and lenalidomide have become the backbone for transplant eligible patients with induction therapy in combination with other agents. Various combinations exist; bortezomib and dexamethasone with lenalidomide, thalidomide, cyclophosphamide, or liposomal doxorubicin. In transplant ineligible patients induction therapies overlap but include mephalan plus dexamethasone with bortezomib, lenalidomide, or thalidomide. As knowledge of the molecular pathways in combination of whole exome sequencing continues to expand, novel therapies will be matched to underlying biology. We discuss these exciting drugs, their mechanism of action, pathways, and their incorporation into ongoing clinical trials to improve overall syrvival. Examples of cell surface and extracellular targets include EGFR, CS-1, IGF-1R, CD40, CD38, CD138, PD-1 and PD-L1 respectively. Of the novel agents, a humanized IgG1 monoclonal antibody to CD38 SAR650984 (SAR) showed a favorable toxicity profile and encouraging single agent activity in an early phase clinical trial. OSI-906 an oral IGF-1R kinase inhibitor in combination with bortezomib was cytotoxic to MM cell lines in a dose-dependent manner suggesting a high degree of synergy for combination therapy. A phase I trial evaluating OSI-906 in combination with bortezomib plus dexamethasone is underway. Of the intracellular targeted agents novel proteosome inhibitors, Bcl2 inhibitors, HSP90 inhibitors, AKT inhibitors, mTOR inhibitors, p38 MAPK inhibitors, autophagy inducers, HDAC inhibitors, aurora kinase and CDK inhibitors have shown promising in vivo activity. TGO2 a multi-kinase inhibitor of CDK 1, 2, 9, JAK2, FLT3, in addition to MAPK, ERK5 in MM cell lines resulted in arrest and rapid apoptosis. TGO2 is under evaluation in phase I clinical trials alone or in combination with carfilzomib. Finally, chimeric antigen receptors (CARs) which are synthetic trans-membrane proteins are being utilized to redirect autologous T-cells with specificity for surface antigens on MM cells. Current targets are the Kappa light chain, CD138, and Lewis Y antigen. CARs targeting BCMA, CS1, and CD38 are in pre-clinical investigation. Initial CARs therapy would focus on R/R MM, while consolidation strategies after first-line therapy or in conjunction with autologous stem cell transplantation are promising.

Keywords: Multiple myeloma, risk factors, diagnosis, therapeutic targets, signaling pathways, molecular pathology

Introduction

Multiple myeloma (MM) is a stem cell malignancy arising from a single plasma cell clone that secretes a monoclonal immunoglobulin [1]. MM accounts for approximately 1% of neoplastic diseases and 10% of all hematological malignancies. [2] The median age at diagnosis is 65 years and is slightly more common in men of African American origin with 2-3 fold increase in incidence compared to Caucasians. [3,4] The development of MM requires the accumulation of activating mutations and loss of tumor suppressors that result in unregulated cell growth, survival, migration, and drug resistance. This genetic step wise evolution starts with the earliest form of the plasma cell dyscrasia, myoclonal gammopathy of underdermined significicance (MGUS), through smoldering myeloma to MM. Two distinct pathogenetic pathways are involved in the development of MM: non-hyperdiploid MM (<48 or >75 chromosomes) which has a high incidence of immunoglobulin heavy chain translocations [t(4;14), t(11;14) and t(14;16)] in addition to loss of 13/13q14 or hyperdiploid MM (48-74 chromosomes) which is associated with multiple trisomies involving chromosomes 3, 5, 7, 9, 11, 15, 19 and 21, but a low incidence of both primary translocations involving the IgH locus at 14q32 and chromosome 13/13q14 loss. [5] Secondary karyotypic mutations develop as MM progress and typically result in activating mutations in KRAS, NRAS, BRAF, FAM46C, TP53 and DIS3, and disruption of the Rb pathway. Progression from MGUS to MM may largely be due to increased MYC expression as this is absent in MGUS and largely increased in MM. [6] TP53 deletions occur around 10% of untreated patients with an increasing prevalence as the disease progresses. [7] An additional molecular transition marker for MGUS to MM is the presence of activating NRAS, or KRAS in newly diagnosed myeloma. [8]. Activating BRAF mutations are described in 4% of myeloma suggesting an additional targetable pathway. [9]. NF-κB expression is highly upregulated in MGUS and MM and is one of the most important drivers to continued survival and resistance.

Mutations in the NF-κB pathway decrease dependence of MM on BM microenvironment and results in constitutive activation of NF-κB thus cell survival and proliferation. [10] Figure 1.

MM is diagnosed by the presence of a serum and/or urine monoclonal protein, at least 10% clonal bone marrow plasma cell infiltrate, and evidence of MM related organ damage: hypercalcemia (serum calcium >11.5mg/dl), renal insufficiency (serum Cr>2mg/dL), anemia (hemoglobin <10g/dl or >2g/dl below lower limit of normal), and bone disease (lytic lesions, severe osteopenia, plasmacytoma, or pathological fractures). Initial workup for diagnosis includes medical history and physical examination and laboratory testing: CBC, CMP, serum and urine protein electrophoresis, IEF, serum quantitative immunoglobulins, serum and urine free light chain, and bone marrow biopsy examination and aspirate. Marrow samples are analyzed by FISH to detect t(11;14), t(4;14), t(14;16), t(6;14), t(14;20), hyperdiploidy, del 13, and del 17p [34]. MM related osteolytic bone lesions exhibit lack of new bone formation and are the major cause of morbidity. Plain radiographs including chest, whole spine, humeri, fermora, pelvis, and skull are recommended for initial evaluation. PET/CT and MRI are more sensitive in detecting bone involvement and are typically reserved to evaluate symptomatic areas not detected on plain radiographs, doubt of extent of disease on plain radiograph, compression fractures, patients with neurological deficits that may have cord compression, or when solitary plasmacytoma or smoldering myeloma is suspected [11].

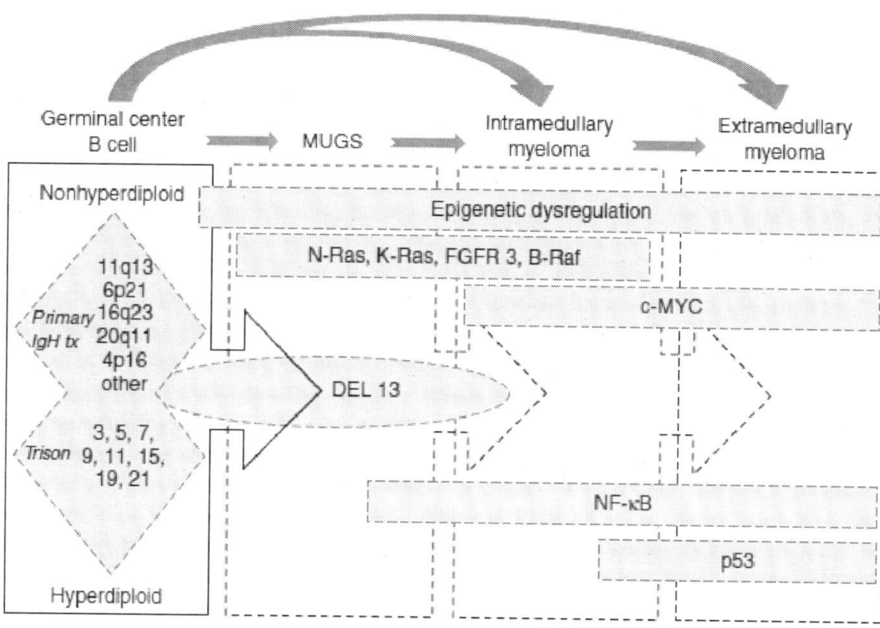

Figure 1.

Risk Stratification

Clinical outcomes depend on multiple risk factors which include performance status, age, stage, cytogentics and response to therapy. Staging models including Durie-Salmon staging (DSS) and International Staging System (ISS) provide prognostic information, however do not provide clinicians with therapeutic direction. [12,13] Further prognostic factors evaluated in a univarient analysis by the Mayo Clinic identified adverse risk factors including performance status, albumin concentration and age having the highest prognostic value which were not included in the DSS or ISS[2]. Despite the use of the prognostic tools there exist disparities in outcomes for patients with matched staging and risk factors largely due to a lack of incorporation and understanding of disease pathobiology at the time these models were developed. With these disparities in clinical outcomes and the lack of a risk stratification tools that guide initial therapy, The Mayo clinic has developed a risk-stratification tool (mSMART) based on independent cytogentic markers that not only categorizes patients into low, intermediate, and high risk but also help guide initial therapy. [13, 14] [Table 1, 2, and 3]. Risk stratification cytogenetic translocations include t(11;14), t(4;14), t(14;16), t(6;14), t(14;20), hyperdiploidy, and del 17p. With the use of risk adaptive stratification, we are able to individualize therapy and potentially avoid dangers of over treating lower risk patients and under treating higher risk patients. Despite the addition of newer and more effective therapeutic options for MM, the disease remains incurable. The goals of therapy are focused on improving overall survival, progression free survival, duration of complete response, and quality of life.

Risk-Adapted Treatment

Overall survival has increased to > 8 years at the present compared to 2-3 years, a decade ago. [15] This is largely as a result of a better elucidation of disease biology, the use risk adaptive tools, novel therapeutic agents, combination therapy, and autologous stem cell transplantation. FDA approved therapeutic options include immunomodulatory (iMiDs) drugs, proteaosome inhibitors, alkylators, anthracycline, vinca alkaloid, and steroids. Bortezomib and lenalidomide have become the backbone for transplant eligible patients with induction therapy in combination with other agents. Various combinations exist: bortezomib plus dexamethasone plus lenalidomide, thalidomide, cyclophosphamide, or liposomal doxorubicin [Tables 4 and 5]. In transplant ineligible patients induction therapies overlap but include mephalan plus dexamethasone with bortezomib, lenalidomide, or thalidomide.

Treatment approaches to a newly diagnosed MM patient includes risk adaptive tools (cytogenetics) and transplant eligibility. Autologous stem cell transplantation (ASCT) eligibility is determined by performance status, comorbidities, and age (USA 75 years old). [16] ASCT is not curative but improves event free survival and overall survival. [17,18] In transplant eligible patients usually 2-4 cycles of a bortezomid and lenalidomide containing regimen is administered followed by stem cell harvest if good response to induction therapy. Patients may either continue with induction therapy with ASCT in first relapse or ASCT up front. ASCT immediately after induction therapy versus delayed ASCT does not affect overall survival but does prolong progression free survival in addition to a break in treatment related side effects, treatments, and a period of time without symptoms. [19] Tandem ASCT is typically reserved for patients who achieve less than a very good partial response in hopes of a high response rates, however there is an increased risk for treatment related mortality. [20-22]

Table 1. Risk stratification of active multiple myeloma

High risk	Intermediate risk	Standard risk
FISH Del 17p t(14;16) t(14:20) GEP High risk signature	FISH T(4;14) Cytogentic del 13 Hypodiploidy PCLI ≥3%	All others including FISH t(11;14) t(6;14)
FISH ¼ fluorescence in situ hybridization; GEP ¼ gene expression profiling; PCLI ¼ plasma cell labeling index.		

Table 2. Mayo Stratification of Myeloma and Risk-Adapted Therapy treatment algorithm for transplant-eligible patients

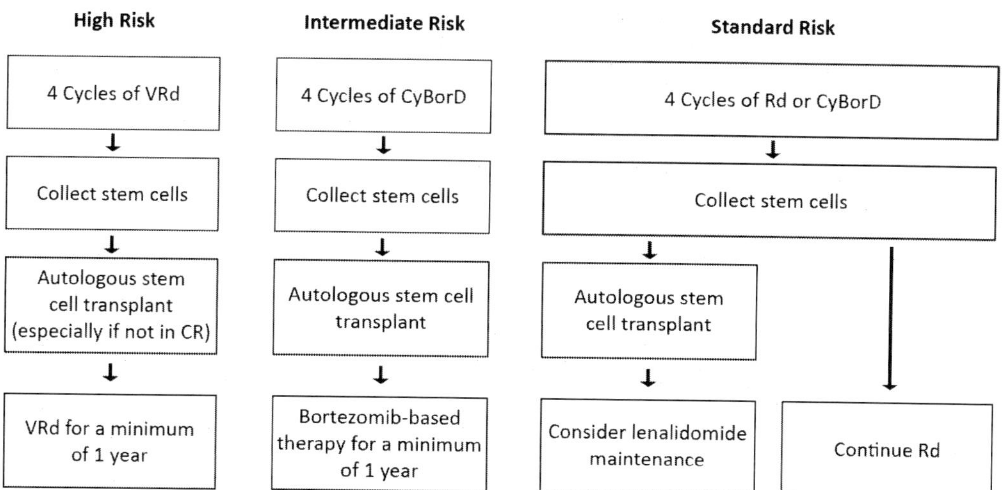

CR=complee remission; CyBorD = cyclophosphamide – bortezomb – dexamethasone; Rd = lenalidomide – dexamethasone; VRd = bortezomb-lenalidomidedexamethasone.

Maintenance Therapy

The role of maintenance therapy post-ASCT remains controversial. Thalidomide was evaluated as maintenance therapy post-ASCT in several trials which does prolong PFS, increase frequency of complete responses, and may improve OS. However, there are significant long term toxicities including peripheral neuropathy and venous thromboembolism (VTE). [23-27] Lenalidomide is an attractive alternative due to less toxic side effects however severe neutropenia, secondary malignancies, and VTE remain a concern. Two phase III trials evaluating lenalidomide maintenance after ASCT have shown improvement in PFS however only one has shown a benefit in OS [28, 29].

Table 3. Mayo Stratification of Myeloma and Risk-Adapted Therapy treatment algorithm for transplant-eligible patients

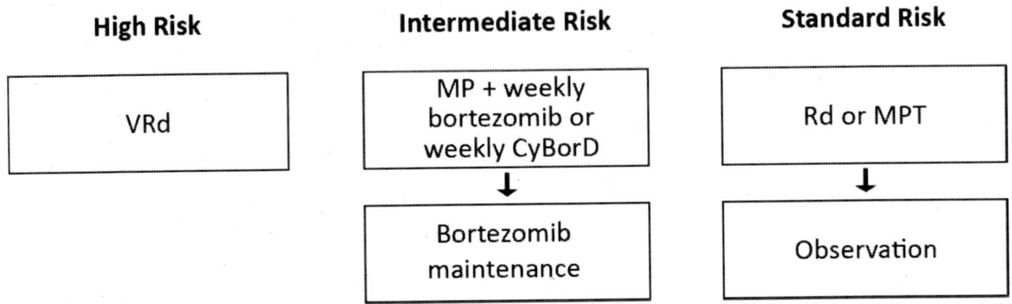

CyBorD = cyclophosphamide – bortezomib – dexamethasone; MP = melphalane – prednisone; MPT = melphalan – prednisone – thalidomide; Rd = lenalidomide – dexamethasone; VRd = bortezomib – lenalidomide – dexamethasone.

Table 4. Therapeutic regimens

Approved front line myeloma regimens	Preferred regimens	Other regimens
Primary therapy for Transplant candidates	Bortezomib/dexamethasone [212] Bortezomib/cyclophosphamide/dexamethasone [88,213] Bortezomib/lenalidomide/dexamethasone [57] Bortezomib/doxorubicin/dexamethasone [31] Bortezomib/thalidomide/dexamethasone [214] Lenalidomide/dexamethasone [86]	Carfilzomib, lenalidomide, and dexamethasone(CRd) [56,215] Carfilzomid, cyclophosphamide, dexamathasone [58] Carfilzomib, Thalidomide, and dexamethasone [216] High dose Dexamethasone Liposomal doxorubicin/vincristine/dexamehtasone [217] Thalidomide/dexamethasone[218,219]
Primary therapy for non-transplant candidates	Bortezomib/dexamethasone Lenalidomide/low-dose dexamethasone [220] Melphalan/prednisone/bortezomib [221,222] Melphalan/prednisone/lenalidomide [30] Melphalan/prednisone/thalidomide [223,224]	High dose Dexamethasone Liposomal doxorubicin/vincristine/dexamehtasone [217] Thalidomide/dexamethasone Melphalan/prednisone [225]

Table 5. FDA approved therapeutic options

Immunomodulator Drugs	Proteosome Inhibitors	Alkylating Agents	Anthracycline	Vinca Alkaloid	Steroids
Thalidomide Lenalidomide Pomalidomide	Bortezombid Carfilzomid	Cyclophosphamide Melphalan	Doxorubicin	Vincristine	Prednisone Dexamethasone

In patients not eligible for ASCT, lenalidomide maintenance therapy was evaluated in a phase III clinica trial after induction with a melphalan containing regimen. Lenalidomide maintenance was found to significantly prolong PFS however no benefit OS was observed. Significant neutropenias were noted in addition to second primary cancers as compared placebo. [30] Bortezomib has been evaluated as maintenance therapy after induction with bortezomib, doxorubicin, and dexamethasone (PAD) compared to vincristine, doxorubicin, and dexamethasone (VAD) followed by thalidomide maintenance in a phase III clinical trial. In high risk patients with increased Cr>2mg/dL, bortezomib induction and maintenance significantly improved PFS to 30 months as compared to 13 months with VAD. A significant OS benefit was noted at 54 months versus 21 months favoring bortezomib. [31] Further clinical trials are needed to delineate the benefit of maintenance therapy with respect to OS along side significant toxicities.

Current Therapies for Newly Diagnosed MM

Transplant Eligible Patients

Induction therapy is initiated for 2-4 cycles before stem cell harvest. Patients then can proceed with frontline ASCT or with induction therapy reserving ASCT until first relapse. A description of induction regimens is provided in FDA approvals. Overall, for transplant eligible patients, providing non alkylator based regimens is important for preserving bone marrow reserve for harvesting stem cells.

Non Transplant Eligible Patients

Treatment options for patients not eligible for ASCT include the same regimens for those who are transplant eligible however melphalan may be incorporated into therapy. Melphalan has been extensively studied and utilized however despite being an active therapy for MM, melphalan-based regimens are falling out of favor due to stem cell damage, secondary myelodysplatic syndromes, acute leukemia, toxicities, and active alternative combination regimens without these toxicities. The same risk adapted drug regimens can be utilized as for transplant in eligible patients.

Novel Targeted Therapies for MM

With better understanding of disease biology therapeutic options include immunomodulatory (iMiDs) drugs and proteasome inhibitors in the treatment paradigm instead of non-specific chemotherapy to pathway specific agents. Despite the effectiveness these therapeutic options have limitations as MM cells possess escape mechanisms of drug resistance and alternate pathway activation. These targetable pathways and consequences of therapeutic intervention are currently under investigation.

Intracellular Targeting Agents

1. Proteasome Inhibitors

The ubiquitin-proteasome pathway (UPP) is important in maintaining normal cellular homeostasis by degrading the majority of regulatory proteins such as cylins, caspases, BCL2 and NF-κB which mediate cell cycle progression, apoptosis, and DNA repair. [32-34] NF-κB is a DNA binding transcription factor that upregulates transcription of IL-6, IGF-1, and VEGF. IL-6 upregulation results in paracrine MM cell growth by bone marrow stromal cells (BMSC). IGF-1 upregulation results in stimulation of cell proliferation and survival. NF-κB upregulation is induced by various cytokines, MM cell binding to BMSCs, and by TNF-α. TNF-α induced upregulation of NF-κB results in increased expression of adhesion molecules, ICAM1 and VCAM1 on MM cells and BMSCs. NF-κB inhibition and activation depends on a regulatory protein, inhibitor of kappaBalpha (IκBα). IκBα sequesters NF-κB in the cytoplasm in an inactivated state and interferes directly with its capacity to bind DNA. In response to extracellular stimuli, cytokines, BMSCs, and infection, IκBα is phosphorylated, then ubiquinated leading to proteosomal degradation. When IκBα is degraded, NF-κB is activated to translocate to the nucleus. [35] Failure of anticancer treatment is largely due to resistance of tumor cell to apoptosis. NF-κB plays an important role in mediating cell survival and inhibiting apoptosis via its activation by oxidative stress, cytokines, and apoptotic stimuli such as anti-cancer therapies. Tumors are largely dependent on proteasome activity compared to normal cells, thus are more sensitive to apoptosis by proteasome inhibition. [36-37] Tumor susceptibility may be that malignant cells rapidly proliferate and accumulate defective proteins at a much higher concentration than normal cells which increases their dependence on preteasome activity for disposal. With proteasome inhibition, accumulation of defective proteins results in cellular dysfunction and trigger of apoptosis[38]. Proteasome inhibition blocks activation of NF-κB by preventing degradation of IκB resulting in apoptosis, stabilization of cyclin-dependent kinase inhibitors reducing MM cell adherence to BMSCs, blocking proangiogenic mediators, overcoming apoptotic regulators such as BCL-2 and over-expression of tumor suppressor TP53. [39]

Bortezomib (Bz) is the first proteasome inhibitor approved by the FDA for use in MM. It is a β5 reversible dipeptidyl boronic acid that inhibits the chymotryptoc-like activity of the 26s proteasome. It also blocks the NF-κB pathway by inhibition of the degradation of NF-κB inhibitor IκBα. Bz leads to downregulation of survival and growth factor pathways and upregulation of pro-apoptotic pathways. [37,40-42] Bz efficacy has been well established in phase I-III trials. In phase I trials the maximum tolerated dose (MTD) IV was 1.3mg/m^2 based on adverse events (AEs) of diarrhea and peripheral neuropathy (PN). [43] The phases II study (CREST) lead to the FDA approval of Bz in R/R MM. In this study Bz was administered at a dose of 1.0 or 1.3mg/m^2 IV with or without dexamethasone. Of the 193 patients, 35% achieved a response, CR in 7 and near CR in 12. At 1 and 5 year follow-up OS was 82% and 32% respectively in the 1.0mg/m^2 group(n=28), and 81% and 45% respectively in the 1.3mg/m^2 group (n=26). [44,45] These findings were confirmed in a phase III trial of Bz in comparison to high dose dexamethasone in relapsed MM with a response rate of 43% and CR of 9%.[46]

Since its initial approval, Bz has been studied with numerous combinations including dexamethasone, thalidomide, melphalan, lenalidomide and many new agents under investigation that will be discussed. Frontline use of Bz in various combinations of other novel therapies have been confirmed in numerous studies where it is superior in response rates and in high risk disease in both transplant eligible and ineligible patients. Despite its efficacy the majority of patients develop resistance to Bz by unclear mechinisms, however this may be due in part to increased or altered proteasome subunit expression. The β5-

proteasome subunit, the major target of Bz, is over-expressed and develop mutations that induces Bz resistance in in vitro models. [47] PN is a well documented toxicity of intravenous Bz. Efforts to decrease PN in clinical trials includes weely administration with success in addition to subcutaneous (subQ) administration. In a phase III trial an exploratory analysis was performed comparing twice-weekly Bz compared to once-weekly Bz. The 3-year PFS, CR, and OS were not statisctically different however in the once-weekly Bz patients in comparison to twice-weekly Bz patients had a reduction in PN of 16% to 3% that was statistically significant (P<0.001). This also resulted in a reduction in discontinuation rate and prolonged the time on therapy. [48] A phase I clinical trial performed to assess safety, efficacy, pharmacokinetics and pharmacodynamics of IV Bz versus subQ Bz. Patients either received Bz 1.mg/m^2 IV or subQ on days 1,4,8, and 11 for up to eight 21-day cycles. The median number of cylces given was identical in both arms. Safety was comparible in both arms as well as AEs: grade 3–4 PN, developed in 17% of patients and 25% thrombocytopenia, in both arms. In the subQ arm, mainly erythema at the injection site was the most significant side effect (51%). Efficacy was also comparible between both arms with ≥PR rates of 42% and 58% for the IV and subQ routes, respectively. [49]. A phase III clinical trial in R/R MM patients was conducted to confirm safety and efficacy of the new route giving the standard dose of Bz either IV or subQ. Both groups received a median of eight cycles. The ≥PR rate was 52% in both groups, including 22% and 20% CRs in the IV and subQ arms, respectively. No differences in OS observed between the groups. Concerning PN, rates of any grade (38% and 53%), and of grade 2 (24% and 41%) and 3 (6% and 16%) severity were significantly lower with subQ versus IV route. [50] Currently Bz is approved for subQ administration due to equivalent clinical efficacy and advantages in reduction in PN and tolerability.

Carfilzomib (Cb) is an irreversible proteasome inhibitor of the epoxyketone class FDA approved for 2nd line treatment of MM. It is currently approved at a dose of 27 mg/m^2 IV on days 1, 2, 8, 9, 15, 16, of a 28-day cycle starting in cycle 2. The 1st cycle has the same dosing schedule however 20mg/m^2 is the starting dose. It is a potent inhibitor of chymotrypsin-like activity of the 20s proteasome (β5) and has potent equivalent potency against LMP7, however has minimal cross-reactivity with other protease classes. It also displays minimal activity against off-target enzymes, including serine proteases, unlike Bz[47]. Preclinical data sugges that Cb inhibited proliferation and inuced apoptosis in Bz-resistant MM cell lines. [51] A phase II single arm trial assessed the viability of Cb as a single agent in heavily pretreated R/R MM pts in a Bz-resistant population. [52] Of the 39 patients evaluated 26% showed a response (5 minorR, 5 PR) with a median of TTP of 6.2 months. 10% were able to complete 12 cycles while PN was noted in < 10% of the patients. Common AEs included fatigue (65%), anemia (65%), thrombocytopenia (46%), neutropenia (20%), nausea (37%), upper respiratory infection (37%), increased Cr (<10%), and diarrhea (33%). A phase IIb study followed 266 patients with R/R MM, who were required to have had at least 2 prior therapies including Bz, and either thalidomide or lanalidomide, and an alkylating agent. [53] Cb was administered as a single agent at 20mg/m^2 IV twice weekly for 3 of 4 weeks in cycle 1, then 27 mg/m^2 for≤ 12 cycles. ORR was 24% with a median duration of response of 7.4 months. As in the prior phase II study, 11% of patients completed 12 cycles and had similar AEs. 77% of patients experienced grade 1 or 2 PN at baseline while new onset PN was infrequent. A large ongoing phase II open label single arm study is evaluating single agent Cb in R/R MM Bz-naïve patients at two different doses 20mg/m^2 or 27mg/m^2 [54] Cohort 1, scheduled to receive intravenous Cb 20 mg/m^2 for all treatment cycles, and Cohort 2, scheduled to receive 20 mg/m^2 for cycle 1 and then 27 mg/m^2 for all subsequent cycles. Preliminary results show an ORR (≥PR) of 42.4% in cohort 1 and 52.2% in cohort 2. Median duration of response was 13.1 months to not-reached (NR). Median time TTP was 8.3 months to NR. Most common AEs (grade 1-3, no grade 4) were fatigue (62%) and nausea (48.8%). This study highlights Cb as a steroid sparing agent in patients with multiple comorbidities.

Carfilzomib was evaluated for its potential impact on high risk cytogenic abnormalities. A prospective trial evaluated the impact of cytogentic abnormalities on outcomes during the phase 2 PX-171-003-A1 study of single agent Cb in R/R MM. Cytogentic profiles were available in 229 patients, 27.1% had high risk cytogenetics [(del 17p13, t(4;14) or t(14;16)] by interphase FISH or del 13 or hypodiploidy by metaphase cytogenitics and 72.9% had standard-risk profiles. ORR were similar between the subgroups 25.8% vs. 24.6%, P=0.85. Time to event end points revealed a trend of shorter duration in high risk paitents, median duration of response (5.6 months vs. 8.3 months) and OS (9.3 vs. 19 months, P=0.0003). These results suggest that single agent Cb has the potential to partially overcome high risk cytogenetics in heavily pre-treated MM patients. [55]

Cb is being studied in the R/R setting including both Bz naïve and refractory patients with various combinations including dexamethasone, lenalidomide, pomalidomide, cyclophosphamide, and new targeted therapies such as PI3K inhibitors, HDAC inhibitors, and kinesin spindle protein inhibitor with promising results. Cb upfront therapy in treatment naïve MM pts was studied in a phase II trial evaluating its efficacy in combination with lenalidomide and dexamethasone followed by 2 yrs of lenalidomide maintenance. There were 63% CR, 26%, VGPR, 8% PR, and 2% SD. PFS 83.3% after median followup of 10 months. No grade 3 or higher AEs occurred, with the most common being electrolyte disturbances (18%), LFT elevations (13%), lymphopenia (63%), anemia (16%), luekopenia (13%). [56] In comparison, the combination of Bz, lenalidomide, and dexamethasone in treatement niave patients was evaluated in a phase II study with all patients achieving at least a PR and 74% achieving VGPR and 29% achieving a CR. Estimated 18-months PFS and OS was 75% and 97%. The most common toxicities included sensory neuropathy (80%) and fatigue (64%), with only 27%/2% and 32%/3% grade 2/3, respectively. [57] Its combination with cyclophosphamide and dexamethasone followed by maintenance Cb was evaluated in a phase II trial for newly diagnosed MM, 35% had unfavorable cytogentics, 31% frail, and a median age of 71 yr. After 9 cycles of induction, 96% of pts achieved at lease a PR, 76% VGPR, 64% CR/nCR including 24% stringent-CR. 1 year PFS 86% and 1 year OS 87%. Grade 4 hematological AE included neutropenia (5%). PN (11%) however only Grade 1 or 2. 20% required dose reduction and 11% required drug discontinuation. Nearly half of the pts continued to maintenance Cb and after 6 months PR rate was 100%, including 68% CR/nCR [58]. In comparison, the combination of Bz, cyclophosphamide, and dexamethasone after 4 cycles resulted in a VGPR 41%, CR 22% for an ORR 63% and a 1 year PFS 93%. Grade 3 and above PN was 9%. [59]

Combination of Cb and selective PI3Kδ inhibition (TGR-1202) was evaluated either alone or in combination in MM cell lines to evaluate cell death and effect on mTOR signaling pathway. TGR-1202 alone did not cause significant cell death in MM cell lines. Combination of both therapies resulted in apoptosis in all cell lines. In a particular cell line U266, Cb and TGR-1202 induced 16% and 14% MM cell apoptosis respectively and in combination apoptosis increased to 75%. To evaluate the impact of the combination on the mTOR pathway which is a known reciprocal feedback loop when PI3K is blocked, TGR-1202 alone did not have an obvious effect on the mTOR pathway, however the combination significantly inhibited phosphor-mTOR, suggesting total pathway blockade. These results support the rationale for future clinical studies of TGR-1202 in combination with carfilzomib. [60]

Marizomib (Mb) is a non-peptidic potent orally active irreversible inhibitor of the three main proteolytic activities of the 20s proteasome, that overcomes Bz resistance in vitro. [61-63] It potently activates apoptosis by a caspase-8 dependent mechanism. Mb also induces cytotoxic effects by way of oxidative stress. [64] Phase I trials evaluating its efficacy in R/R MM in Bz treated pts have been conducted to establish Mb MTD. The MTD was $0.4mg/m^2$ over a 60-min infusion or $0.5mg/m^2$ over a 120-min infusion. DLTs included reversible cognitive changes, transient hallucinations, and loss of balance. Drug related AEs included fatigue, GI, dizziness, and headeache. PN or thrombocytopenia was not evident. [65] Three of the 15 patients treated with the active dose range demonstrated a PR. Of the treated patients 19% experienced PR, and 57% SD. Bz and Mb are two distinct PIs that trigger uniquely the apoptotic signaling pathway and in combination have been shown to have a synergistic anti-MM activity in vivo. [66] Further preclinical studies evaluating Mb in combination with lelanidomide or HDAC inhibitors have shown synergistive anti-tumor activity in MM cell lines. [67-68]

Ixazomib (MLN2238, Ib) is a dipeptidic boronic acid PI that is orally bioavailable that preferentially binds and inhibits the chymotrypsin-like proteolytis (β5) site of the 20s proteasome. Bz and Ib have similar selectivity and potency however the proteasome binding kinetics are different. Both exhibit time dependent reversible proteasome inhibition however Ib has a shorter proteasome dissociation half-life and improved PK, PD, and anti-tumor activity compared to Bz. [69] Treatment of MM cells in vivo and ex vivo mouse models with Ib predominantly inhibits chymotrypsin-like activity of the proteasome and induces accumulation of ubiquitinated proteins. Ib is effective in inhibiting growth and inducing apoptosis in MM cells without affecting the viability of normal cells. A head to head analysis of Ib versus Bz showed a significantly longer survival times in mice treated with Ib. Immunostaining Ib treated mice showed growth inhibition, apoptosis, and a decrease associated with angiogenesis. Ib triggers apoptosis via activation of caspase-3, 8, and 9, and increases p53, p21, NOXA, PUMA, and E2F; induction of endoplasmic reticulum (ER) stress response proteins Bip, phospho-eIF2-α, and CHOP; and inhibition of NF-κB. Finally, combining Ib with lenalidomide, HDACI suberoylanilide hydroxamic acid, or dexamethasone triggers synergistic anti-MM activity in mouse models. [70]

Oprozomib (ONX 0912, Ob) is an orally bioavailable epoxyketone-based proteasome inhibitor which is a truncated derivative of Cb that maintains the selectivity, potency, and anti-tumor activity of Cb. It selectively inhibits chymotrypsin-like activity of the proteasome inhibiting growth and induces apoptosis in MM cells resistant to conventional and Bz therapies. [71] It specifically is associated with activation of caspase-8, caspase-9, caspase-3 and poly (ADP) ribose polymerase (PARP), as well as inhibition of migration of MM cells and angiogenesis. Ob also enhances anti-MM activity of Bz, Ld, dexamethasone, or pan-HDAC inhibitor. Ob is effective at decreasing both MM growth and MM-associated bone disease via: direct killing of MM cells; inhibition of osteoclasts differentiation and resorption; and enhancement of osteoblast formation and function is also observed in Ob. [72] With Ob's anti-MM effect, enhanced activity with other conventional therapies, and effects on osteoclasts, osteoblasts, and bone marrow environment suggest further clinical investigation in early clinical trials.

Delanzomib (CEP-18770, Db), unlike Bz is a orally bioavailable reversible PI in the peptide boronic acid class inhibitor of the chymotrypsin-like activity of the proteasome that downregulates NF-κB and expression of several NF-κB downstream effectors. [73] In vitro it has strong anti-angiogenic activity and potently represses RANKL-induced osteoclastogenesis. Favorable cytotoxicity profile was observed toward normal human epithelial cells, bone marrow progenitors, and BMSC. Db in combination with melphalan or Bz induces synergistic inhibition of MM cell viability in vitro. In MM xenograft models Db in addition to melphalan completely prevented growth of both melphalan sensitive and resistant tumors. In combination with Bz, Db induced complete regression of Bz sensitive tumors and markedly delayed progression of Bz resistant MM. It also exhibited marked anti-MM effects in xenograft models as a single agent. [74] A phase I trial conducted to evaluate PK and PD of Db (CEP-18770) administered on days 1, 4, 8, and 11 of a 21d cycle and found a MTD of 1.5mg/m^2. Skin rash was dose-limiting and occurred in 53% of patients. Other toxicities included asthenia (29%), stomatitis (21%), and pyrexia (16%). No significant PN was observed. Proteasome inhibition in the peripheral blood was dose related. [75] A phase I/II trial for R/R MM patients evaluated Db in a dose escalating weekly schedule (days 1, 8, 15) in 28 day cycles. MTD was found to be 2.1mg/m^2 with a similar toxicity profile. Two patients achieved SD that lasted more than 6 months. The phase II portion of the study was prematurely stopped due to lack of efficacy. [76] Further clinical trials of Db may be warranted given its potential synergistic effects with other agents in MM.

2. *Immunomodulatory Drugs* (IMiDs)

FDA approved immunomodulatory (IMiDs) drugs include thalidomide, lenalidomide and recently approved pomalidomide. Their mechanism of action to date is not clearly understood however multiple mechanisms are proposed which include anti-angiogenesis, anti-proliferation, induction of apoptosis, stimulatation of NK-cell anti-MM immunity, direct downregulation of key functions of tumor cells, cytokine inhibition, anti-inflammatory effects, and indirectly by modulating cell adhesion interaction of MM cells in their bone marrow microenvironment. [77-78] Previously described mechanisms of action for IMiDs include activation of caspase-8, enhance MM cell sensitivity to Fas-induced apoptosis, and downregulate NF-κB activity as well as expression of cellular inhibitor of apoptosis protein-2 and FLICE inhibitory protein. IMiDs also block the stimulatory effect of IGF-1 on NF-κB activity and potentiate the activity of TNF-related apoptosis-inducing ligand (TRAIL/Apo2L). IMiDs may also directly block the NF-κB pathway allowing for apoptosis via the caspase-8/death receptor pathway. [79] IMiDs affect cell adhesion directly via down-regulation of pro-survival cytokines TNF-α, IL-6, IL-8, and VEGF. [80] Lenalidomide (Ln) and pomalidomide (Pn) have been shown to increase p21(WAF-1) expression which in turn causes cell cycle arrest in plasma cells independent of P53, suggesting efficacy in cancers with P53 mutations or deletions. [81] Recently a more concrete mechanism of action for IMiDs cytotoxicity and tertragenetic effects has been proposed. The fist breakthrough was revealed when thalidomide was shown to bind cereblon, which is a substrate-recognition component of a cullin-dependent ubiquitin ligase, and inhibits cereblons auto-ubiquitination activity. In MM cell lines resistant to IMiDs they often have down-regulated cereblon, while

IMiDs responsive MM cell lines have high cereblon concentrations. It appears that IMiDs are not cereblon antagonist but alter the substrate specificity of cereblon. Two independent papers have found 2 targets of Ln bound cereblon, IKZF1 and IKZF3 which are part of the Ikaros family zinc finger proteins. IKZF1 and IKZF3 are key B-cell transcription factors which are selectively ubiquinated and degraded by the Ln bound cerebron. In addition, a single amino acid substitution of IKZF3 conferred resistance to Ln-induced degradation and rescued Ln-induced inhibition of cell growth. The Ln immune stimulatory upregulation effect of IL-2 is now better understood as depletion of IKZF1 and IKZF3 causes upregulation of IL-2 in T-cells. [82-83] The importance of this pathway was confirmed by knockdown in MM cell lines of IKZF1 or IKZF3 which was sufficient for cytotoxicity. MM unresponsiveness to Ln as a result of low levels of cereblon supports that cytotoxic effects of Ln are dependent upon cereblons action on IKFZ1 and IKZF3.

Thalidomide is the first in the IMiDs drug class to be approved for use in MM based on its antiangiogenic properties. In R/R MM, thalidomide monotherapy produces response rate of 30% and in combination with dexamethasone response rates of 40-50%. [84] Significant toxicities include VTE and neuropathy. Currently it is approved in the front line setting for transplant eligible and ineligible patients in various combinations.

Lenalidomide (Ln) a 2nd generation IMiD was FDA and EMEA approved based on a phase III trial showing the combination of Ln with high dose dexamethasone (Dex) was superior to Dex alone in R/R MM. [85] Progression was delayed by 11.3 months vs 4.7 months in combination. CR or PR was noted in 60.2% in combination vs 24% Dex alone. Overall survival was improved with a HR of 0.66 p=0.3. Grade 3 or 4 AEs were observed in 10% of patients in combination including neutropenia 29.5% vs 2.3%, thrombocytopenia 11.4% vs 5.7%, and VTE 11.4% vs 4.6% in dexamethasone alone. The combination of Ln and either high or low dose Dex was evaluated in a phase III trial. [86] The combination of Ln plus low dose Dex was associated with improved survival and lower toxicity. In a recent meta-analysis, Ln and Dex was compared to thalidomide and Dex and patients receiving Ln plus Dex had a longer time to progression, PFS, and OS. In addition the use of Ln and Dex in R/R MM who had prior treatment with thalidomide experienced higher ORR, TTP, PFS as compared to those receiving placebo plus Dex. [87] In a phase I/II trial evaluating the combination of Ln, Bz and Dex in newly diagnosed MM patients. [57] Ln 25mg (d1-14), Bz 1.3mg/m^2 (d1,4,8,11), and Dex 40mg (d 1,2,4,5,8,9,11,12) was given on a Q3week cycle. PR was noted in 100% and 74% and 67% achieving VGPR or better. 42% proceeded to undergo transplantation. With a median follow up of 21 months, the estimated 18-months PFS and OS with and without transplantation were 75% and 97% respectively. Toxicities included neuropathy (80%) and fatigue (64%). Grade 3/4 hematological toxicities included lymphopenia (14%), neutropenia (9%), and thrombocytopenia (6%). 32% patients also reported neuropathic pain. Thrombosis was rare (6%) overall and no treatment related mortality was observed. Ln in combination with Bz has been evaluated in various combinations as either a three or four drug regimen with Dex, cyclophosphamide, and/or anthracycline with promising results [59,86,88] The role of Ln in maintenance therapy after stem cell transplantation was evaluated in two studies. [89,90] Both studies show a significant TTP advantage, but only a slight OS advantage observed in one study compared to no OS benefit in the other. A recent meta-analysis evaluating the impact of thalidomide or Ln as maintenance therapy post stem cell transplant found that thalidomide with corticosteroids maintenance did results in significant OS benefit (HR 0.72) while Ln maintenance showed no benefit. [91] Significant PFS advantage was noted with both IMiDs (HR 0.49). Ln maintenance has been evaluated in transplant ineligible patients in a phase III trial using melphalan, prednisone, and Ln for induction followed by Ln maintenance versus placebo. [30] After median follow up of 30 months a significant PFS was noted in the maintenance arm of 31 months versus 13 months. There was no difference in OS. Without a clear OS benefit in transplant eligible and ineligible patients and taking into consideration of costs, toxicities, and potential risks of secondary malignancies, the role of Ln maintenance is yet to be determined.

Table 6. Pomalidomide studies compared to historical

Phase	Tx	Responses	AE	Reference
I/II	Pomalidomide, Bz, and dexamethasone(PVD) in R/R MM 14 pts	83% ORR: 1sCR, 3 CR, 3 VGPR and 3 PR	leukopenia and thrombocytopenia; however, the majority of these were grade 1-2. In 14 evaluable patients Grade ≥3 AEs included neutropenia (5), leukopenia (3), lung infection (1), lymphopenia (1) and atrial flutter (1)	[226]
I	PVD R/R MM	ORR 75%, 30% VGPR or better	grade 3/4 adverse events (AEs) were neutropenia (29%) and thrombocytopenia (19%).	[227]
I/II	Cb, Pom, dex in R/R MM	1 CR, 18 VGPR, 24 PR, 11 MR, 11 SD, and 2 PD for an ORR of 64% and a ≥MR rate of 81%	Grade ≥3 AEs >20% of patients included fatigue (48%), neutropenia (40%), anemia (34%), thrombocytopenia (34%), and diarrhea (20%)	[228]
II	Pom, dex, +/- cyclophosphamide in lenalidomide R/R MM	ORR 48.5%, clinical benefit rate (MR and better) was 68.2%. PFS 6.4 mo. Duration of response 10.4 mo.	grade ¾ AEs neutropenia (30%), febrile neutropenia (13%), pneumonia (13%), thrombocytopenia (11%) thromboembolic events were noted in 4%.	[229]
I/II	Pom, dex, and pegylated doxorubicin	ORR and clinical benefit was 43.5% and 48.3% respectively.SD 20.7%, PD 27.6%	≥ grade 3 (G3) neutropenia (37.5%), leukopenia (37.5%), lymphopenia (25%), anemia (9.4%), hyponatremia (9.4%), thrombocytopenia (6.3%), and duodenal ulcers (3.4%)	[230]
II	Thalidomide,dex in R/R MM	ORR 46%	AEs somnolence 26%, constipation 37%, PN 27%, VTE 5%	[84]
III	Lenalidomide,dex in R/R MM	TTP 11.3, ORR 60.2%, CR 15.9%	≥ grade 3 AEs neutropenia 29.5%, thrombocytopenia 11.4%, VTE 11.4%	[85]
II	Thalidomide, cyclophosphamide, dex in R/R MM	CR 17%, PR 62%, MR 11%, SD 6%, PD 4%. Objective RR 90%. 2 year OS and EFS 73% and 34%, respectively	Grade I/II neuropathy 49%, constipation 57%	[231]
II	Thalidomide, liposomal doxorubicin, dex in R/R MM	CR 26%, 6% near CR, 6% VGPR, 38% PR, 16% MR, 8%PD. ORR 92%. Median EFS 17 mo.	Grade 3/4 AEs: neutropenia 50%, febrile neutropenia 36% pts, VTE 12%, PN 2%	[232]
I/II	Lenalidomide, cyclophosphamide, and dexamethasone in R/R MM	CR 29%, VGPR 7%, PR 45%, ORR 81%. 2 yr PFS 56%. 30 mo OS 80%.	Grade ¾ hematological complications 26%, infections 3%, VTE 6%.	[233]
I/II	Lenalidomide, adriamycin, and dexamethasone in R/R MM	ORR 73%, CR 77%, VGPR 74%. TTP 45 weeks, 1 yr OS 88%	Grade ¾ AEs; neutropenia 48%, thrombocytopenia 38%, VTE 4.5%, neutropenic infections 10.5%	[234]

Pomalidomide (Pom) is a 3rd generation IMiD that inhibits TNF-α up to 50,000 times greater than thalidomide in in vitro assays and roughly 10 times more potent than Ln92-95. Like other IMiDs it mechanism of action is similar.[96,97]. Pom has been shown to prevent and treat MM bone disease by favorably altering osteoclastic activity by inhibiting osteoclast formation via the RANKL pathway [98,99] A phase I trial evaluated the MTD of Pom to be 4mg/day. In these R/R MM pts 42% achieved minimal response or better, 21% PR or better, and 3% a CR. Median DR, PFS, and OS were 4.6, 4.6 and 18.3 months. PN and VTE were low ≤ 5%. DLTs were grade 4 neutropenia. [100] A phase II trial was conducted combining Pom alone or in combination with low-dose Dex in R/R MM pts. [101] This study evaluated pts with ≥2 prior therapies including Ln and Bz. At a median follow-up of 14.2 mo, median PFS was 4.2 and 2.7 mo, ORR 33% and 18%, median DR 8.3 months and 10.7 mo, and median OS 16.5 and 13.6 months for Pom alone versus Pom with low-dose Dex respectively. Grade 3-4 neutropenia occurred in 41% (Pom+LoDEX) and 48% (Pom), and no grade 3-4 neuropathy was reported. A phase III trial compared Pom with either LoDex or HDex in R/R MM pts who had not responded to Bz and Ln. [102] After median follow-up of 10.0 mo, median PFS with Pom plus LoDex was 4.0 months versus 1.9 months with Hdex (HR 0.48; p<0.0001). This benefit was observed irrespective of age, gender, cytogenetic risk, or previous treatment with anti-myeloma therapy. Median PFS was also significantly prolonged, irrespective of whether pts had received up to ≥3 prior treatments. Treatment with Pom plus LoDex was superior with respect to ORR (31% vs 10%) and OS (12.7 months versus 8.1mo) as compared to Pom plus HDex. The most common grade 3-4 AEs Pom plus LoDex and HDex groups were neutropenia (48% versus 16%), anaemia (33% versus 37%), and thrombocytopenia (22% versus 26%). Pom has been evaluated in phase I/II trials in combination with Bz, Cb, cyclophosphamide, or pegylated liposomal doxorubicin in R/R MM pts, results are listed in Table 6. Currently a phase III trial is underway evaluating the combination of Pom plus Bz plus Dex versus Bz plus LdDex in pts with R/R MM. [95]

3. Bcl2 Inhibitors

Bcl2 family proteins BCLXL, BCLW, and MCL-1 are anti-apoptotic factors that help cells evade programmed cell death particularly in cancer cells. High Bcl2 levels are often found in most lymphoid malignancies, CLL, and multiple myeloma. [103] Bcl2 pro-apoptotic proteins include "multidomain" BAX, BAK, and BOK which have three BH3 domains (BH1-3) and Bim, Bid, Bad, NOXA, and PUMA which share homology with only the BH3 domain and are defined as BH3-only proteins. [104] BAX and BAK activation leads to homo-oligomerization causing the formation of pores resulting in apoptosis and cell death. BH3-only proteins act as direct activators of BAK/BAX or as sensitizers by displacing inhibitory proteins from BAK/BAX. Bcl2 anti-apoptotic family member proteins bind BH3 domains preventing BAK/BAX homo-oligomerization and BH3-only protein activation.

Several small molecule inhibitors have been developed that mimic the BH3 domain interacting with BH3-only proteins activating apoptosis cascade via displacing inhibitory proteins of BAX and BAK or activating pro-apoptotic BH3-only molecules. ABT-199 is the first-in-class orally bioavailable Bcl-2-selective BH3 mimetic. In a preclinical model, ABT-199 was evaluated in human MM cell lines (HMCLs) and was found to have activity in HMCLs with the CCND1 translocation. Cells harboring the CCND1 translocation were noted to have abnormal p53, indicating that ABT-199 induced cell death is independent of the p53 status. ABT-199 was also shown to have highly selective binding to only the Bcl2 hydrophobic groove. Senstativity to cytotoxic effects of HMCLs were associated with higher expression of Bcl2. There was significant variability in HMCLs sensitivity to ABT-199 whith sensitivity being restricted to the CCND1 subgroup. A particular cell line harboring del17p with t(11;14) was found to be highly sensitive to ABT-199 indicating that it may be able to overcome poor prognostic impact of del 17p of t(11;14) pts. Currently, two phase I clinical trials are underway evaluating ABT-199 in R/R MM as a single agent and in combination with Bz and Dex. [105,106]

4. HSP90 Inhibitors

Heat shock proteins (HSPs) are molecular chaperones that facilitate normal protein folding and guard the proteome from misfolding, aggregation and degradation thus preventing acculumation of misfolded proteins and restoring normal homeostasis. [107] HSP expression is increased in response to proteotoxic stressors including heat, heavy metals, hypoxia, and acidosis. Tumor survival is dependent on HSP over-expression to achieve homeostasis in a hostile environment. HSP also participate in many higher-order functions, such as post-translational regulation of signaling molecules, assembly/disassembly of transcription complexes, and processing of immunogenic peptides by the immune system. HSP90 and its co-chaperones inhibit cell apoptosis via modulating activity of many proto-oncogenes such as AKT, TNF-receptors, and NF-κB function. Oncogenic mutations of HSPs targets require much higher requirements of HSP90 function to maintain cellular viability. HSP90 is a key chaperone for maintaining signal transduction proteins for MM cell growth, survival and drug resistance. [108] HSP90 inhibitors interrupt its chaperone function leading to accumulation of misfolded proteins, endoplasmic reticulum stress, and ultimately apoptosis.

Tanespimycin (KOS-953) is a HSP90 inhibitor that acts through inhibition of the ATPase activity of HSP90. Pre-clinical models have shown Bz induces HSP90 in MM cells along with up-regulation of stress response gene transcripts suggesting a rationale for combining HSP90 inhibitors with Bz. In pre-clinical models, tanespimycin has demonstrated cytotoxicity against MM cells exerting pleiotropic effects including reduced activity of Akt, anti-apoptotic caspase-8 and 9, suppression of protective BMSCs, and inhibition of osteoclastogenesis and angiogenesis. Tanespimycin has been shown to have a synergistic affect with Bz to induce apoptosis in MM cell lines resistant to doxorubicin and Bz. Pre-clinical data suggest that tanespimycin may also be protective against PN associated with Bz. The combination of tanespicycin plus Bz dramatically increases the intracellular load of ubiquinated proteins in MM cells. A phase I/II trial evaluating safety and tolerability tanespimycin in combination with Bz found 3% CR, 12% PR, 12% MR for a combined ORR 27%. Response rates where dependent on prior Bz exposure: CR+PR was 24% in Bz-naïve pts, 9% in Bz-pre-treated pts, and 13% in Bz-refractory pts; ORR was 48%, 22%, and 13% respectively. [109] Median PFS for Bz-naïve pts 7.2 mo, Bz-pre-treated pts 3.7 mo, and Bz-refractory pts 1.6 months. Median OS for all pts was 18 months. Median OS for Bz-naïve pts was NR, median OS 17.7 months for Bz-pre-treated pts, and 13.8 months for Bz-refractory pts. PN was observed in 21% pts of which most had PN at the time of enrollment. Reduction in the rate of PN was observed which was consistent with in vivo rat models suggesting tanespimycin protects against Bz-induced PN. Most common AEs (all grades) were diarrhea (60%), nausea (49%), thrombocytopenia (40%), transient elevations of AST (28%) and dizziness (28%). Most toxicity was grade 1 or 2. Further clinical trials are pending its activity in MM. [110]

Only limited clinical efficacy has been achieved with HSP90 inhibitors in clinical trials. HSP70 has been described to interact functionally with HSP90 complex. Importantly, HSP70 is up-regulated by PI3K dependent signaling. Specific HSP72/HSP73 knockout or inhibition decreases HSP90-chaperone clients affecting multiple oncogenic signaling pathways. HSP72/HSP73 inhibition in combination with HSP90 inhibition (AUY 922) is synergistic in induction of MM cell death. Inhibition of the PI3K/AKT/GSK3β pathway with PI103 decreased expression of heat shock transcription factor 1 and down-regulated constitutive and inducible HSP70 expression. The combination of PI103 and HSP90 inhibitor (AUY 922) resulted in additive cytotoxicity, thus treatment with PI3K inhibitors might represent an alternative therapeutic option to target HSP70. [111] Other HSP90 inhibitors include Ganetespib, AT13387 and retaspimycin and are currently under early clinical trial in MM evaluation. [112]

5. PI3K/AKT/mTOR Pathway

The *PI3K/AKT/mTOR* pathway is central to cellular regulation of apoptosis, proliferation, motility and energy metabolism. AKT is a serine-threonine kinase which is activated by PI3K in response to extracellular growth factors within the BMSC. AKT activation induces MM cell growth and survival through GSK-3β and mTOR phosphorylation. AKT activation is implicated with advanced stage and poor prognosis in MM pts and therapy related resistance. PI3K/AKT/mTOR pathway has been shown to be frequently activated in MM cell lines. Supporting the activation of PI3K/AKT/mTOR pathway is deletion or mutation of PTEN resulting in hyperactivation of AKT enhancing tumor progression. Activating mutations of AKT often are implicated in cell survival and tumorgenicity. [111,113,114]

BAY80-6946 is a PI3K inhibitor that has been shown in a pre-clinical model in vivo and ex vivo to be highly efficacious in 4 MM cell lines by inhibiting cell cycle progression and increases apoptosis in a dose-dependent manner. It abrogated the stimulation conferred by IGF-1 in addition to decreasing AKT phosophylation. These results elucidate the potential benefit of targeting the PI3K pathway and support the use of *BAY80-6946 in clinical trials. [115]*

MK-2206 is a pan-AKT inhibitor and has shown anti-tumor cytotoxicity in a pre-clinical model. mTORC1 inhibitors have shown little efficacy largely due to the reactivation of AKT due to rapamycin induced mTORC2 activity. The up-regulation of AKT prompted the combination of MK-2206 with rapamycin however up-regulation of pErk is now a resistance mechanism in MM cells. Pre-treatment with MEK1/2 inhibior UO126 in combination with rapamycin and MK-2206 provided strong synergy in killing MM cells supporting clinical investigation of MK-2206. [116]

Mammalian Targets of Rapamycin (mTOR) Inhibitors

The mammalian target of rapamycin (mTOR) is a central regulator of cell growth, survival, and metabolism. [117] mTOR forms two distinct multiprotein complexes, mTOR complex-1 (mTORC1) and mTOR complex-2 (mTORC2). mTORC1 plays a critical role in regulation of protein synthesis and growth which is activated by the PI3K/AKT pathway and inactivated by tuberous sclerosis complex (TSC). mTORC2 is activated by growth factors which activate downstream mediators that control mobility, invasion, and cytoskeletal assembly in addition to AKT feedback activation mediated by mTORC2 following mTORC1 inhibition. mTORC1 is sensitive to rapalogues such as rapamycin, everolimus and temsiroliums however mTORC2 is considered to be resistant to rapamycin. [118] DEPTOR is an mTOR-interacting protein whose expression is suppressed by mTORC1 and mTORC2. [119] DEPTOR alterations of expression has been described in human cancers including MM that harbor cylinD1/D3 or c-MAF/MAFB translocations where it is highly expressed. DEPTOR over-expression suppresses S6K1 and relieves feedback inhibition from mTORC1 to PI3K signaling, thus activating AKT. Additional pathway of resistance has been described via rapamycin induced hyperactivation of AKT through the loss of the mTORC1/S6K1/IRS-1/PI3K negative feedback loop. [120,121] Rapamycin induces IGF-I activation which abrogates antiproliferative effects of rapamycin via AKT activation. This process is regulated by S6K1 and IRS-1 interaction. A regulator protein S6K1 is responsible for inactivation of IRS-1 which is responsible for induction of AKT activity via IGF-1R signaling. S6K1 is inhibited by rapamycin thus leading to increased levels of IRS-1 and consequent AKT activation.

Temsirolimus is a signal transduction inhibitor that interacts with the ubiquitous intracellular FK506-binding protein 12 which specifically inhibits mTOR. A phase II trial was conducted evaluating 16 pts with R/R MM given temsirolimus 25mg IV weekly until progression. [122] One PR and 5 MR were observed for a RR 38%. Median TTP was 138 days. Grade 3-4 toxicities included fatigue (n=3), neutropenia (n=2), thrombocytopenia (n=2), interstitial pneumonitis, stomatitis, and diarrhea (n=1). In a phase I/II trial of weekly Bz plus temsirolimus was evaluated in R/R MM pts. The phase I portion enrolled 20 pts and 43 pts in the phase II portion. [123] The MTD was determined to be 1.6 mg/m2 Bz on days 1, 8, 15, and 22 in combination with 25 mg temsirolimus on days 1, 8, 15, 22, and 29, for a cycle of 35 days. The phase II study revealed PR or better in 33% pts. In the phase I study common AEs grade 3-4 were thrombocytopenia (n=13), lymphopenia (n=10), neutropenia (n=9), leukopenia (n=7), anemia (n=5). Three deaths were reported during the phase I/II trial which included H1N1 influenza, cardiac amyloid, and ventricular arrhythmia unrelated to treatment. Temsirolimus in combination with Ln was administered to R/R MM pts in a phase I trial evaluating tolerability and possible interactions. [124] PK analyais indicated increased doses of temsirolimus resulted in statistically significant changes in clearance, Tmax, and AUC-time curves, when administered with constant doses of Ln due to Ln being a substrate of ABCB1 (P-glycoprotein [Pgp]). This study reported clinically significant P-gp-based drug-drug interaction with Ln.

Pan-PI3K/mTor inhibitors (*BEZ235* and *NVP-BGT226*) are in clinical development. NVP-BGT226 inhibits MM cell lines [nM range] in a time and dose-dependent manner. Inhibition of growth, cell cycle progression, and induction of apoptosis is noted with NVP-BGT226 treated MM cells. Inhibition of AKT phosphorylation was observed in a time and dose-dependent manner. Stimulatory effects of IGF-1, IL-6, and conditioned medium from HS-5 stromal cells on MM cell growth were completely abrogated by NVP-BGT226. [125] In a pre-clinical model, BEZ235 was tested on a panel of MM cell lines sensitive and resistant to conventional cytotoxic chemotherapeutic agents. BEZ235 induced rapid commitment to and induction of cell death in a number of cell lines. In addition, BEZ235 was able to target MM cells in the presence of exogenous IL-6, IGF-1, stromal cells, or osteoclast, which are known to protect against various anti-MM agents. In vivo xenograft studies revealed significant reduction in tumor burden and survival in BEZ235-treated human MM tumor-bearing mice. [126] Anti-MM activity of pan-PI3K/mTOR inhibitors in pre-clinical models warrants further investigation in early phase clinical trials.

6. P38 MAPK Inhibitors

P38 Mitogen-activated protein kinase (MAPK) functions in the generation of signals that are critical to controlling normal and malignant hematopoiesis and survival via cytokines and growth factors such as IL-6 and other inflammatory mediators implicated in MM. [127]. P38 MAPK has been shown to be activated in the MM microenvironment. Inhibitors of p38 MAPK block production inflammatory cytokines IL-6, VEGF, IL-1β, which promote cell proliferation, survival, and drug-resistance in MM cells.

SCIO-469 a p38α-selective inhibitor was evaluated in mouse xenograft models of human MM cell lines. Oral treatment with SCIO-469 (10, 30, 90mg/kg) twice daily in mice with palpable tumors, resulted in significantly reduced tumor growth in a dose-dependent manner. This response was also noted in SD-282 an analog of SCIO-469. Dex plus SCIO-469 elicited anti-tumor activity in Dex sensitive tumors at much lower doses than typically observed suggesting potential for combination therapy. Early phase clinical trials are underway evaluating safety and efficacy of SCIO-469 in R/R MM pts. [128,129]

LY2228820 (LY) is a p38 MAPK inhibitor with modest cytotoxicity against MM cell lines in addition to significantly enhancing Bz toxicity by down-regulating Bz-induced heat shock protein 27 phosphorylation. [130] LY was shown to inhibit IL-6 secretion, and macrophage inflammatory protein-1α secretion a chemokine that promotes osteoclast formation. LY inhibits osteoclast formation in vitro and osteoclastogenesis in vitro in a SCID-hu MM model via modulating the cytokine network within MM BM microenvironment. This pre-clinical study suggests that LY may be a novel agent to improve MM pt outcome both by enhancing the effect of Bz and by reducing skeletal events.

7. Autophagy Inhibitors

Plitidepsin (Aplidin) is an extremetly potent inducer of apoptosis studied in vitro and also exhibits strong anti-tumor activity in xenograft models in multiple solid and hematologic tumors. In addition to its cytotoxic properties it also exhibits a strong anti-angiogenic activity. In a pre-clinical model accessing the activity of Aplidin in vitro and in vivo in human MM cell lines revealed inhibition of DNA synthesis, cell cycle progression arrest, decrease in cyclin D1 and CDK4 expression, and induction of apoptosis by lowering mitochondrial membrane potential, by inducing cytochrome c release and activation of caspase-9 and caspase-3. [131] In vivo testing in xenograft mice produced a reduction in serum paraprotein concentration by 42% and a decrease in BM invasion with myeloma cells by 35%. An open-label, single-arm, phase II trial anti-tumor activity and safety of plitidepsin was evaluated in R/R MM pts at a dose of 5mg/m^2 over 3hr IV every 3 weeks. [132] Those with suboptimal response to single agent plitidepsin were given Dex 20mg/day on days 1-4 every 2 weeks. 47 patients were evaluable for efficacy. ORR was 13% with plitidepsin alone and 22% plus Dex. Anemia (29%) and thrombocytopenia (18%) were the most grade ¾ hematologic toxicities. Non hematological *AE* included Fatigue (16%), muscular toxicity (6%), transient elevation of alanine aminotransferase/aspartate aminotransferase (27%) and creatine phosphokinase (23%). Single agent plitidepsin has limited but reproducable activity in R/R MM patients with increased activity with Dex and is not a promising combination for further development.

Curcumin is the active component in the plant curcuma longa (turmeric) which has been shown to inhibit the proliferation of multiple myeloma cells throught the downregulation of IL-6 and NF-κB. It also suppresses proliferation, induces apoptosis in MM cells in addition to inhibiting osteoclastogenesis through the suppression of RANKL signaling. [133,134] A phase I trial was performed evaluating the effect of curcumin on plasma cells and osteoclast in pts with MGUS. [135] Patients were administered 4 grams/day of oral curcumin. Blood counts, β2 microglobulin, serum paraprotein, and immunoglobulin electrophoresis (IEPG and EPG) were followed with treatment. Results revealed that curcumin was able to decrease paraprotein load in a select group (those having a praprotein level of >20 g/l) of MGUS pts. 50% of these pts had a 12% to 30% reduction in paraprotein levels. 27% pts on curcumin also had a 25% decrease in urinary N-telopeptide of type I collagen. An open-label double-blind placebo-controlled cross-over extension study was performed evaluating cercumin in pts with MGUS and smoldering myeloma. [136]. Nineteen pts with MGUS and 17 pts with smoldering myeloma (SM) were enrolled into two groups: Group A given 4g curcumin at the start of the study and crossed over to placebo at 3 months Group B given 4g placebo initially and crosse over to curcumin at 3 months. All pts were given the option after completion of the 4g arms, to enter the open-label, 8g extension study for a further 3 months 25 pts completed the 4g cross-over study and 18 pts completed the 8g extension study. Four and 8 g daily decreased the free light-chain ratio (rFLC) (−35 and −36%), involved free light-chain (iFLC) (−8 and −10%), and the difference between clonal and non-clonal light-chain (dFLC) (−9 and −11%) in both MGUS and SM pts. Significant reductions were also seen in both total serum protein (P = 0.04) and random urinary protein concentrations (P = 0.04), but not in the serum paraprotein concentration. Patients with abnormal light chain benefitted from curcumin therapy with an increased benefit at higher doses of 8g/day. UDPYD, a marker of bone resoprtion was also noted to decrease in the curcumin arm while increase in the placebo arm. This study suggests that curcumin therapy might have the potential to slow the disease progression in MGUS and SM patients.

8. Histone Deacetylase (HDAC) Inhibitors

Gene expression is controlled by acetylation of specific lysine residues found in histones. The balance of histone acetylation depends on the activity of two enzymes: histone acetyltransferases and histone deacetylases. Hyperacetylation results in more relaxed state of chromatin which enhances accessibility of the transcription machinery and accessory proteins for translation. Hypoacetylation leads to a more compact chromatin state resulting in gene silencing. Acetylation is not reserved only for histones but also various proteins involved in transcription, translation, splicing, DNA repair, cell cylce progression, protein folding, cytoskeleton dynamics, signal transduction, and metabolism. Some of these proteins include p53, HSP90, tubulin, NF-κB, HIF-1α, RUNX3, STAT-3, E2F1, Ku70 and c-MYC, thus acytelation functions as a broad post-translation modification regulating protein functions. [137] Numerous epigenetic alterations have been described in MM involving alterations in DNA acetylation resulting in decreased DNA transcription, including transcription of tumor suppressor genes. [138] Histone deacetylase inhibitors (HDACi) are responsible for deacetylation of proteins (histone and non-histone) thus negatively impact epigenetic mechanisms and post-translational modification of proteins. HDACi impact on chromatin results in hyperacetylation of histones thus impacting genes expression. In MM cell lines, HDACi results in up- or down-regulation of gene expression. MM pathways affected by HDACi include cell cycle progression, apoptosis, cytokine signaling, adhesion and migration, proteasomal degradation, drug resistance and DNA damage. HDACi ultimately affect a combination of gene expression and degregulation of proteins primarily through the modulation of acetylation. The best characterized pathways involved in HDACi include pro-apoptotic and cell cycle arrest via: up-regulation of pro-apoptotic or down-regulation of anti-apoptotic Bcl2 family memebers, downregulation of inhibitors of apoptosis (IAP), and mitochondrial changes which release apoptosis inducing factor (AIF) and cytochrome-c into the cytosol.

Interestingly HDACi have been shown to downregulate members of the proteasome pathway, including genes encoding the subunits of the 26s proteasome and ubiquitin conjugating enzymes in vitro. [139] It also appears that HDACi enhances the cytotoxic effects of Bz in vitro and in vivo. This synergy is a result of disruption of protein degredation following inhibition of proteasome and aggresome pathways by Bz and HDACi respectively. The unfolded protein response (UPR) is responsible for coping with the accumulation of proteins that need to be degraded as a result of proteasome inhibition by Bz. UPR activation is dependent upon HDAC. Further synergy between Bz and HDAC inhibitors included disruptions in interactions between NF-κB, IκB, and HSP90 pathways. HDACi impact is also seen on its effect on the BM microenvironment with down-regulation of genes involved in cytokine signaling such ast IGF-1, IGF-1 receptor, and IL-6R.

Vorinostat: Phase I clinical trials evaluating the use of HDACi in R/R MM patients have resulted in acceptable toxicity profiles however single agent activity was modest with only minimal response or stabilization of disease. [140-144] Based on pre-clinical models of combined synergy of proteasome inhibitors with of HDACi, multiple trials have been conducted in R/R and newly diagnosed MM pts. In a phase I trial combining vorinostat with Bz in R/R MM pts demonstrated PR 27%, MR 6%, and 59% disease stabilization. All pts reported AEs, 89% were mild to moderate. Thirty-eight percent of pts experienced serious AEs, 41% were considered drug related. The MTD was not reached. A phase I clinical trial was carried out Ln, Bz, and Dex (RVD) plus vorinostat as front-line therapy in 30 MM pts145. The MTD of vorinostat was determined to be 200mg in combination with RVD. The most common G1 or higher toxicities included thrombocytopenia (n=30), constipation (n=25), diarrhea (n=20), fatigue (n=19), nausea (n=16), and neuropathy (n=8). Grade 3 toxicities that occurred in ≥10% of pts were thrombocytopenia (n=8), fatigue (n=5), neutropenia (n=3), cardiovascular (n=3) and neuropathy (n=3). The ORR (PR or better) was 100%, VGPR or better 52% and CR 28%. For pts who completed 4 cycles, VGPR and CR rates were 60% and 32% respectively and pts who completed 8 cycles, the rates were 64% (VGPR) and 55% (CR). At a median follow up of 11.5 month (range 1 – 31 months) there has been only one pt with progressive disease (asymptomatic relapse from CR). Currently an additional phase II trial evaluating vorinostat plus bortezomib in R/R MM pts is pending results [146,147] (Table 7).

Table 7. HDAC inhibitor comparison chart

Phase	Tx	Responses	AE	Reference
I	Vorinostat +VRD in newly diagnosed MM	ORR 100%, VGPR or better 52%, CR 28%	Grade 3 and 4 AEs thrombocytopenia 27%, fatigue 17%, neutropenia 10%, cardiovascular 10%, and PN 10%	[145]
I/II	VRD newly diagnosed MM	PR 100%, ORR 74% and VGPR 67%	Grade ¾ AEs lymphopenia 14%, neutropenia 9%, and thrombocytopenia 6%, VTE 6%	[57]
III	Bz + vorinostat or placebo in R/R MM	PFS 7.63 mo in Bz +vorinostat and 6.83 mo in Bz and placebo	Grade ¾ AEs Vorinostat arm vs placebo: thrombocytopenia 45% vs 24%, neutropenia 28% vs 25%, anemia 17% vs 13%	[235]
Ib	Panobinostat + Bz R/R MM	Responses in all cohorts 68%, Bz refractory 62%	Grade ¾ AEs: thrombocytopenia 78%, neutropenia 60%, anemia 16%	[149]
II	Panobinostat + Bz R/R MM	ORR 34.5%, PFS 5.4 mo	Grade ¾ AEs: thrombocytopenia 63.6%, fatigue 20%, diarrhea 20%	[150]
I/II	Panobinostat+Cb R/R MM with high risk cytogenetics	ORR 64%, ≥VGPR 30%, PR 30%, MR%, SD 26%, PD 5%	Grade ¾ AEs: Thrombocytopenia 30%, neutropenia(Gr 3 20%, Gr 4 2%), nausea 9%	[152]

A phase III trial (VANTAGE 088) was carried out evaluating the combination of Bz with vorinostat or placebo in R/R MM pts. [147] Bz was administered in 21 day cycles (1.3 mg/m^2 IV on days 1, 4, 8, and 11) plus oral vorinostat (400 mg) or matching placebo once-daily on days 1-14. Median PFS was 7.63 monthsin the vorinostat group and 6.83 months in the placebo group (hazard ratio [HR] 0·77, 95% CI 0·64-0·94; p=0·0100). The most common grade 3-4 adverse events in the vorinostat group versus placebo group were thrombocytopenia (45% versus 24%), neutropenia (28% versus 25%), and anaemia (17% versus 13%).

Panobinostat is a potent pan-deacetylase inhibitor that disrupst the aggresome and HSP90 function by inhibition of HDAC6 resulting in cytotoxic misfolded/unfolded protein aggregates and MM cell death. [148] The combination of panobinostat and Bz were evaluated in a phase Ib study in R/R MM and Bz pre-treated pts for safety and dosing schedule. [149] Results revealed a panobinostat dose of 20mg plus 1.3mg/m^2 of Bz. No grade ¾ PN was observed, however grade ¾ thrombocytopenia (n=30), neutropenia (n=23), diarrhea (n=23), nausea (n=18), pyrexia (n=17) and fatigue (n=16) was observed. Responses were observed in 68% of pts across all cohorts and in 62% of pts who were Bz refractory. Results revealed tolerability and activity and suggests that panobinostat may reverse Bz resistance. PANORAMA 2 was a phase II trial evaluating panobinostat plus Bz in R/R MM pts refractory to Bz within the 60 days of last Bz treatment. [150] ORR was 34.5% with a clinical benefit rate of 52.7%. Median exposure and PFS were 4.6 and 5.4 months, respectively. Common grade 3/4 adverse events, regardless of study drug relationship, included thrombocytopenia (63.6%), fatigue (20.0%), and diarrhea (20.0%). The results of this study suggest that panobinostat can recapture responses in heavily pre-treated, Bz-refractory MM pts. PANORAM 1 is a phase III trial that is currently ongoing evaluating Panobinostat or placebo plus Bz and Dex in R/R MM pts. [150]

A phase II trial evaluated melphalan, thalidomide, and prednisone in combination with panobinostat in pts with R/R MM. At least a PR was observed in 38.5% of patients. The MTD of panobinostat plus MPT could not be determined due to high rates of DLTs experienced with panobinostat at doses of 10mg and 15mg. Grade ¾ AEs included neutropenia (71%) and thrombocytopenia (35.5%). The combination of MPT and panobinostat three times weekly for three weeks followed by a 9-day rest peioriod was not well tolerated in patients with R/R MM, suggesting alternative dosing schedules of this combination. [151]

In a phase I/II multicenter trial the combination of panobinostat plus Cb in R/R MM patients was evaluated. A total of 44 pts were accrued. Most pts were ISS stages 2 and 3, 38% had adverse prognostic cytogenetics, including 23% with del17p. The median number of prior therapies was 3, including 89% with Bz, 89% with IMiDs, and 34% prior ASCT. Forty five percent of pts experienced ≥ grade 3 hematologic-related AEs, the most common being G3 thrombocytopenia (30%) and neutropenia (20% G3 and 2% G4). Thirty four percent of pts experienced ≥ grade 3 non-hematologic AEs, the most common being fatigue (11% G3) and nausea/vomiting (9% G3). The most salient of all grade AEs were nausea, vomiting (39% G1, 20% G2, 9% G3, 0 G4) and thrombocytopenia (14% G1, 27% G2, 30% G3, 0 G4). PN was rare mostly G1 and G2 and no G3/4. The final treatment doses were determined to be 30mg and 20/45 mg/$m^2$of Cb. The median panobinostat dose delivered was 23.4mg and 40.8mg/m^2 of Cb. ORR was 64% with 31% ≥VGPR and 30% PR. In addition, there were 5% MR, 26% SD and 5% PD. ORR for Bz exposed pts, Bz refractory pts and dual Bz and IMiD refractory pts was 60%, 67% and 66%, respectively. With a median follow up of 6.3 months, PFS at 6 and 12 months was 63% and 41% respectively. OS was 83% at 6 and 12 months and median TTP 8.6 months. The combination of panobinostat plus Cb was well tolerated and showed promising activity in this high risk R/R MM population. Given the dose reductions, the MTD was not reached and further studies evaluating correct dose levels will need to be explored. [152]

Belinostat is an HDACi that induces a concentration-dependent increase in acetylation of histones H3 and H4 resulting in alteration in cell-cycle survival regulatory proteins in various tumor types. It also has been shown to induce apoptosis and increase expression of cyclin-dependent kinase inhibitor p21 and p27 which are negative regulators of tumor growth. In a pre-clinical model, belinostat was combined with Bz and was found to trigger reactive oxygen species (ROS) generation that was accompanied by p53, H2AX and p38-mitogent-activated protein kinase phosphorylation. [153] The combination also resulted in synergistic inhibition of osteoclast formation. MM cell death was mediated via ROS DNA damage. In a phase I trial of safety of belinostat in advanced hematological malignancies including MM found the MTD to be 1000mg/m^2/d days 1-5 of a 21 day cycle. [144] No CR or PR was noted in heavily pre-treated (median 4 prior regimens) pts. Of the four MM pts, one achieved disease stabilization. The most common treatment-related adverse events (all grades) were nausea (50%), vomiting (31%), fatigue (31%) and flushing (31%). No grade 3 or 4 hematological toxicity compared with baseline occurred except one case of grade 3 lymphopenia. A Phase II Study of belinostat in combination with Bz in pts with R/R MM was terminated for unknown reasons. [154] Clinical Trial of belinostat in combination with Dex in R/R MM pts has completed but results are pending. [155]

Romidepsin is a cyclic tetrapeptide HDACi that is FDA approved for cutaneous and peripheral T-cell lymphoma. Romidepsin has been shown to have activity against MM cell lines in pre-clinical models by way of up-regulation of tumor suppressor genes, down-regulation of anti-aopototic molecules, and induction of apoptosis in a dose-dependent fashion. Additional mechanisms of action include disruption of of HSP90 function and activity not just limited to class 1 HDACs but broader activity including class 2 HDACs. Romidepsin has also been shown to overcome Bz resistance in MM cell lines via HDAC inhibition and by decreasing trasciptional expression via caspase-8 dependent degradation of Sp1 protein, the most potent transactivator of class I HDAC genes. [156] A phase I clinical trial evaluated the combination of romidepsin, Bz, and Dex in R/R MM pts. [157] The MTD of romidepsin was 10mg/m^2 IV (days 1, 8, and 15) every 28 days with standard Bz and Dex. AEs included grade ≥ 3 thrombocytopenia (64%) and PN (76%). Overall responses greater than a minimal response was 72%, 8% CR, 52% PR including 28% with VGPR. Median TTP was 7.3 months, and median OS was >36 months. Currently multiple ongoing clinical trials are evaluating romidepsin in various combinations for R/R MM pts.

IFT2357 is a pan-HDAC inhibitor of the hydroxamate family that was shown in a pre-clinical study to modulate genes related to transcription regulation, cell cycle, and apoptosis in MM cell lines. IFT2357 is able to down-modulated IL-6Rα (CD126) transcripts and protein resulting in decreased signaling by IL6-R measured by STAT3 phosphorylation in the presence and absence of IL-6. [158] It has also been shown to be a potent inducer of apoptosis of MM cell lines in addition to decrease production of IL-6, VGEF, and IFNγ by mesenchymal stromal cells. [159] In a phase II trial the safety and efficacy of IFT2357 alone or in combination with Dex was evaluated in 19 R/R MM pts. [142] The MTD was determined to be 100mg twice daily. Median duration of treatment was 6 weeks. Three pts experienced grade 3–4 gastro-intestinal toxicity and 3 had transient electrocardiographic abnormalities. Thrombocytopenia occurred in all but one pt (grade 3/4 in 10 pts). At completion of the study, 5 PD, and 9 died of progressive MM. An additional phase II high pulse dose clinical trial of orally administered IFT2375 in R/R MM patients has been terminated for unknown reasons. [160]

AR-42 is a novel orally bioavailable, phenylbutyrate-based HDAC inhibitor and in a pre-clinical study was found to suppress gp10 expression, and both constitutive and inducible STAT3 activation. This correlated with downregulation of STAT3 downstream, cell survival and proliferation factors, Bcl-xL, and cyclin D1, leading to induction of apoptosis and G1 and G2 cell cycle arrest in MM cell lines suggesting further clinical clinical development in MM. [161] Currently a phase I clinical trial evaluating the safety of AR-42 is recruiting patients with R/R MM, CLL, or lymphoma. [162]

9. Cell Cyle Kinase Inhibitors

Cyclin-dependent kinases (CDKs) are a family of serine threonine protein kinases that are activated by regulatory cyclins whose activity is critical for cell cycle regulation and transcription. CDKs specifically regulate cell cycle progression via G1 phase-specific transcription by phosphorylating the Rb protein, promoting DNA replication during S phase, and mitosis regulation. [163] They also aid in mRNA transcription functions. There is evidence that dysregulated and/or increased expression of cyclin D1, D2 or D3 occurs early in MM tumorgenesis thus predisposing MM cells to proliferative stimuli. [164-166] Inhibition of CDKs involved in cell cycle progression, such as CDK 4 and 6 with PD 0332991 demonstrates only cell cycle growth arrest. [167] Whereas using multi-targeted CDK inhibitors and drugs that target transcriptional CDKs such as Seliciclib, UCN-01, P276000, and AT7519 were able to achieve MM cell cytotoxicity. Of interest is CDK inhibitors that block transcriptional type CDKs in MM, specifically RNAPII inactivation. RNA polymerase

II inactivation leads to p53 activation and thus a decrease in a number of anti-apoptotic proteins. RGB-286638 is a novel compound of the indenopyrazole family of CDKIs with potent activity specifically against transcriptional-type CDKs in MM cells. In a pre-clinical model RGB-286638 was shown to be a potent CDK9 inhibitor in addition to multiple other CDKs resulting in trascriptional arrest and caspase-dependent apoptosis in MM cell lines [196]. It was also found to inhibit RNAPII resulting in increased p53 levels through nucleolar fragmentation and depletetion of mdm2.

TG02 is a novel orally bioavailable multikanse inhibitor that inhibits cell cycle regulators CDK1 and CKD2 in addition to transcriptional regulators CDK7 and CDK9. It is also a potent inhibitor of MAPK ERK5 which supports MM proliferation and survival after being stimulated by activating cytokines such as IL-6. In a pre-clinical model TG02 was shown to inhibit proliferation and survival of MM cell lines and selectively induce apoptosis of primary patient derived malignant plasma cells. [168] TG02 also exhibited single agent activity in xenograft mouse models and enhanced *in vivo* activity of Bz and Ln. Signaling analysis revealed blocked activity of CDKs 1, 2, and 9 as well as MAPK ERK5 leading to cell-cycle arrest and rapid commitment to apoptosis through depletion of cell survival factors such as Mcl-1. Currently a phase I clinical trial evaluating TG02 in pts with advanced hematological malignancies including MM is actively recruiting. [169]

Dinaciclib (SCH727965) is an inhibitor of CDK 1, 2, 5, and 9. Treatment of MM cell lines with Dinaciclib led to a concentration-dependent inhibition of growth associated with rapid induction of G2/M cell cycle arrest and apoptotis. [170] Xenograft MM models treated with dinaciclib led to tumor regression associated with reduced Rb protein phosphorylation and Bcl2 expression. Dinaciclib also induces p53 expression in addition to downregulating expression of anti-apoptotic factors Mcl-1 and XIAP. To confirm the role of p53 activation and induction of cell death with dinaciclib a knockdown p53 model completely abolished the induction of apoptosis following treatment with dinaciclib. In a separate preclinical study, Dinaciclib exhibits anti-MM effects via dysregulation of the IRE1/XBP-1 arm of the unfolded protein response. [171] Currently Phase I clinic trials are underway evaluating dinaciclib alone or in combination with standard MM therapies. [172,173]

Palbociclib (PD-0332991) is an orally active small molecule that inhibits CDK 4 and 6. In a pre-clinical model it was shown to induce rapid G1 cell cycle arrest in human MM cell lines and in xenograft models. [174] Induction of cell cycle G1 arrest by PD-0332991 sensitizes MM cells to killing by Bz. A phase I trail evaluating Palbociclib in combination with Bz and Dex in R/R MM pts has been completed with results pending. [175]

Aurora Kinase Inhibitors

Cell proliferation is dependent on activation of each cell cycle phase requiring intricate regulation of cell cycle check points and repairing genetic damage. These cell cycle check points are regulated by aurora kinases, cyclins, and cyclin-dependent kinases. Aurora kinases are serine/threonine kinases that localize to centrosomes and centromeres during the mitotic phase of the cell cycle. Defective chromatid segregation causes genetic instability leading to tumorgenesis. Three members of the Aurora family are aurora-A, -B, and -C. Aurora-A and C localizes to centrosomes in early S phase and aurora-B localizes to the spinle mizone during anaphase. Defectuve Aurora-A may result in aneuploidy which is characteristic of tumors.

Aurora-A expression is regulated by tomor suppressor gene p53. Dysregulated over-expression of Aurora-A and -B are often found in tumor cells and has been associated with centrosome amplication and worse prognosis in MM. [176] In a pre-clinical study inhibition of Aurora-A gene expression via siRNA in MM cells results in apoptosis. [177]

Alisertib (MLN8237) is a small molecule Aurora-A kinase inhibitor that was evaluated in a pre-clinical model with MM cell lines which resulted in mitotic spindle abnormalities, mitotic arrest, and inhibition of cell proliferation through apoptosis and senescence. It up-regulates p53 and tumor supressor genes p21 and p27. Alisertib in combination with dexamethasone, doxorubicin, or Bz resulted in syndergistic/additive anti-MM activity *in vitro*. In MM mouse models alisertib significantly increased OS and decreased tumor burden[176]. Currently phase I/II trials are investigating alisertib in R/R MM pts as a single agent or in combination with Bz. [178,179]

ENMD-2076 is an orally active Aurora-A and B kinase inhibitor that was evaluated in vitro and in vivo and showed significant cytotoxicity againts MM cell lines. It inhibited Aurora-A and B and induced G2/M cell cycle arrest. It was also shown to inhibit the PI3K/AKT pathway, downregulate survivin and X-linked inhibitor of apoptosis. Treating xenograft MM mouse model with ENMD-2076 resulted in a dose-dependint inhibition of tumor growth in addition to reduction in pHisH3, Ki-67, angiogenesis, pFGFR3, and significant increase in cleaved caspase-3. In this pre-clinical model ENMD-2076 showed significant activity agains MM cells *in vitro* and *in vivo* and acts on multiple pathways improtant for MM cell growth and survival. [180] In a phase I clinical trial, ENMD-2076 was evaluated as a single agent in R/R MM pts. Nine patients were enrolled and no DLT was observed. All pts treated at dose level 1 had PD, 1 pt in dose level 2 had SD, and 2 pts on dose level 3 had SD with 21% and 19% reduction in serum M-protein after the 1st cycle. Grade 3 AEs included hypertension (n=1), asymptomatic elevation of lipase (n=2), and thrombocytopenia (n=1).

AT9283 is a small-molecule multi-targeted kinase inhibitor with potent activity against Aurora A, Aurora B, and Janus kinase 2/3. In a pre-clinical model AT9283 was evaluated *in vitro* and *in vivo* MM mouse models alone and in combination with Ln. AT9283 inhibited cell growth and induced apoptosis *in vitro* by way of increasing polyploid DNA content, decreasing pHisH3, and pAurora A. Its activity resulted in inhibition or STAT3 tyrosin phosphorylation in MM cells. Treating xenograft mice with AT9283 resulted in decreased MM cell growth and prolonged survival. AT9283 combined with Ln resulted in synergistic cytotoxicity in MM cells which was attribitued to increased inhibition of phosphorylated STAT3 and phosphorylated extracelluar signal-regulated kinase. [181] A phase II trial evaluating the safety and efficacy of single agent AT9283 in R/R MM patients is currently underway [182]

Cell Surface Receptor Targets in Multiple Myeloma

MM have several cell surface receptor targets, which are important for cell cycle progression, survival, programmed cell death and MM-BMSC interactions. Their selective elaboration on MM cell surface makes them attractive targets. Therapeutic monoclonal antibodies, small molecule inhibitors to receptor kinases and antibody drug conjugates are in various stages of clinical development.

EGFR (HER1): The epidermal growth factor receptor (EGFR, HER1) is a member of the ErbB family of receptor tyrosine kinases. The role of mutated EGFR in the malignant cell survival, proliferation and metastasis of several malignancies has been established. Ligand binding leads to EGFR activation resulting in EGFR homo- or hetero-dimerization (HER2, HER3, HER4) stimulating the tyrosine kinase activity which initiates cell signaling via MAPK and PI3/AKT pathways promoting cell cycle progression, survival and migration. [183] Heparing binding epidermal growth factor (HB-EGF) is elaborated by mononuclear cells particularly monocytes and stromal cells within MM bone marrow microenvironment. HB-EGF stimulates HER1 and HER4 expressed on MM cells delivering a proliferate signal via the PI3K/AKT pathway. A Pan-HER inhibitor blocked the HB-EGF induced MM cell growth when cultured within the bone marrow environment which expresses HB-EGF and induced apoptosis of the pt's MM cells causing 55% reduction in the number of viable myeloma cells. Addition of Dex caused a 84% reduction in viable MM cells. Addition of anti-IL-6 demonstrated a similar additive benefit. [184] *Cetuximab* has been evaluated in a phase II trial in R/R MM and was found to be safe and feasible. It showed moderate efficacy in heavily pre-treated pts in combination with dexamethasone. [185] Combining cetuximab with other active drugs may yield promising results.

Interleukin 6: IL-6 is an inflammatory cytokine that plays an important role in immune response and hematopoiesis. It acts through IL-6R which is a highly glycosylated single polypeptide chain with a molecular weight of 80 kd. IL-6 is produced by a paracrine mechanism by BMSCs. Adhesion of MM cells to BMSCs and osteoblasts play an important role in the transcription and secretion of IL-6 by the BMSCs and osteoblasts. [186] Results from studies with MM cell lines have shown that a minority of MM cells produce IL-6 by an autocrine mechanism. IL-6 is involved in the proliferation of plasmablastic cells in the bone marrow and in the differentiation of these cells in to mature plasma cells. It is also a potent growth factor for MM cells not only *in vitro* but also *in vivo*. IL-6 has been shown to overcome apoptosis of MM cells, and upregulates cellular expression Bcl-XL protein in particular MM cell line (IL-6 dependent B9 myeloma cells). The involvement of retinoblastoma protein in MM cell growth has been reported. IL-6 has been demonstrated to promote MM cell growth via phosphorylation of RB. [187] *Siltuximab*, an anti IL-6 chimeric monoclonal antibody (Mab) was evaluated in a phase 2 trial in combination with Dex in R/R MM pts who had received $\geq$2 prior therapies one of which was bortezomib. No responses were observed with single agent siltuximab however, combination with Dex showed 23% PR and responses were seen in the Dex refractory group. Hematological toxicity was common but manageable. [188] Siltuximab has been tested in combination with Ln and Bz in phase I/II trial (NCT01531998) the results of which have not been reported yet. Siltuximab holds great promise for treatment of MM and should be tested in phase III trials in combination with other active agents. FDA recently approved it for use in Castleman's disease.

CS1: CS1 is a cell surface glycoprotein and a member of the immunoglobulin gene superfamily and is highly expressed on MM cells. CS1 is detected in sera obtained from MM pts, however not present in the sera of healthy subjects. It is postulated to have role in the adhesion to the MM-BMSCs. *Elotuzumab* (HuLuc63) is a humanized Mab that targets CS1 thus inhibiting MM-BMSC adhesion in a dose-dependent manner and can interrupt MM adhesion to BMSCs overcoming the protective effect provided by the BM microenvironment. Elotuzumab was also shown to be toxic to MM cells by inducing ADCC even against autologous tumor cells from pts with MM that are sensitive or resistant to conventional therapies. Elotuzumab has shown significant activity against the MM cells *in vitro* when combined with Bz plus Ln. The effect of elotuzumab was also seen in human MM xenograft models in mice. [189] Currently Elotuzumab is undergoing clinical trials in combination with Bz and Ln.

CD40: CD40 is a transmembrane protein and a member of the TNFR superfamily. It is recognized as a critical regulator of cellular and humoral immunity via its expression on B-lymphocytes, dendritic cells and monocytes. [190] It is also expressed on the cell surface of other normal cells including endothelial cells, fibroblasts, hematopoietic progenitors, platelets and basal epithelial cells. CD40 ligand (CD40) is the chief ligand described for CD40 and is expressed primarily by activated T lymphocytes and platelets. CD40-CD40L interaction plays a role in the regulation of atherosclerosis, graft rejection, coagulation, infection control and autoimmunity. Almost all B-cell malignancies and ~70% of solid tumors express CD40. The consequences of CD40 signaling are multifaceted and many even have biologically opposed roles. CD40-CD40L interaction induces activation and proliferation of B-lymphocytes but triggers apoptosis of carcinoma cells including MM cells depending on their p53 status. [191] The effect of CD40 signaling causes the activation of NF-κB, p38 MAPK, c-jun-NH2-kinase, JAK/STAT and PI3 kinase pathways. [192] Studies show that CD40 stimulation has a role in MM cell homing and migration but also causes growth arrest and apoptosis in MM cells, the exact mechanism of which is unclear.

Anti-CD40 Mab has shown to block IL-6 secretion induced by MM cell adhesion to BM stromal cells, as IL-6 is a key growth and survival factor for human MM cells, blockage of its secretion causes abrogation of MM cell growth in the bone marrow micro-environment. [193] Yu-Zu Tai et al., tested *dacetuzumab* (SGN-40), a humanized Mab on MM cell lines and patient cells. They showed significant growth arrest and apoptosis in the presence of the *de novo* protein synthesis inhibitor CHX. Dacetuzumab induced cytotoxicity is associated with up-regulation in cytotoxic TNF ligands (i.e., FasL, TRAIL and TNF-α) and suppresses expression of IL-6R protein and mRNA associated with inhibition of growth and survival of MM cells induced by IL-6 but not by IGF-1. Dacetuzumab was evaluated in a phase 1 study of 44 advanced MM pts. Adverse events included cytokine release syndrome, non-infectious ocular inflammation, and elevated hepatic enzymes. 20% of patients showed a best response of stable disease. [194]

CD38: CD 38 is a transmembrane glycoprotein with an extracellular domain and cytoplasmic tail and functions in receptor mediated adhesion and signaling. It is expressed on the normal hematopoietic and lypmphoid tissues, however, has a relatively high expression on MM cells. It is therefore considered a potential therapeutic target in the treatment of MM. *Daratumumab*, a Mab directed against the CD38 has shown activity against CD38 expressing lymphoma and MM cell lines. It also showed activity against patient derived MM cells. The mechanism of cytotoxicity includes ADCC and CDC in MM cells. [195] Daratumumab is currently undergoing a phase I/II study in R/R MM pts. It is used as a single agent and in combination with Ln (NCT01615029).

SAR650984 is an unconjugated humanized IgG1 Mab that binds selectively to CD38 and has been evaluated in a phase I trial, the MTD was not reached and the safety was predictable and manageable. This agent demonstrated encouraging single agent activity in heavily pre-treated R/R MM pts. [196] A phase Ib study is ongoing and is recruiting R/R MM pts to determine the MTD, safety profile, PK and clinical activity in combination with Ln plus LD-dex (NCT01749969).

PD-1 and PD-L1: Natural killer (NK) cells play a key role in the innate immune system and have shown to exert anti-tumor activity against malignant plasma cell clones in MM. This NK versus MM is attenuated by activating and inhibitory receptors on the NK cell surface, which interact with ligands on the MM cell surface. Programmed death-1 (PD-1), which is a member of the B-7 family of co-signaling molecules and associates with ligands, PD-L1 and PD-L2 and plays a key role in downregulating the T-cell immune response. [197] PD-1 and PD-L1 Mabs are currently undergoing trials in different tumors with encouraging results. It has been shown that NK cells from MM pts express PD-1, whereas normal NK cells do not and primary MM cells express the receptor. [198] *Pidilizumab* (CT-011) is a novel IgG1 humanized Mab which modulates the immune response by interacting with PD-1. It has been shown to be safe and well tolerated in a phase I trial and single agent activity is observed. [199] Ln in part causes T-cells to secrete IL-2 thus enhancing the NK-cell versus MM effect. [200] Given the complimentary mechanism of action of these drugs, the combination was tested on MM cell lines and patient MM cells in combination with NK cells. It was shown that Ln downregulates expression of PD-L1 on primary MM cells which is independent of a direct apoptotic effect and enhances the NK cell migration toward malignant plasma cells. The cytotoxicity conferred by Pidilizumab was increased and particularly against the PD-L1 bearing CD138+ malignant plasma cells clone in MM pts because CD 138-, PD-L1- normal cellular marrow elements were spared in autologous killing assays. Based on these findings a phase I/II trial of Pidilizumab plus Ln is recruiting R/R MM pts (NCT02077959). Currently Pidilizumab in combination with dendritic cell vaccine is recruiting in a phase II trial in MM pts in the post-transplant setting (NCT01067287). *Nivolumab*, a fully humanized Mab against PD-1 and *ipilumab*, a Mab targeting CTLA4 are being evaluated alone and in combination in a phase I trial in pts with hematologic malignancies (NCT01592370).

CD138: CD138 (syndecan-1) is an integral membrane protein which acts as a receptor for the extracellular matrix. It is expressed on the differentiated plasma cells and is a primary diagnostic marker for MM. The extracellular domain of CD138 binds to soluble extracellular molecules via its heparin sulfate chains, which include EGF, FGF, HGF and to soluble extracellular molecules such as collagen and fibronectin. [201] This makes CD138 an attractive therapeutic target. Ikeda et al., tested a series of immunoconjugates composed of the murine/human chimeric anti-CD138 antibody nBT062 conjugated with potent cytotoxic maytansinoid moieties. The Mab-ADC nBT062-SPDB-DM4 was potent when tested on MM cell lines, and showed little or no toxicity in CD138 negative cell lines and PMBC from healthy volunteers were exposed to this agent. *In vitro* studies showed that G2/M cell cycle arrest followed by apoptotic cell death thus causing inhibition of proliferation of MM cells. These antibodies also demonstrate that they can block the adhesion of MM cells to BMSCs suggesting that the immunoconjugates may function to overcome cell adhesion-mediated drug resistance to conventional treatments. At this time there are no clinical trials, which are enrolling to evaluate this drug.

Cellular Immune Therapy: Chimeric Antigen Receptos (CARs)

T-lymphocytes express CARs which are synthetic transmembrane proteins that confer an alternative specificity for particular antigens. [202] Two main components of CARs are the extracelluar domain that recognizes the cell-surface antigent and the intracellular signaling domain that initiates signal transduction required for T-cell activation. The extracellular antigen recogniztion domain is comprised of a heavy and light chain immunoglobulin antibody specific to a particular antigetn. Antigen binding to the CAR results in T-cell activation primarily through the zeta chain of the CD3 complex. CARs are separated into 1st, 2nd, and 3rd generation based on the number of intracellular singaling domains they contain. It is important to note T-cell activagtion requires other co-stimulatory signals from the antigen presenting cell (APC) which includes CD28 and 4-1BB and conversly CTLA-4 and PD-1 are checkpoint signals that suppress T-cell activation. These checkpoint signals are often manipulated by tumors to induce immune tolerance thuse evading immune mediated destruction. First generation CARs, those without costimulatory signaling domain, exhibited limeted activity in-vivo cell expansion and levels. Second generation CARs, those with CD28 costimulatory intracellular domain, have resulted in a significant in-vivo expansion and persistance. The addition of the costimaltory signaling 4-1BB domain with CD28 has show promising pre-clinical results. To stimulate the T-cell to be receptive to an antigen independent of an MHC bearing APC cell requires modification of the APC. This is done by developing a artificial APC by conjugating anti-CD3 and anti-CD28 antibodies to them which inturn provides simultaneious activating (CD3) and costimulatory (CD28) signals to cultured T-cells. The ideal CAR is one that is highly specific to cell-surface antigen to that tumor type as CARs developed in the past for HER2/neu and carbonic anhydrase IX have lead to fatal complications in patients as they also expressed these antigens at low levels in normal tissues.[203,204] Three principles are used in developing CAR-Tcells: (a) The target must be expressed on the surface, (b) Off-tumor expression of the target, evan at low levels, must not be present in an essential organ or cell type (i.e., hematopoetic stem cells), (c) To avoid antigen escape, all the tumor cells must express the target, or, alternatively, the target must be essential for maintenance of the tumorigenic phenotype. [205]. Two potential CAR modified T-cells targets for MM include the kappa immunogobulin light chain and CD138.

Kappa light chain target is of interest given that mature B-cell malignancies are typically light chain restricted to either kappa or lamba but not both. Targeting one of the light chains is attractive as normal B-cells expressing the uninvolved light chain would be left behind. This was explored in pre-clinical study with B-cell malignancies with ant-kappa light chain CD28 linked CAR which showed cytotoxic activity against Igκ positive tumor cell lines *in vitro* and *in vivo.* [206] As MM advances, immunoglobulin production is down-regulated and may be a potential mechanism of resistance thus altering the effect of CARs [207]. Currently a phase I clinical trial is underway evaluating Kappa-CD28 T lymphocytes in CLL, B-NHL or MM. [208]

CD138 is a cell membrane heparin sulfate proteoglycan which is expressed on both neoplastic and non-neoplastic plasma cells. In a preclinical model using anti-CD138 CAR against humans MM cell lines and mouse models showed significant anti-tumor activity toward CD138-positive MM cells. [209] Currently a phase I/II clinical trial is recruiting R/R MM patients to evaluate the safety and efficacy of a anti-CD138 CAR. [210]

B-cell maturation antigen (BCMA) is a member of the TNFR family that is expressed on terminally differentiated B-cells and promotes pro-survival signals to mature B-cells, plamsa cells and MM cells. Its targets include B-cell activator of the TNF family (BAFF) and a proliferation inducing ligand (APRIL). BCMA is postulated to play a critical role in protecting MM cells from apoptosis within the tumor microenvironment. In a pre-clinical study BCMA expression was exclusively found on plasma cells and novel anti-BCMA CARs were developed from MM cells from 5 patients. The anti-BCMA-CARs exhibited BCMA-specific functions including cytokine production, proliferatin, cytotoxicity, and *in vivo* tumor eradication. [211]

Additional T-Cell CARs targeting Le^y, CD38, and CS1 antigens have been evaluated however of concern in the case of Le^y not all myeloma harbor this antigen and also share it with epithelial and gastric tissue. Likewise CS1 and CD38 antigents are not exclusive to MM cells but are expressed by other hematopoietic cells and B- and T-cells respectively and thus potentially increasing off target toxicities.

A summary of the intracellular and extracellular pathways and their respective targeted drugs are shown in Figure 2.

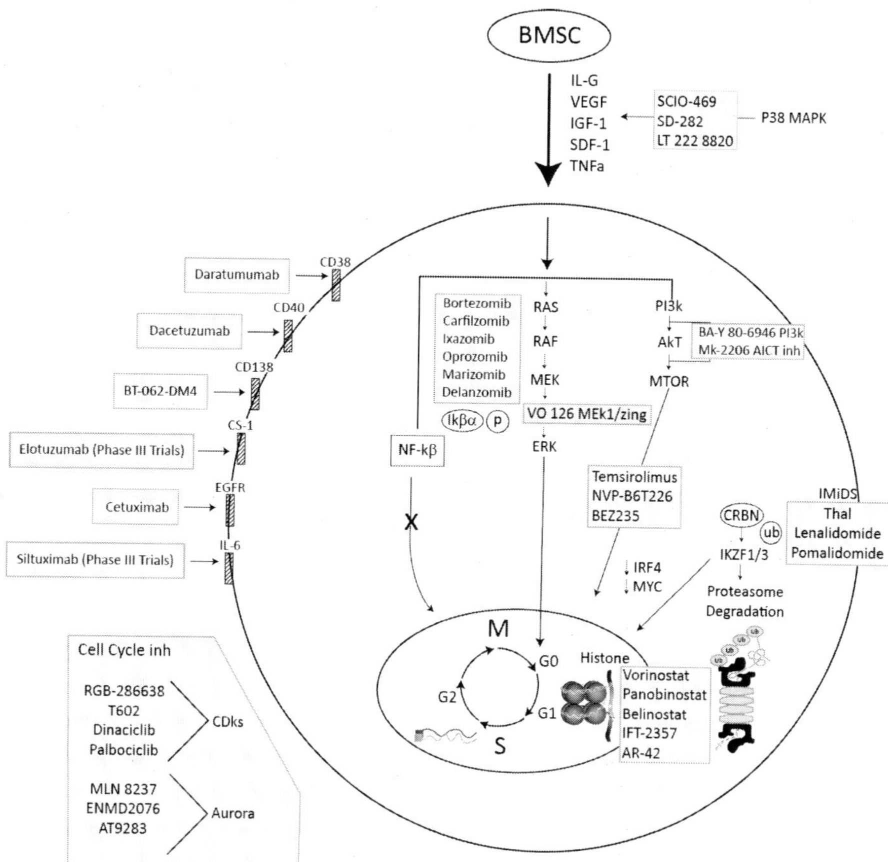

Conclusion

The process of MM tumorgenesis, development of drug resistance and multiple escape pathways is a complex process. Multiple pathways with embedded mutations provide a degree of impact on disease progression, cell survival and resistance indicative of tumor heterogeniety. Current risk stratification and diagnostic paradigm is most likely to change in the near future due to technological advances such as next generation sequencing and proteome analysis. Extensive genomic analysis by next generation sequencing of paired tumor to normal samples from over 200 MM patients has identified mutated oncogenes, gene copy number alterations and tumor suppressors by homozygous deletions and loss of heterozygosity. Eleven genes (65% pts) are recurrently mutated in MM, 5 of which were previously identified (KRAS, NRAS, FAM46C, DIS3, TP53). Additionally 4 other genes (BRAF, TRAF3, CYLD, RB1) have also been implicated in MM pathogenesis. PRDM1 a tumor suppressor acts as a transcriptional repressor to promote plasma cell survival. EGR1 known to interfere with JUN-induced MM growth has recurrent somatic hypermutations. Mutations are also identified in the Interferon regulatory factor IRF4 a survival factor and SP140 a lymphoid restricted tumor suppressor. The study demonstrated no significant associations between specific mutations and clinical features, tumor ploidy or history of previous therapy. A 3-gene set pathway level pattern of mutations retain significance. They are the NF-κB pathway, histone modifying enzymes and the coagulation cascade (51% pts). Eighteen percent of pts lack functional mutations and are likely to be driven by other mechanisms including dysregulated over-expression of to be discovered genes. Evidence of clonal heterogeneity by estimating cancer cell fraction (CCF) identified on average 3 subclones in addition to the major clone in a given MM patient. Moreover, mutations are present in subclones and also multiple mutations within the same pathway (KRAS, NRAS, BRAF) implicating combination therapy with a BRAF and MEK inhibitor [REF]. Hence, the future MM patient will have a comprehensive molecular pathologic profile prior to been assigned the optimal rational combination therapy.

Survival pathways such as HSP90, P38 MAPK, CDK, Aurora Kinase and HDAC, and PI3K/AKT/ mTOR equip MM crucial to escape pathways to overcome drug resistance. Despite promising pre-clinical models many of these new targeted agents have little to no clinical activity but have significant toxicities. Pre-clinical models unfortunately are not able to fully replicate MM in its true environment but do aid a viewing portal to particular aspect of its complex and heterogenetic disease pathogenesis. In our opinion HDACi are unique in that they have synergy with and may reverse Bz resistance by way of down-regulating genes encoding the proteasome complex and disrupting interactions between NF-κB, IκB, and HSP90. Clinical trials suggest that HDACi are able to recapture responses in Bz R/R MM pts. Despite improved outcomes with combining multiple agents the added toxicities must be weighed against clinical benefit. The most promising HDACis are vorinostat, panobinostat and romidepsin based on clinical trials. HSP 90 inhibitors are interesting in that they have a protective effect on PN development though clinically do not add much response to Bz R/R MM patients. Despite promising pre-clinical data some of these novel therapies do not have impressive clinical response rates in the R/R setting however more clinical trial may be warrented in treatment naïve patients to prevent drug resistance. Unlike IMiDs and PIs that have a broad mechanism of action and inhibit key driving pathways, novel inhibitors are targeting specific escape or regulatory pathways that may not impact clinical responses enough individually. It is not yet known the appropriate combination and timing of targeted therapy despite knowing there potential clinical relevance. Combining these targeted therapies for maximum clinical benefit must also be carefully weighed against the increased toxicities that have been observed.

Targeting the extracellular receptors on MM cells is actively being pursued and many agents are currently in various stages of clinical development. Elotuzumab, targets IL-6 involved in proliferation of plasma cells whereas targeting CD-40 with Dacetuzumab also causes a decrease in secretion of IL-6 along with apoptosis. These newer agents have been shown to be safe when administered as single agents and are now being tested in combination with drugs like Bz and Ln, in R/R MM pts. In the coming years we predict that these agents will be incoporated to reverse drug resistance to active agents and be part of multidrug regimens with increased efficacy with a safe toxicity profilre in therapy of MM. In addition, immune checkpoint Mabs and CAR therapy provide an interesting opportunity to re-direact the immune system to target R/R MM.

Acknowledgment

Acknowledged contribution: Donna McDonnell and Karen Axley

References

[1] Smith A, Wisloff, Finn et al.: Criteria for the classification of monoclonal gammopathies, multiple myeloma and related disorders: a report of the International Myeloma Working Group. *Br. J. Haematol.* 121:749, 2003.

[2] Rajkumar SV: Multiple myeloma: 2013 update on diagnosis, risk-stratification, and management. *Am. J. Hematol.* 88:226-35, 2013.

[3] Kyle RA, Gertz MA, Witzig TE, et al.: Review of 1027 patients with newly diagnosed multiple myeloma. *Mayo Clin. Proc.* 78:21-33, 2003.

[4] Landgren O, Weiss BM: Patterns of monoclonal gammopathy of undetermined significance and multiple myeloma in various ethnic/racial groups: support for genetic factors in pathogenesis. *Leukemia* 23:1691-7, 2009.

[5] Misso G, Zappavigna S, Castellano M, et al.: Emerging pathways as individualized therapeutic target of multiple myeloma. *Expert Opin. Biol. Ther.* 13 Suppl 1:S95-109, 2013.

[6] Avet-Loiseau H, Attal M, Moreau P, et al.: Genetic abnormalities and survival in multiple myeloma: the experience of the Intergroupe Francophone du Myelome. *Blood* 109:3489-95, 2007.

[7] Lode L, Eveillard M, Trichet V, et al.: Mutations in TP53 are exclusively associated with del(17p) in multiple myeloma. *Haematologica* 95:1973-6, 2010.

[8] Chng WJ, Gonzalez-Paz N, Price-Troska T, et al.: Clinical and biological significance of RAS mutations in multiple myeloma. *Leukemia* 22:2280-4, 2008.

[9] Chapman MA, Lawrence MS, Keats JJ, et al.: Initial genome sequencing and analysis of multiple myeloma. *Nature* 471:467-72, 2011.

[10] Demchenko YN, Kuehl WM: A critical role for the NFkB pathway in multiple myeloma. *Oncotarget* 1:59-68, 2010.

[11] Rajkumar SV: Multiple myeloma: 2012 update on diagnosis, risk-stratification, and management. *Am. J. Hematol.* 87:78-88, 2012.

[12] Durie BG, Salmon SE: A clinical staging system for multiple myeloma. Correlation of measured myeloma cell mass with presenting clinical features, response to treatment, and survival. *Cancer* 36:842-54, 1975.

[13] Dispenzieri A, Rajkumar SV, Gertz MA, et al.: Treatment of newly diagnosed multiple myeloma based on Mayo Stratification of Myeloma and Risk-adapted Therapy (mSMART): consensus statement. *Mayo Clin. Proc.* 82:323-41, 2007.

[14] Mikhael JR, Dingli D, Roy V, et al.: Management of newly diagnosed symptomatic multiple myeloma: updated Mayo Stratification of Myeloma and Risk-Adapted Therapy (mSMART) consensus guidelines 2013. *Mayo Clin. Proc.* 88:360-76, 2013.

[15] Kumar SK, Rajkumar SV, Dispenzieri A, et al.: Improved survival in multiple myeloma and the impact of novel therapies. Blood 111:2516-20, 2008.

[16] Rajkumar SV: Treatment of multiple myeloma. *Nat. Rev. Clin. Oncol.* 8:479-91, 2011.

[17] Child JA, Morgan GJ, Davies FE, et al.: High-dose chemotherapy with hematopoietic stem-cell rescue for multiple myeloma. *N. Engl. J. Med.* 348:1875-83, 2003.

[18] Attal M, Harousseau JL: Randomized trial experience of the Intergroupe Francophone du Myelome. *Semin. Hematol.* 38:226-30, 2001.

[19] Fermand JP, Katsahian S, Divine M, et al.: High-dose therapy and autologous blood stem-cell transplantation compared with conventional treatment in myeloma patients aged 55 to 65 years: long-term results of a randomized control trial from the Group Myelome-Autogreffe. *J. Clin. Oncol.* 23:9227-33, 2005.

[20] Attal M, Harousseau JL, Facon T, et al.: Single versus double autologous stem-cell transplantation for multiple myeloma. *N. Engl. J. Med.* 349:2495-502, 2003.

[21] Cavo M, Tosi P, Zamagni E, et al.: Prospective, randomized study of single compared with double autologous stem-cell transplantation for multiple myeloma: Bologna 96 clinical study. *J. Clin. Oncol.* 25:2434-41, 2007.

[22] Kumar A, Kharfan-Dabaja MA, Glasmacher A, et al.: Tandem versus single autologous hematopoietic cell transplantation for the treatment of multiple myeloma: a systematic review and meta-analysis. *J. Natl. Cancer Inst.* 101:100-6, 2009.

[23] Attal M, Harousseau JL, Leyvraz S, et al.: Maintenance therapy with thalidomide improves survival in patients with multiple myeloma. *Blood* 108:3289-94, 2006.

[24] Spencer A, Prince HM, Roberts AW, et al.: Consolidation therapy with low-dose thalidomide and prednisolone prolongs the survival of multiple myeloma patients undergoing a single autologous stem-cell transplantation procedure. *J. Clin. Oncol.* 27:1788-93, 2009.

[25] Barlogie B, Tricot G, Anaissie E, et al.: Thalidomide and hematopoietic-cell transplantation for multiple myeloma. *N. Engl. J. Med.* 354:1021-30, 2006.

[26] Morgan GJ, Jackson GH, Davies FE, et al.: Maintenance Thalidomide May Improve Progression Free but Not Overall Survival; Results from the Myeloma IX Maintenance Randomisation. *ASH Annual Meeting Abstracts 112*:656-, 2008.

[27] Ludwig H, Adam Z, Tothova E, et al.: Thalidomide maintenance treatment increases progression-free but not overall survival in elderly patients with myeloma. *Haematologica* 95:1548-54, 2010.

[28] Attal M, Lauwers-Cances V, Marit G, et al.: Lenalidomide maintenance after stem-cell transplantation for multiple myeloma. *N. Engl. J. Med.* 366:1782-91, 2012.

[29] McCarthy PL, Owzar K, Hofmeister CC, et al.: Lenalidomide after stem-cell transplantation for multiple myeloma. *N. Engl. J. Med.* 366:1770-81, 2012.

[30] Palumbo A, Hajek R, Delforge M, et al.: Continuous lenalidomide treatment for newly diagnosed multiple myeloma. *N. Engl. J. Med.* 366:1759-69, 2012.

[31] Sonneveld P, Schmidt-Wolf IG, van der Holt B, et al.: Bortezomib induction and maintenance treatment in patients with newly diagnosed multiple myeloma: results of the randomized phase III HOVON-65/ GMMG-HD4 trial. *J. Clin. Oncol.* 30:2946-55, 2012.

[32] Adams J: The proteasome: structure, function, and role in the cell. *Cancer Treat Rev.* 29 Suppl 1:3-9, 2003.

[33] Adams J: The proteasome: a suitable antineoplastic target. *Nat. Rev. Cancer* 4:349-60, 2004.

[34] Hideshima T, Richardson PG, Anderson KC: Mechanism of action of proteasome inhibitors and deacetylase inhibitors and the biological basis of synergy in multiple myeloma. *Mol. Cancer Ther.* 10:2034-42, 2011.

[35] Jacobs MD, Harrison SC: Structure of an IkappaBalpha/NF-kappaB complex. *Cell* 95:749-58, 1998.

[36] Jeremias I, Kupatt C, Baumann B, et al.: Inhibition of nuclear factor kappaB activation attenuates apoptosis resistance in lymphoid cells. *Blood* 91:4624-31, 1998.

[37] Moreau P, Richardson PG, Cavo M, et al.: Proteasome inhibitors in multiple myeloma: 10 years later. *Blood* 120:947-59, 2012.

[38] Boccadoro M, Morgan G, Cavenagh J: Preclinical evaluation of the proteasome inhibitor bortezomib in cancer therapy. *Cancer Cell Int.* 5:18, 2005.

[39] Hideshima T, Ikeda H, Chauhan D, et al.: Bortezomib induces canonical nuclear factor-kappaB activation in multiple myeloma cells. *Blood* 114:1046-52, 2009.

[40] Conticello C, Giuffrida R, Adamo L, et al.: NF-kappaB localization in multiple myeloma plasma cells and mesenchymal cells. *Leuk. Res.* 35:52-60, 2011.

[41] Mitsiades N, Mitsiades CS, Poulaki V, et al.: Molecular sequelae of proteasome inhibition in human multiple myeloma cells. *Proc. Natl. Acad. Sci. U S A* 99:14374-9, 2002.

[42] Jakubowiak AJ, Kendall T, Al-Zoubi A, et al.: Phase II trial of combination therapy with bortezomib, pegylated liposomal doxorubicin, and dexamethasone in patients with newly diagnosed myeloma. *J. Clin. Oncol.* 27:5015-22, 2009.

[43] Richardson PG, Barlogie B, Berenson J, et al.: A phase 2 study of bortezomib in relapsed, refractory myeloma. *N. Engl. J. Med.* 348:2609-17, 2003.

[44] Jagannath S, Barlogie B, Berenson JR, et al.: Updated survival analyses after prolonged follow-up of the phase 2, multicenter CREST study of bortezomib in relapsed or refractory multiple myeloma. *Br. J. Haematol.* 143:537-40, 2008.

[45] Richardson PG, Sonneveld P, Schuster MW, et al.: Bortezomib or high-dose dexamethasone for relapsed multiple myeloma. *N. Engl. J. Med.* 352:2487-98, 2005.

[46] Jain S, Diefenbach C, Zain J, et al.: Emerging role of carfilzomib in treatment of relapsed and refractory lymphoid neoplasms and multiple myeloma. *Core Evid.* 6:43-57, 2011.

[47] Palumbo A, Bringhen S, Rossi D, et al.: Bortezomib-melphalan-prednisone-thalidomide followed by maintenance with bortezomib-thalidomide compared with bortezomib-melphalan-prednisone for initial treatment of multiple myeloma: a randomized controlled trial. *J. Clin. Oncol.* 28:5101-9, 2010.

[48] Moreau P, Coiteux V, Hulin C, et al.: Prospective comparison of subcutaneous versus intravenous administration of bortezomib in patients with multiple myeloma. *Haematologica* 93:1908-11, 2008.

[49] Moreau P, Pylypenko H, Grosicki S, et al.: Subcutaneous versus intravenous administration of bortezomib in patients with relapsed multiple myeloma: a randomised, phase 3, non-inferiority study. *Lancet Oncol.* 12:431-40, 2011.

[50] Kuhn DJ, Chen Q, Voorhees PM, et al.: Potent activity of carfilzomib, a novel, irreversible inhibitor of the ubiquitin-proteasome pathway, against preclinical models of multiple myeloma. *Blood* 110:3281-90, 2007.

[51] Jagannath S, Vij R, Stewart AK, et al.: An open-label single-arm pilot phase II study (PX-171-003-A0) of low-dose, single-agent carfilzomib in patients with relapsed and refractory multiple myeloma. *Clin. Lymphoma Myeloma Leuk.* 12:310-8, 2012.

[52] David S. Siegel M, PhD, Thomas Martin, MD, Michael Wang, MD et al. : Results of PX-171-003-A1, An Open-Label, Single-Arm, Phase 2 (Ph 2) Study of Carfilzomib (CFZ) In Patients (pts) with Relapsed and Refractory Multiple Myeloma (MM) *ASH* 2010.

[53] Vij R, Wang M, Kaufman JL, et al.: An open-label, single-arm, phase 2 (PX-171-004) study of single-agent carfilzomib in bortezomib-naive patients with relapsed and/or refractory multiple myeloma. *Blood* 119:5661-70, 2012.

[54] Jakubowiak AJ, Siegel DS, Martin T, et al.: Treatment outcomes in patients with relapsed and refractory multiple myeloma and high-risk cytogenetics receiving single-agent carfilzomib in the PX-171-003-A1 study. *Leukemia* 27:2351-6, 2013.

[55] Korde N ZA, KwokM, et al. : Phase II clinical and correlative study of carfilzomib, lenalidomide, and dexamethasone (CRd) in newly diagnosed Multiple Myeloma(MM) patients[abstract]. *Blood*, 2012.

[56] Richardson PG, Weller E, Lonial S, et al.: Lenalidomide, bortezomib, and dexamethasone combination therapy in patients with newly diagnosed multiple myeloma. *Blood* 116:679-86, 2010.

[57] Sara Bringhen M, Chiara Cerrato, MD, Maria Teresa Petrucci, MD: A Phase II Study with Carfilzomib, Cyclophosphamide and Dexamethasone (CCd) For Newly Diagnosed Multiple Myeloma. *ASH,* 2013.

[58] Kumar SK, Flinn I, Noga SJ, et al.: Bortezomib, dexamethasone, cyclophosphamide and lenalidomide combination for newly diagnosed multiple myeloma: phase 1 results from the multicenter EVOLUTION study. *Leukemia* 24:1350-6, 2010.

[59] Claire Torre YG, MD, PhD, Lawrence H. Boise, PhD, et al.: Combined Carfilzomib and Selective PI3Kδ Inhibition (TGR1202) Results In Enhanced Myeloma Cell Apoptosis. *ASH*, 2013.

[60] Feling RH, Buchanan GO, Mincer TJ, et al.: Salinosporamide A: a highly cytotoxic proteasome inhibitor from a novel microbial source, a marine bacterium of the new genus salinospora. *Angew. Chem. Int. Ed. Engl.* 42:355-7, 2003.

[61] Chauhan D, Catley L, Li G, et al.: A novel orally active proteasome inhibitor induces apoptosis in multiple myeloma cells with mechanisms distinct from Bortezomib. *Cancer Cell* 8:407-19, 2005.

[62] Lawasut P, Chauhan D, Laubach J, et al.: New proteasome inhibitors in myeloma. *Curr. Hematol. Malig. Rep.* 7:258-66, 2012.

[63] Allegra A, Alonci A, Gerace D, et al.: New orally active proteasome inhibitors in multiple myeloma. *Leuk. Res.* 38:1-9, 2014.

[64] Paul G. Richardson M, Andrew Spencer, MD2, Paul Cannell, MBBS, FRCPA, FRACP3, Simon J. Harrison, MBBS MRCP (uk) MRCPath (uk) PhD4, Laurence

Catley, MBBS, FRCPA, FRACP5, Craig Underhill, MBBS, FRACP6, Todd M. Zimmerman, MD7, Craig C. Hofmeister, MD8, Andrzej J Jakubowiak, MD, PhD9, Jacob P. Laubach, MD10, Michael A. Palladino, PhD11, Angie M. Longenecker, RN, BSN11*, Ana Lay11*, Sandra Wear, RN12*, G. Kenneth Lloyd, PhD11*, Alison L. Hannah, MD11, Steve Reich, MD11*, Matthew A. Spear, MD11 and Kenneth C. Anderson, MD13: Phase 1 Clinical Evaluation of Twice-Weekly Marizomib (NPI-0052), a Novel Proteasome Inhibitor, in Patients with Relapsed/Refractory Multiple Myeloma (MM) ASH, 2011.

[65] Chauhan D, Singh A, Brahmandam M, et al.: Combination of proteasome inhibitors bortezomib and NPI-0052 trigger in vivo synergistic cytotoxicity in multiple myeloma. *Blood* 111:1654-64, 2008.

[66] Chauhan D, Singh AV, Ciccarelli B, et al.: Combination of novel proteasome inhibitor NPI-0052 and lenalidomide trigger in vitro and in vivo synergistic cytotoxicity in multiple myeloma. *Blood* 115:834-45, 2010.

[67] Millward M, Price T, Townsend A, et al.: Phase 1 clinical trial of the novel proteasome inhibitor marizomib with the histone deacetylase inhibitor vorinostat in patients with melanoma, pancreatic and lung cancer based on in vitro assessments of the combination. *Invest New Drugs* 30:2303-17, 2012.

[68] Kupperman E, Lee EC, Cao Y, et al.: Evaluation of the proteasome inhibitor MLN9708 in preclinical models of human cancer. *Cancer Res.* 70:1970-80, 2010.

[69] Chauhan D, Tian Z, Zhou B, et al.: In vitro and in vivo selective antitumor activity of a novel orally bioavailable proteasome inhibitor MLN9708 against multiple myeloma cells. *Clin. Cancer Res.* 17:5311-21, 2011.

[70] Chauhan D, Singh AV, Aujay M, et al.: A novel orally active proteasome inhibitor ONX 0912 triggers in vitro and in vivo cytotoxicity in multiple myeloma. *Blood* 116:4906-15, 2010.

[71] Zhou HJ, Aujay MA, Bennett MK, et al.: Design and synthesis of an orally bioavailable and selective peptide epoxyketone proteasome inhibitor (PR-047). *J. Med. Chem.* 52:3028-38, 2009.

[72] Piva R, Ruggeri B, Williams M, et al.: CEP-18770: A novel, orally active proteasome inhibitor with a tumor-selective pharmacologic profile competitive with bortezomib. *Blood* 111:2765-75, 2008.

[73] Sanchez E, Li M, Steinberg JA, et al.: The proteasome inhibitor CEP-18770 enhances the anti-myeloma activity of bortezomib and melphalan. *Br. J. Haematol.* 148:569-81, 2010.

[74] Gallerani E, Zucchetti M, Brunelli D, et al.: A first in human phase I study of the proteasome inhibitor CEP-18770 in patients with advanced solid tumours and multiple myeloma. *Eur. J. Cancer* 49:290-6, 2013.

[75] Ocio EM, Mateos MV, San-Miguel JF: Novel agents derived from the currently approved treatments for MM: novel proteasome inhibitors and novel IMIDs. *Expert Opin. Investig. Drugs* 21:1075-87, 2012.

[76] Mitsiades N, Mitsiades CS, Poulaki V, et al.: Apoptotic signaling induced by immunomodulatory thalidomide analogs in human multiple myeloma cells: therapeutic implications. *Blood* 99:4525-30, 2002.

[77] Hideshima T, Chauhan D, Shima Y, et al.: Thalidomide and its analogs overcome drug resistance of human multiple myeloma cells to conventional therapy. *Blood* 96:2943-50, 2000.

[78] Lacy MQ: New immunomodulatory drugs in myeloma. *Curr. Hematol. Malig. Rep.* 6:120-5, 2011.

[79] Chauhan D, Hideshima T, Rosen S, et al.: Apaf-1/cytochrome c-independent and Smac-dependent induction of apoptosis in multiple myeloma (MM) cells. *J. Biol. Chem.* 276:24453-6, 2001.

[80] Escoubet-Lozach L, Lin IL, Jensen-Pergakes K, et al.: Pomalidomide and lenalidomide induce p21 WAF-1 expression in both lymphoma and multiple myeloma through a LSD1-mediated epigenetic mechanism. *Cancer Res.* 69:7347-56, 2009.

[81] Lu G, Middleton RE, Sun H, et al.: The myeloma drug lenalidomide promotes the cereblon-dependent destruction of Ikaros proteins. *Science* 343:305-9, 2014.

[82] Kronke J, Udeshi ND, Narla A, et al.: Lenalidomide causes selective degradation of IKZF1 and IKZF3 in multiple myeloma cells. *Science* 343:301-5, 2014.

[83] von Lilienfeld-Toal M, Hahn-Ast C, Furkert K, et al.: A systematic review of phase II trials of thalidomide/dexamethasone combination therapy in patients with relapsed or refractory multiple myeloma. *Eur. J. Haematol.* 81:247-52, 2008.

[84] Dimopoulos M, Spencer A, Attal M, et al.: Lenalidomide plus dexamethasone for relapsed or refractory multiple myeloma. *N. Engl. J. Med.* 357:2123-32, 2007.

[85] Rajkumar SV, Jacobus S, Callander NS, et al.: Lenalidomide plus high-dose dexamethasone versus lenalidomide plus low-dose dexamethasone as initial therapy for newly diagnosed multiple myeloma: an open-label randomised controlled trial. *Lancet Oncol.* 11:29-37, 2010

[86] Yang B, Yu RL, Chi XH, et al.: Lenalidomide treatment for multiple myeloma: systematic review and meta-analysis of randomized controlled trials. *PLoS One* 8:e64354, 2013.

[87] Kumar S, Flinn I, Richardson PG, et al.: Randomized, multicenter, phase 2 study (EVOLUTION) of combinations of bortezomib, dexamethasone, cyclophosphamide, and lenalidomide in previously untreated multiple myeloma. *Blood* 119:4375-82, 2012.

[88] McCarthy PL OK, Anderson KC, et al.: Phase III intergroup study of lenalidomide versus placebo maintenance therapy following single autologous hematopoietic stem cell transplantation (AHSCT) for multiple myeloma: CALGB 100104 *ASH*, 2010.

[89] Michel Attal M, Valerie cances Lauwers1*, Gerald Marit, Service: Maintenance Treatment with Lenalidomide After Transplantation for MYELOMA : Final Analysis of the IFM 2005-02. *ASH Annual Meeting Abstracts*, 2010.

[90] Ye X, Huang J, Pan Q, et al.: Maintenance therapy with immunomodulatory drugs after autologous stem cell transplantation in patients with multiple myeloma: a meta-analysis of randomized controlled trials. *PLoS One* 8:e72635, 2013.

[91] Shortt J, Hsu AK, Johnstone RW: Thalidomide-analogue biology: immunological, molecular and epigenetic targets in cancer therapy. *Oncogene* 32:4191-202, 2013.

[92] Ruchelman AL, Man HW, Zhang W, et al.: Isosteric analogs of lenalidomide and pomalidomide: synthesis and biological activity. *Bioorg. Med. Chem. Lett.* 23:360-5, 2013.

[93] Richardson PG, Mark TM, Lacy MQ: Pomalidomide: new immunomodulatory agent with potent antiproliferative effects. Crit Rev Oncol Hematol 88 Suppl 1:S36-44, 2013.

[94] NCT01734928: Safety and Efficacy of Pomalidomide, Bortezomib and Low-dose Dexamethasone in Subjects with Relapsed or Refractory Multiple Myeloma.
[95] Zhu YX, Braggio E, Shi CX, et al.: Cereblon expression is required for the antimyeloma activity of lenalidomide and pomalidomide. *Blood* 118:4771-9, 2011.
[96] Zhu YX, Kortuem KM, Stewart AK: Molecular mechanism of action of immune-modulatory drugs thalidomide, lenalidomide and pomalidomide in multiple myeloma. *Leuk. Lymphoma* 54:683-7, 2013.
[97] Anderson G, Gries M, Kurihara N, et al.: Thalidomide derivative CC-4047 inhibits osteoclast formation by down-regulation of PU.1. *Blood* 107:3098-105, 2006.
[98] Bolzoni M, Storti P, Bonomini S, et al.: Immunomodulatory drugs lenalidomide and pomalidomide inhibit multiple myeloma-induced osteoclast formation and the RANKL/OPG ratio in the myeloma microenvironment targeting the expression of adhesion molecules. *Exp. Hematol.* 41:387-97.e1, 2013.
[99] Richardson PG, Siegel D, Baz R, et al.: Phase 1 study of pomalidomide MTD, safety, and efficacy in patients with refractory multiple myeloma who have received lenalidomide and bortezomib. *Blood* 121:1961-7, 2013.
[100] Richardson PG, Siegel DS, Vij R, et al.: Pomalidomide alone or in combination with low-dose dexamethasone in relapsed and refractory multiple myeloma: a randomized phase 2 study. *Blood* 123:1826-32, 2014.
[101] San Miguel J, Weisel K, Moreau P, et al.: Pomalidomide plus low-dose dexamethasone versus high-dose dexamethasone alone for patients with relapsed and refractory multiple myeloma (MM-003): a randomised, open-label, phase 3 trial. *Lancet Oncol.* 14:1055-66, 2013.
[102] Scarfo L, Ghia P: Reprogramming cell death: BCL2 family inhibition in hematological malignancies. *Immunol. Lett.* 155:36-9, 2013.
[103] Tsujimoto Y, Cossman J, Jaffe E, et al.: Involvement of the bcl-2 gene in human follicular lymphoma. *Science* 228:1440-3, 1985.
[104] NCT01794507: A Study Evaluating ABT-199 in Multiple Myeloma Subjects Who Are Receiving Bortezomib and Dexamethasone as Standard Therapy.
[105] NCT01794520: A Phase I Study Evaluating ABT-199 in Subjects with Relapsed or Refractory Multiple Myeloma.
[106] Whitesell L, Lindquist SL: HSP90 and the chaperoning of cancer. *Nat. Rev. Cancer* 5:761-72, 2005.
[107] Chanan-Khan AA, Borrello I, Lee KP, et al.: Development of target-specific treatments in multiple myeloma. *Br. J. Haematol.* 151:3-15, 2010.
[108] Richardson PG, Chanan-Khan AA, Lonial S, et al.: Tanespimycin and bortezomib combination treatment in patients with relapsed or relapsed and refractory multiple myeloma: results of a phase 1/2 study. *Br. J. Haematol.* 153:729-40, 2011.
[109] NCT00546780: A Study of Tanespimycin (KOS-953) in Patients with Multiple Myeloma in First Relapse.
[110] Chatterjee M, Andrulis M, Stuhmer T, et al.: The PI3K/Akt signaling pathway regulates the expression of Hsp70, which critically contributes to Hsp90-chaperone function and tumor cell survival in multiple myeloma. *Haematologica* 98:1132-41, 2013.
[111] Siegel D, Jagannath S, Vesole DH, et al.: A phase 1 study of IPI-504 (retaspimycin hydrochloride) in patients with relapsed or relapsed and refractory multiple myeloma. *Leuk. Lymphoma* 52:2308-15, 2011.

[112] Fresno Vara JA, Casado E, de Castro J, et al.: PI3K/Akt signalling pathway and cancer. *Cancer Treat Rev*. 30:193-204, 2004.

[113] Zollinger A, Stuhmer T, Chatterjee M, et al.: Combined functional and molecular analysis of tumor cell signaling defines 2 distinct myeloma subgroups: Akt-dependent and Akt-independent multiple myeloma. *Blood* 112:3403-11, 2008.

[114] Glauer J, Pletz N, Schon M, et al.: A novel selective small-molecule PI3K inhibitor is effective against human multiple myeloma in vitro and in vivo. *Blood Cancer J*. 3:e141, 2013.

[115] Ramakrishnan V, Kimlinger T, Haug J, et al.: Anti-myeloma activity of Akt inhibition is linked to the activation status of PI3K/Akt and MEK/ERK pathway. *PLoS One* 7:e50005, 2012.

[116] Shor B, Gibbons JJ, Abraham RT, et al.: Targeting mTOR globally in cancer: thinking beyond rapamycin. *Cell Cycle* 8:3831-7, 2009.

[117] Briest F, Grabowski P: PI3K-AKT-mTOR-signaling and beyond: the complex network in gastroenteropancreatic neuroendocrine neoplasms. *Theranostics* 4:336-65, 2014.

[118] Peterson TR, Laplante M, Thoreen CC, et al.: DEPTOR is an mTOR inhibitor frequently overexpressed in multiple myeloma cells and required for their survival. *Cell* 137:873-86, 2009.

[119] Huang J, Manning BD: A complex interplay between Akt, TSC2 and the two mTOR complexes. *Biochem. Soc. Trans*. 37:217-22, 2009.

[120] O'Reilly KE, Rojo F, She QB, et al.: mTOR inhibition induces upstream receptor tyrosine kinase signaling and activates Akt. *Cancer Res*. 66:1500-8, 2006.

[121] Farag SS, Zhang S, Jansak BS, et al.: Phase II trial of temsirolimus in patients with relapsed or refractory multiple myeloma. *Leuk. Res*. 33:1475-80, 2009.

[122] Ghobrial IM, Weller E, Vij R, et al.: Weekly bortezomib in combination with temsirolimus in relapsed or relapsed and refractory multiple myeloma: a multicentre, phase 1/2, open-label, dose-escalation study. *Lancet Oncol*. 12:263-72, 2011.

[123] Hofmeister CC, Yang X, Pichiorri F, et al.: Phase I trial of lenalidomide and CCI-779 in patients with relapsed multiple myeloma: evidence for lenalidomide-CCI-779 interaction via P-glycoprotein. *J. Clin. Oncol*. 29:3427-34, 2011.

[124] Baumann P, Schneider L, Mandl-Weber S, et al.: Simultaneous targeting of PI3K and mTOR with NVP-BGT226 is highly effective in multiple myeloma. *Anticancer Drugs* 23:131-8, 2012.

[125] McMillin DW, Ooi M, Delmore J, et al.: Antimyeloma activity of the orally bioavailable dual phosphatidylinositol 3-kinase/mammalian target of rapamycin inhibitor NVP-BEZ235. *Cancer Res*. 69:5835-42, 2009.

[126] Medicherla S, Reddy M, Ying J, et al.: p38alpha-selective MAP kinase inhibitor reduces tumor growth in mouse xenograft models of multiple myeloma. *Anticancer Res*. 28:3827-33, 2008.

[127] NCT00095680: Extension Study of the Efficacy and Safety of Oral SCIO-469 in Relapsed, Refractory Patients with Multiple Myeloma.

[128] NCT00087867: Study of Oral SCIO-469 in Relapsed, Refractory Patients with Multiple Myeloma.

[129] Ishitsuka K, Hideshima T, Neri P, et al.: p38 mitogen-activated protein kinase inhibitor LY2228820 enhances bortezomib-induced cytotoxicity and inhibits osteoclastogenesis in multiple myeloma; therapeutic implications. *Br. J. Haematol*. 141:598-606, 2008.

[130] Caers J, Menu E, De Raeve H, et al.: Antitumour and antiangiogenic effects of Aplidin in the 5TMM syngeneic models of multiple myeloma. *Br. J. Cancer* 98:1966-74, 2008.
[131] Mateos MV, Cibeira MT, Richardson PG, et al.: Phase II clinical and pharmacokinetic study of plitidepsin 3-hour infusion every two weeks alone or with dexamethasone in relapsed and refractory multiple myeloma. *Clin. Cancer Res.* 16:3260-9, 2010.
[132] Bharti AC, Donato N, Singh S, et al.: Curcumin (diferuloylmethane) down-regulates the constitutive activation of nuclear factor-kappa B and IkappaBalpha kinase in human multiple myeloma cells, leading to suppression of proliferation and induction of apoptosis. *Blood* 101:1053-62, 2003.
[133] Bharti AC, Takada Y, Aggarwal BB: Curcumin (diferuloylmethane) inhibits receptor activator of NF-kappa B ligand-induced NF-kappa B activation in osteoclast precursors and suppresses osteoclastogenesis. *J. Immunol.* 172:5940-7, 2004.
[134] Golombick T, Diamond TH, Badmaev V, et al.: The potential role of curcumin in patients with monoclonal gammopathy of undefined significance--its effect on paraproteinemia and the urinary N-telopeptide of type I collagen bone turnover marker. *Clin. Cancer Res.* 15:5917-22, 2009.
[135] Golombick T, Diamond TH, Manoharan A, et al.: Monoclonal gammopathy of undetermined significance, smoldering multiple myeloma, and curcumin: a randomized, double-blind placebo-controlled cross-over 4g study and an open-label 8g extension study. *Am. J. Hematol.* 87:455-60, 2012.
[136] Maes K, Menu E, Van Valckenborgh E, et al.: Epigenetic modulating agents as a new therapeutic approach in multiple myeloma. *Cancers* (Basel) 5:430-61, 2013.
[137] Ocio EM, Mateos MV, Maiso P, et al.: New drugs in multiple myeloma: mechanisms of action and phase I/II clinical findings. *Lancet Oncol.* 9:1157-65, 2008.
[138] Mitsiades CS, Mitsiades NS, McMullan CJ, et al.: Transcriptional signature of histone deacetylase inhibition in multiple myeloma: biological and clinical implications. *Proc. Natl. Acad. Sci. U S A* 101:540-5, 2004.
[139] DeAngelo DJ, Spencer A, Bhalla KN, et al.: Phase Ia/II, two-arm, open-label, dose-escalation study of oral panobinostat administered via two dosing schedules in patients with advanced hematologic malignancies. *Leukemia* 27:1628-36, 2013.
[140] Niesvizky R, Ely S, Mark T, et al.: Phase 2 trial of the histone deacetylase inhibitor romidepsin for the treatment of refractory multiple myeloma. *Cancer* 117:336-42, 2011.
[141] Galli M, Salmoiraghi S, Golay J, et al.: A phase II multiple dose clinical trial of histone deacetylase inhibitor ITF2357 in patients with relapsed or progressive multiple myeloma. *Ann. Hematol.* 89:185-90, 2010.
[142] Richardson P, Mitsiades C, Colson K, et al.: Phase I trial of oral vorinostat (suberoylanilide hydroxamic acid, SAHA) in patients with advanced multiple myeloma. *Leuk. Lymphoma* 49:502-7, 2008.
[143] Gimsing P, Hansen M, Knudsen LM, et al.: A phase I clinical trial of the histone deacetylase inhibitor belinostat in patients with advanced hematological neoplasia. *Eur. J. Haematol.* 81:170-6, 2008.
[144] Jonathan L. Kaufman M, Jatin J. Shah, M.D, Jacob P. Laubach, MD: Lenalidomide, Bortezomib, and Dexamethasone (RVD) in Combination with Vorinostat As Front-Line Therapy for Patients with Multiple Myeloma (MM): Results of a Phase 1 Study. *ASH Annual Meeting Abstracts*, 2012.

[145] David S. Siegel M, PhD, Meletios Athanasios Dimopoulos, MD, Sung-Soo Yoon, MD, PhD: Vantage 095: Vorinostat in Combination with Bortezomib in Salvage Multiple Myeloma Patients: Final Study Results of a Global Phase 2b Trial *ASH Annual Meeting Abstracts*, 2011.

[146] Dimopoulos M, Siegel DS, Lonial S, et al.: Vorinostat or placebo in combination with bortezomib in patients with multiple myeloma (VANTAGE 088): a multicentre, randomised, double-blind study. *Lancet Oncol.* 14:1129-40, 2013.

[147] Dokmanovic M, Clarke C, Marks PA: Histone deacetylase inhibitors: overview and perspectives. *Mol. Cancer Res.* 5:981-9, 2007.

[148] J. F. San-Miguel OS, D. S. Siegel: Phase Ib study of oral panobinostat (LBH589) plus intravenous bortezomib in patients (Pts) with relapsed (Rel) or Rel and refractory (Ref) multiple myeloma (MM). ASH Annual Meeting Abstracts, 2010.

[149] Richardson PG, Schlossman RL, Alsina M, et al.: PANORAMA 2: panobinostat in combination with bortezomib and dexamethasone in patients with relapsed and bortezomib-refractory myeloma. *Blood* 122:2331-7, 2013.

[150] Offidani M, Polloni C, Cavallo F, et al.: Phase II study of melphalan, thalidomide and prednisone combined with oral panobinostat in patients with relapsed/refractory multiple myeloma. *Leuk. Lymphoma* 53:1722-7, 2012.

[151] Jesus Berdeja M, Michael Savona, MD, Joseph R Mace, MD: A Single-Arm, Open-Label, Multi-Center Phase I/II Study Of The Combination Of Panobinostat and Carfilzomib In Patients (pts) with Relapsed Or Relapse/Refractory Multiple Myeloma (MM) *ASH Annual Meeting Abstracts*, 2013.

[152] Feng R, Oton A, Mapara MY, et al.: The histone deacetylase inhibitor, PXD101, potentiates bortezomib-induced anti-multiple myeloma effect by induction of oxidative stress and DNA damage. *Br. J. Haematol.* 139:385-97, 2007.

[153] NCT00431340: A Phase II Study of Belinostat in Combination with Bortezomib in Patients with Relapsed, Refractory Multiple Myeloma.

[154] NCT00131261: Clinical Trial of PXD101 in Patients with Advanced Multiple Myeloma.

[155] Harrison SJ, Quach H, Link E, et al.: A high rate of durable responses with romidepsin, bortezomib, and dexamethasone in relapsed or refractory multiple myeloma. *Blood* 118:6274-83, 2011.

[156] Kikuchi J, Wada T, Shimizu R, et al.: Histone deacetylases are critical targets of bortezomib-induced cytotoxicity in multiple myeloma. *Blood* 116:406-17, 2010.

[157] Todoerti K, Barbui V, Pedrini O, et al.: Pleiotropic anti-myeloma activity of ITF2357: inhibition of interleukin-6 receptor signaling and repression of miR-19a and miR-19b. *Haematologica* 95:260-9, 2010.

[158] Golay J, Cuppini L, Leoni F, et al.: The histone deacetylase inhibitor ITF2357 has anti-leukemic activity in vitro and in vivo and inhibits IL-6 and VEGF production by stromal cells. *Leukemia* 21:1892-900, 2007.

[159] NCT00792506: Phase II High Pulse Dose Clinical Trial of Orally Administered ITF2357 In Patients with Relapsed/Refractory Multiple Myeloma.

[160] Zhang S, Suvannasankha A, Crean CD, et al.: The novel histone deacetylase inhibitor, AR-42, inhibits gp130/Stat3 pathway and induces apoptosis and cell cycle arrest in multiple myeloma cells. *Int. J. Cancer* 129:204-13, 2011.

[161] NCT01129193: AR-42 in Treating Patients with Advanced or Relapsed Multiple Myeloma, Chronic Lymphocytic Leukemia, or Lymphoma.

[162] Cirstea D, Hideshima T, Santo L, et al.: Small-molecule multi-targeted kinase inhibitor RGB-286638 triggers P53-dependent and -independent anti-multiple myeloma activity through inhibition of transcriptional CDKs. *Leukemia* 27:2366-75, 2013.

[163] Bergsagel PL, Kuehl WM: Molecular pathogenesis and a consequent classification of multiple myeloma. *J. Clin. Oncol.* 23:6333-8, 2005.

[164] Canavese M, Santo L, Raje N: Cyclin dependent kinases in cancer: potential for therapeutic intervention. *Cancer Biol. Ther.* 13:451-7, 2012.

[165] Kramer A, Schultheis B, Bergmann J, et al.: Alterations of the cyclin D1/pRb/p16(INK4A) pathway in multiple myeloma. *Leukemia* 16:1844-51, 2002.

[166] Baughn LB, Di Liberto M, Wu K, et al.: A novel orally active small molecule potently induces G1 arrest in primary myeloma cells and prevents tumor growth by specific inhibition of cyclin-dependent kinase 4/6. *Cancer Res.* 66:7661-7, 2006.

[167] Alvarez-Fernandez S, Ortiz-Ruiz MJ, Parrott T, et al.: Potent antimyeloma activity of a novel ERK5/CDK inhibitor. *Clin. Cancer Res.* 19:2677-87, 2013.

[168] NCT01204164: Phase I Study of TG02 Citrate in Patients with Advanced Hematological Malignancies.

[169] Desai BM, Villanueva J, Nguyen TT, et al.: The anti-melanoma activity of dinaciclib, a cyclin-dependent kinase inhibitor, is dependent on p53 signaling. *PLoS* One 8:e59588, 2013.

[170] Nguyen TK, Grant S: Dinaciclib (SCH727965) inhibits the unfolded protein response through a CDK1- and 5-dependent mechanism. *Mol. Cancer Ther.* 13:662-74, 2014.

[171] NCT01096342: Dinaciclib in Treating Patients with Relapsed or Refractory Multiple Myeloma.

[172] NCT01711528: Dinaciclib, Bortezomib, and Dexamethasone in Treating Patients with Relapsed Multiple Myeloma.

[173] Menu E, Garcia J, Huang X, et al.: A novel therapeutic combination using PD 0332991 and bortezomib: study in the 5T33MM myeloma model. *Cancer Res.* 68:5519-23, 2008.

[174] NCT00555906: An Investigational Drug, Palbociclib (PD-0332991), Is Being Studied In Combination with Velcade And Dexamethasone In Patients with Multiple Myeloma. Patients Must Have Received Prior Treatment for Multiple Myeloma.

[175] Gorgun G, Calabrese E, Hideshima T, et al.: A novel Aurora-A kinase inhibitor MLN8237 induces cytotoxicity and cell-cycle arrest in multiple myeloma. *Blood* 115:5202-13, 2010.

[176] Evans R, Naber C, Steffler T, et al.: Aurora A kinase RNAi and small molecule inhibition of Aurora kinases with VE-465 induce apoptotic death in multiple myeloma cells. *Leuk. Lymphoma* 49:559-69, 2008.

[177] NCT00697346: Study of MLN8237 in Patients with Advanced Hematological Malignancies.

[178] NCT01034553: Aurora A Kinase Inhibitor MLN8237 and Bortezomib in Treating Patients with Relapsed or Refractory Multiple Myeloma.

[179] Wang X, Sinn AL, Pollok K, et al.: Preclinical activity of a novel multiple tyrosine kinase and aurora kinase inhibitor, ENMD-2076, against multiple myeloma. *Br. J. Haematol.* 150:313-25, 2010.

[180] Santo L, Hideshima T, Cirstea D, et al.: Antimyeloma activity of a multitargeted kinase inhibitor, AT9283, via potent Aurora kinase and STAT3 inhibition either alone or in combination with lenalidomide. *Clin. Cancer Res.* 17:3259-71, 2011.

[181] NCT01145989: A Study of AT9283 in Patients with Relapsed or Refractory Multiple Myeloma.

[182] Mendelson J BJ: Epidermal growth factor receptor targeting in cancer. *Seminars of oncology* 33:369-385, 2006.

[183] Mahtouk K, Jourdan M, De Vos J, et al.: An inhibitor of the EGF receptor family blocks myeloma cell growth factor activity of HB-EGF and potentiates dexamethasone or anti-IL-6 antibody-induced apoptosis. *Blood* 103:1829-37, 2004.

[184] von Tresckow B, Boll, Boris, Eichenauer, Dennis A., Peine, Denissa, Knop, Stefan, Goebeler, Mariele, Chemnitz, Jens M., Hallek, Michael, Engert, Andreas, Hubel, Kai: A phase II clinical trial of anti-EGFR antibody cetuximab in patients with refractory or relapsed multiple myeloma: Final Results. *ASH annual meeting abstracts* 118:3695, 2011.

[185] Teoh G, Anderson KC: Interaction of tumor and host cells with adhesion and extracellular matrix molecules in the development of multiple myeloma. *Hematol. Oncol. Clin. North Am.* 11:27-42, 1997.

[186] Urashima M, Ogata A, Chauhan D, et al.: Interleukin-6 promotes multiple myeloma cell growth via phosphorylation of retinoblastoma protein. *Blood* 88:2219-27, 1996.

[187] Voorhees PM, Manges RF, Sonneveld P, et al.: A phase 2 multicentre study of siltuximab, an anti-interleukin-6 monoclonal antibody, in patients with relapsed or refractory multiple myeloma. *Br. J. Haematol.* 161:357-66, 2013.

[188] Tai YT, Dillon M, Song W, et al.: Anti-CS1 humanized monoclonal antibody HuLuc63 inhibits myeloma cell adhesion and induces antibody-dependent cellular cytotoxicity in the bone marrow milieu. *Blood* 112:1329-37, 2008.

[189] Grewal IS, Flavell RA: CD40 and CD154 in cell-mediated immunity. *Annu. Rev. Immunol.* 16:111-35, 1998.

[190] Teoh G, Tai YT, Urashima M, et al.: CD40 activation mediates p53-dependent cell cycle regulation in human multiple myeloma cell lines. Blood 95:1039-46, 2000

[191] Dadgostar H, Zarnegar B, Hoffmann A, et al.: Cooperation of multiple signaling pathways in CD40-regulated gene expression in B lymphocytes. *Proc. Natl. Acad. Sci. U S* A 99:1497-502, 2002.

[192] Urashima M, Chauhan D, Uchiyama H, et al.: CD40 ligand triggered interleukin-6 secretion in multiple myeloma. *Blood* 85:1903-12, 1995.

[193] Hussein M, Berenson JR, Niesvizky R, et al.: A phase I multidose study of dacetuzumab (SGN-40; humanized anti-CD40 monoclonal antibody) in patients with multiple myeloma. *Haematologica* 95:845-8, 2010.

[194] de Weers M, Tai YT, van der Veer MS, et al.: Daratumumab, a novel therapeutic human CD38 monoclonal antibody, induces killing of multiple myeloma and other hematological tumors. *J. Immunol.* 186:1840-8, 2011.

[195] Martin III TG SS, Glenn M, Zheng W, Daskalakis N, Mikhael JR: SAR650984, A CD38 monoclonal antibody in patients with selected CD38+ hematological malignancies-data from a dose escalation phase 1 study. *Blood* 122, 2013.

[196] Keir ME, Butte MJ, Freeman GJ, et al.: PD-1 and its ligands in tolerance and immunity. *Annu. Rev. Immunol.* 26:677-704, 2008.

[197] Benson DM, Jr., Bakan CE, Mishra A, et al.: The PD-1/PD-L1 axis modulates the natural killer cell versus multiple myeloma effect: a therapeutic target for CT-011, a novel monoclonal anti-PD-1 antibody. *Blood* 116:2286-94, 2010.
[198] Berger R, Rotem-Yehudar R, Slama G, et al.: Phase I safety and pharmacokinetic study of CT-011, a humanized antibody interacting with PD-1, in patients with advanced hematologic malignancies. *Clin. Cancer Res.* 14:3044-51, 2008.
[199] Schafer PH, Gandhi AK, Loveland MA, et al.: Enhancement of cytokine production and AP-1 transcriptional activity in T cells by thalidomide-related immunomodulatory drugs. *J. Pharmacol. Exp. Ther.* 305:1222-32, 2003.
[200] Dhodapkar MV, Abe E, Theus A, et al.: Syndecan-1 is a multifunctional regulator of myeloma pathobiology: control of tumor cell survival, growth, and bone cell differentiation. *Blood* 91:2679-88, 1998.
[201] Garfall AL, Fraietta JA, Maus MV: Immunotherapy with chimeric antigen receptors for multiple myeloma. *Discov. Med.* 17:37-46, 2014.
[202] Morgan RA, Yang JC, Kitano M, et al.: Case report of a serious adverse event following the administration of T cells transduced with a chimeric antigen receptor recognizing ERBB2. *Mol.Ther.* 18:843-51, 2010.
[203] Lamers CH, Sleijfer S, Vulto AG, et al.: Treatment of metastatic renal cell carcinoma with autologous T-lymphocytes genetically retargeted against carbonic anhydrase IX: first clinical experience. *J. Clin. Oncol.* 24:e20-2, 2006.
[204] Maus MV, June CH: Zoom Zoom: racing CARs for multiple myeloma. *Clin. Cancer Res.* 19:1917-9, 2013.
[205] Vera J, Savoldo B, Vigouroux S, et al.: T lymphocytes redirected against the kappa light chain of human immunoglobulin efficiently kill mature B lymphocyte-derived malignant cells. *Blood* 108:3890-7, 2006.
[206] Leung-Hagesteijn C, Erdmann N, Cheung G, et al.: Xbp1s-negative tumor B cells and pre-plasmablasts mediate therapeutic proteasome inhibitor resistance in multiple myeloma. *Cancer Cell* 24:289-304, 2013.
[207] NCT00881920: Kappa-CD28 T Lymphocytes, Chronic Lymphocytic Leukemia, B-cell Lymphoma or Multiple Myeloma, CHARKALL.
[208] Jiang H, Zhang W, Shang P, et al.: Transfection of chimeric anti-CD138 gene enhances natural killer cell activation and killing of multiple myeloma cells. *Mol. Oncol.* 8:297-310, 2014.
[209] NCT01886976: Treatment of Chemotherapy Refractory Multiple Myeloma by CART-138.
[210] Carpenter RO, Evbuomwan MO, Pittaluga S, et al.: B-cell maturation antigen is a promising target for adoptive T-cell therapy of multiple myeloma. *Clin. Cancer Res.* 19:2048-60, 2013.
[211] Harousseau JL, Attal M, Leleu X, et al.: Bortezomib plus dexamethasone as induction reatment prior to autologous stem cell transplantation in patients with newly diagnosed multiple myeloma: results of an IFM phase II study. *Haematologica* 91:1498-505, 2006.
[212] Reeder CB, Reece DE, Kukreti V, et al.: Cyclophosphamide, bortezomib and dexamethasone induction for newly diagnosed multiple myeloma: high response rates in a phase II clinical trial. *Leukemia* 23:1337-41, 2009.

[213] Cavo M, Tacchetti P, Patriarca F, et al.: Bortezomib with thalidomide plus dexamethasone compared with thalidomide plus dexamethasone as induction therapy before, and consolidation therapy after, double autologous stem-cell transplantation in newly diagnosed multiple myeloma: a randomised phase 3 study. *Lancet* 376:2075-85, 2010.

[214] Jakubowiak AJ, Dytfeld D, Griffith KA, et al.: A phase 1/2 study of carfilzomib in combination with lenalidomide and low-dose dexamethasone as a frontline treatment for multiple myeloma. *Blood* 120:1801-9, 2012.

[215] Joseph R. Mikhael M, Craig B. Reeder, MD2, Edward N. et al.: A Phase I/II Trial Of Cyclophosphamide, Carfilzomib, Thalidomide and Dexamethasone (CYCLONE) In Patients with Newly Diagnosed Multiple Myeloma: Final Results Of MTD Expansion Cohort *ASH*, 2013.

[216] Rifkin RM, Gregory SA, Mohrbacher A, et al.: Pegylated liposomal doxorubicin, vincristine, and dexamethasone provide significant reduction in toxicity compared with doxorubicin, vincristine, and dexamethasone in patients with newly diagnosed multiple myeloma: a Phase III multicenter randomized trial. *Cancer* 106:848-58, 2006.

[217] Rajkumar SV, Blood E, Vesole D, et al.: Phase III clinical trial of thalidomide plus dexamethasone compared with dexamethasone alone in newly diagnosed multiple myeloma: a clinical trial coordinated by the Eastern Cooperative Oncology Group. *J. Clin. Oncol.* 24:431-6, 2006.

[218] Rajkumar SV, Rosinol L, Hussein M, et al.: Multicenter, randomized, double-blind, placebo-controlled study of thalidomide plus dexamethasone compared with dexamethasone as initial therapy for newly diagnosed multiple myeloma. J. *Clin. Oncol.* 26:2171-7, 2008.

[219] Rajkumar SV, Jacobus S, Callander N, et al.: A Randomized Phase III Trial of Lenalidomide Plus High-Dose Dexamethasone Versus Lenalidomide Plus Low-Dose Dexamethasone in Newly Diagnosed Multiple Myeloma (E4A03): A Trial Coordinated by the Eastern Cooperative Oncology Group. *ASH Annual Meeting Abstracts* 108:799-, 2006.

[220] Mateos MV, Oriol A, Martinez-Lopez J, et al.: Bortezomib, melphalan, and prednisone versus bortezomib, thalidomide, and prednisone as induction therapy followed by maintenance treatment with bortezomib and thalidomide versus bortezomib and prednisone in elderly patients with untreated multiple myeloma: a randomised trial. *Lancet Oncol.* 11:934-41, 2010.

[221] San Miguel JF, Schlag R, Khuageva NK, et al.: Persistent overall survival benefit and no increased risk of second malignancies with bortezomib-melphalan-prednisone versus melphalan-prednisone in patients with previously untreated multiple myeloma. *J. Clin. Oncol.* 31:448-55, 2013.

[222] Facon T, Mary JY, Hulin C, et al.: Melphalan and prednisone plus thalidomide versus melphalan and prednisone alone or reduced-intensity autologous stem cell transplantation in elderly patients with multiple myeloma (IFM 99-06): a randomised trial. *Lancet* 370:1209-18, 2007.

[223] Hulin C, Facon T, Rodon P, et al.: Efficacy of melphalan and prednisone plus thalidomide in patients older than 75 years with newly diagnosed multiple myeloma: IFM 01/01 trial. *J. Clin. Oncol.* 27:3664-70, 2009.

[224] Kyle RA, Rajkumar SV: Multiple myeloma. *N. Engl. J. Med.* 351:1860-73, 2004.

[225] Joseph R. Mikhael M, Vivek Roy, M.D., Paul G. Richardson, MD: A Phase I/II Trial Of Pomalidomide, Bortezomib and Dexamethasone In Patients with Relpased Or Refractory Multiple Myeloma *ASH Annual Meeting Abstracts*, 2013.

[226] Paul G. Richardson M, Craig C Hofmeister, MD2, David Siegel: MM-005: A Phase 1 Trial of Pomalidomide, Bortezomib, and Low-Dose Dexamethasone (PVD) In Relapsed and/Or Refractory Multiple Myeloma (RRMM) *ASH Annual Meeting Abstracts*, 2013.

[227] Jatin J. Shah MD, Edward A. Stadtmauer, MD, Rafat Abonour, MD, et al.: Phase I/II Dose Expansion Of a Multi-Center Trial Of Carfilzomib and Pomalidomide with Dexamethasone (Car-Pom-d) In Patients with Relapsed/Refractory Multiple Myeloma *ASH Annual Meeting Abstracts*, 2013.

[228] Rachid Baz M, Thomas G Martin III, MD, Melissa Alsina, MD: Pomalidomide (Pom) Dexamethasone (D) with or without Oral Weekly Cyclophosphamide (Cy) For Lenalidomide Refractory Multiple Myeloma (LRMM): A Multicenter Randomized Phase II Trial *ASH Annual Meeting Abstracts*, 2013.

[229] James R. Berenson M, James D. Hilger, Ph.D.1, Leonard Klein, MD, et al.: Pomalidomide, Dexamethasone and Pegylated Liposomal Doxorubicin for Patients with Relapsed/Refractory Multiple Myeloma: Results From a Phase 1/2 Trial *ASH Annual Meeting Abstracts*, 2013.

[230] Kyriakou C, Thomson K, D'Sa S, et al.: Low-dose thalidomide in combination with oral weekly cyclophosphamide and pulsed dexamethasone is a well tolerated and effective regimen in patients with relapsed and refractory multiple myeloma. *Br. J. Haematol.* 129:763-70, 2005.

[231] Palumbo A, Facon T, Sonneveld P, et al.: Thalidomide for treatment of multiple myeloma: 10 years later. *Blood* 111:3968-77, 2008.

[232] Schey SA, Morgan GJ, Ramasamy K, et al.: The addition of cyclophosphamide to lenalidomide and dexamethasone in multiply relapsed/refractory myeloma patients; a phase I/II study. *Br. J. Haematol.* 150:326-33, 2010.

[233] Knop S, Gerecke C, Liebisch P, et al.: Lenalidomide, adriamycin, and dexamethasone (RAD) in patients with relapsed and refractory multiple myeloma: a report from the German Myeloma Study Group DSMM (Deutsche Studiengruppe Multiples Myelom). *Blood* 113:4137-43, 2009.

[234] Meletios Athanasios Dimopoulos M, Sundar Jagannath, MD, Sung-Soo Yoon, MD, PhD: Vantage 088: Vorinostat in Combination with Bortezomib in Patients with Relapsed/Refractory Multiple Myeloma: Results of a Global, Randomized Phase 3 Trial *ASH Annual Meeting Abstracts*, 2011.

[235] Meletios Athanasios Dimopoulos M, Sundar Jagannath, MD, Sung-Soo Yoon, MD, PhD: Vantage 088: Vorinostat in Combination with Bortezomib in Patients with Relapsed/Refractory Multiple Myeloma: Results of a Global, Randomized Phase 3 Trial *ASH Annual Meeting Abstracts*, 2011.

In: Multiple Myeloma: Risk Factors, Diagnosis and Treatments ISBN: 978-1-63321-514-6
Editor: Steve Holt

Chapter 2

Development of Proteasome Inhibitors for the Treatment of Multiple Myeloma

Ota Fuchs*
Institute of Hematology and Blood Transfusion,
Prague, Czech Republic

Abstract

Multiple myeloma (MM) is the most common primary bone malignancy, characterized by accumulation of terminally differentiated B-lymphocytes, malignant plasma cells, within bone marrow.

MM remains mostly an incurable disease with high morbidity in the most cases. The introduction of novel agents has improved outcomes for patients with MM during the last years. The ubiquitin-proteasome path-way (UPP) is responsible for degradation of numerous proteins involved in MM cell proliferation, survival, and drug resistance. UPP is a major proteolytic system for proteins mediating the cell cycle and controlling apoptosis including cyclin-dependent kinase inhibitors (p21/CIP1, WAF1 and p27/KIP1), cyclin D, cyclin E, the dual-specificity phosphatase cdc 25, the protein kinase Wee1, p53, inhibitors of apoptosis proteins /IAPs/, caspases, NF-κB inhibitor IκB and others).

Bortezomib (Velcade™, PS-341) is boronate-based dipeptide proteasome inhibitor (PI) that primarily targets the chymotrypsin-like activities of the intracellular proteasome enzyme complex. Bortezomib was approved by the US Food and Drug Administration in 2003 and fully in 2005 in MM patients who have received at least one prior therapy. For optimization of clinical response and disease control bortezomib-based combination strategies (with alkylating agents: melphalan, cyclophosphamide, bendamustine; glucocoticoids: prednisone, dexamethasone; and immunomodulatory drugs) have been effectively used, particularly in relapsed or refractory MM patients who have exhausted the standard therapies or those who are not eligible for autologous stem cell trans-plantation. Bortezomib directly induces apoptosis of tumor cells and reverses drug

* Corresponding author: Ota Fuchs, PhD; U Nemocnice 1, 128 20 Prague 2, Czech Republic; e-mail: Ota.Fuchs@uhkt.cz, telephone: +420221977313, fax: +420221977380.

resistance of MM cells by affecting cytosine circuits, cell adhesion and angiogenesis in bone marrow microenvironment.

However, a considerable proportion of MM patients fail to respond to bortezomib and many MM patients relapse from this drug, either when it is used alone or as bortezomib-based combinations.

Therefore the new PI generation with the higher efficacy of proteasome inhibition, the enhanced antitumor activity and the decreased toxicity was developed.

Keywords: Multiple myeloma; proteasome; proteasome inhibitor; bortezomib; apoptosis

Introduction

Multiple myeloma (MM) is a hematological malignancy characterized by the clonal expansion of monoclonal immunoglobulin-secreting plasma cells in the bone marrow (BM). MM is associated with lytic bone lesions, anemia, immunodeficiency, and renal impairment. MM accounts for more than 10% of all hematologic malignancies and about 1% of all cancers [1]. In 2013, approximately 22,500 individuals in the United States and 6/100,000 in Europe were diagnosed with MM [2]. MM remains mostly incurable despite conventional intensive high dose chemotherapy followed by hematopoietic stem cell transplant. The costs associated with MM are among the highest.

The median age at MM diagnosis is 70 years, with 35% of patients younger than 65 years [3]. MM occurs in men (7 per 100, 000) at a rate 56% higher than women (4.5 per 100, 000). There has been a significant improvement in overall 5-year survival in patients with MM since the 1960s; 12% from 1960 to 1963 to 34% from 1996 to 2003.

Apart from the introduction of bisphosphonates in the 1990s and the development of autologous stem cell transplantation in the mid-1980s, patients with MM were treated mainly by the alkylating agent melphalan and a synthetic corticosteroid drug prednisone or dexamethasone (Decadron). The increasing knowledge of MM biology is already contributing to more specific drug designs. It was shown that as important as the malignant cells themselves is their interaction with the microenvironment in the pathogenesis of MM [4]. Discoveries in the genetic abnormalities associated with MM [5-10] and better understanding of the bone marrow [11, 12] microenvironment have led to new diagnostic, prognostic and treatment strategies. Therefore, drugs with a dual effect on the plasma cells and their bone marrow milieu in MM could be particularly valuable. The introduction of new therapies and the using of autologous stem-cell transplantation have led to increases in overall survival and progression-free survival in patients with MM. However, none of these therapies are curative and nearly all patients relapse.

Novel agents, such as thalidomide, the immunoregulatory drugs of next generation lenalidomide (also known as CC-5013, IMID-3 or Revlimid^{TM}) and pomalidomide (CC-4047), proteasome inhibitors (bortezomib, also known as PS-341 or Velcade^{TM}), histone deacetylase inhibitors (panobinostat, vorinostat and romidepsin) and anti-cell surface glycoprotein CS1 monoclonal antibody Elotuzumab in various combinations can achieve responses in patients who have relapsed and refractory MM [13-27]. However, the median survival remains at 6 years, with only 10% of MM patients surviving at 10 years.

Ubiquitin-Dependent Proteolysis

Ubiquitin-dependent proteolysis regulates the stability and function of key regulatory proteins that regulate the cell cycle, gene transcription, receptor endocytosis, intracellular trafficking, response to extracellular signal, signal transduction, antigen presentation, and control cell growth. Ubiquitin is a highly conserved protein of 76 amino acids that is covalently attached to substrate proteins through an energy-dependent enzymatic mechanism and polyubiquitinated proteins are degraded by a multi-compartmentalized protease called the 26S proteasome [28-31].

For the discovery of ubiquitin and its function in non-lysosomal pathway of protein degradation, the 2004 Nobel Prize in Chemistry was awarded to Drs. Avram Hershko, Aaron Ciechanover and Irwin Rose [32-35].

Schematic representation of the ubiquitin conjugation (ubiquitination, also referred to as ubiquitylation or ubiquitinylation) and of the ubiquitin-proteasome system is shown in Figure 1. Ubiquitination is a posttranslational modification of proteins. Ubiquitin is activated in an ATP-dependent manner by an ubiquitin – activating enzyme known as an enzyme-1 (E1).

Subsequently, ubiquitin is transferred to an ubiquitin-conjugating enzyme-2 (E2). E2, with the help of an ubiquitin-protein ligase (E3) and in some cases in the presence of an accessory factor (E4) [36], specifically attaches ubiquitin to the protein substrate. Only ten E1 enzymes, but about 100 E2 enzymes and 1000 E3 enzymes exist in human cells [37].

E3 ubiquitin ligases determine the specificity of protein substrates and are targets for pharmaceutical intervention. There are two major types of E3 ligases: the RING (really interesting new gene) domain-containing E3s and the Hect (homologous to E6-associated protein carboxyl terminus) domain-containing E3s. RING E3s bring the E2 enzyme in close proximity of the target protein, allowing the E2 to directly ubiquitinate the substrate. However, in the case of Hect E3s, ubiquitin is first transferred onto a conserved cysteine in the Hect domain. Consequently, Hect E3 enzyme ubiquitinates the substrate protein.

Polyubiquitin chain formation results from a linkage between the C terminus of one ubiquitin and a lysine side chain in another. Generated poly-ubiquitin chain (at least four attached ubiquitins) functions as signal for the subsequent degradation of protein substrates in the 26S proteasome.

Eukaryotic proteasomes, model of a barrel-like structure in Figure 2 consist of two outer α-rings and of two inner β-rings, each assembled from seven similar, but distinct, subunits. 19S regulatory complex caps both ends of the 20S proteasome to form 26S proteasome. 19S subunits are involved in the recognition of proteins designated for degradation. Each 19S regulatory complex contains at least seventeen different subunits and is assembled from two main subcomplexes-a base that contains six ATPases (Rpt) plus three non-ATPase subunits (Rpn), and a lid subcomplex that sits on top of the base and consist at least eight non-ATPase regulatory particles (Rpn). 19S regulatory complex recognizes the polyubiquitin proteolytic signal and unfolds substrates [29].

The 19S regulatory complex also takes a role in recycling ubiquitin as it contains deubiquitinating enzymes.

The 20S core exhibits three enzymatic activities (chymotrypsin-like, trypsin-like, and peptidyl-glutamyl peptide-hydrolyzing also named caspase-like) in the inner β-rings.

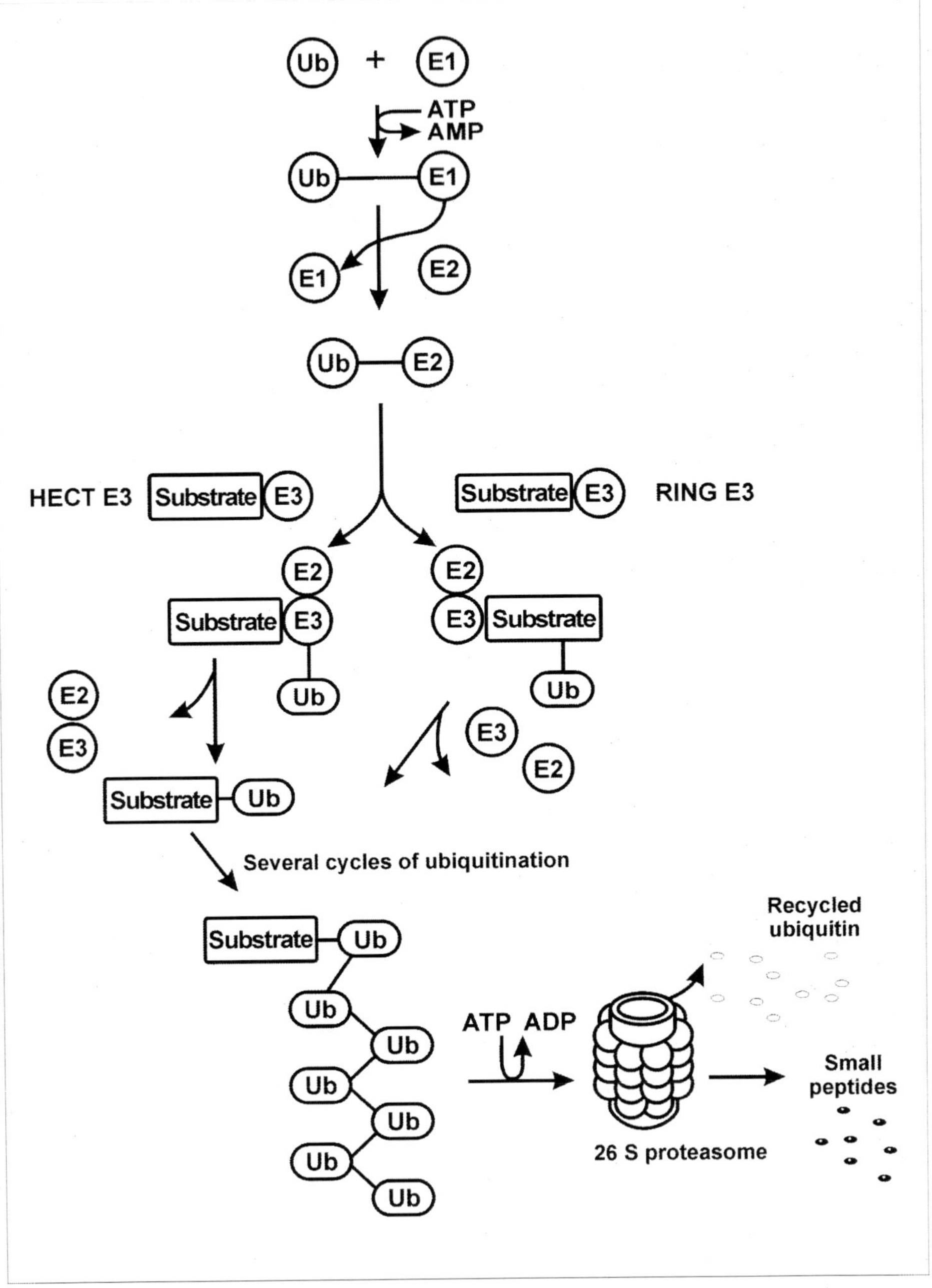

Figure 1. The ubiquitin-proteasome system. Attachment of ubiquitin to the target protein requires three enzymatic steps. Ubiquitin-activating enzymes activate ubiquitin by forming a high energy thiol ester bond between an E1 active site-located cystine residue and the C-terminal glycine residue of ubiquitin. This reaction requires energy provided by the hydrolysis of ATP and forms an activated thiol ester bond to ubiquitin-conjugating enzymes that serve as carrier proteins. Ubiquitin-protein ligases catalyze the covalent attachment of ubiquitin to the target protein by the formation of isopeptide bonds. Multiple cycles of ubiquitination finally result in the synthesis and attachment of polyubiquitin chains that serve as a recognition signal for the degradation of the target protein by the 26S proteasome.

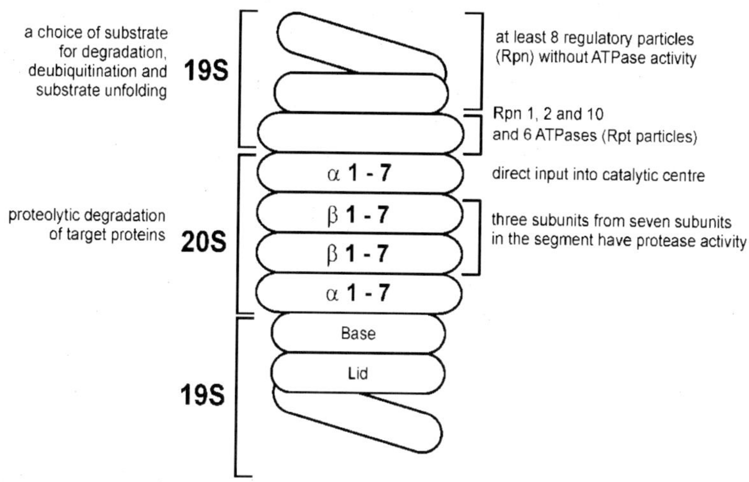

Figure 2. The structure of the 26S proteasome. The 26S proteasome consists of the 20S catalytic core complex and two 19S regulatory complexes capping the 20S complex at both ends. The 20S complex is composed of four axially stacked rings. Each of the outer rings consists of seven polypeptide α subunits that serve as the gates through which proteasome substrates enter, whereas each of the two inner rings is formed by seven proteolytic β subunits, and only three of them, β1, β2, and β5, are proteolytically active and harbor proteolytic sites that face the central cavity of the 20S complex. The 19S complex consists of the base and lid subcomplex. The base subcomplex contains six nonredundant ATPases. The lid subcomplex contains at least eight subunits including deubiquitinating enzymes and receptors for ubiquitinated proteins. The polyubiquitinated target protein enters the 19S regulatory complex and is recognized, deubiquitinated, unfolded, and translocated into the central cavity of the 20S catalytic core complex, where it is degraded by different hydrolytic activities. Ubiquitin is recycled by the ubiquitin carboxy terminal hydrolase. Peptides as a product of degradation are released from the 26S proteasome by diffusion and are used for major histocompatibility class I antigen presentation or are further degraded to single amino acids by cytosolic peptidases.

Many proteins degraded by proteasome are implicated in important cell processes: cell-cycle-regulatory proteins (cyclins A,B,C,D and E, inhibitors of cyclin-dependent kinases - proteins $p21^{WAF1/CIP1}$ and $p27^{KIP1}$, the tumor suppressor p53, inhibitor of NF-κB- protein IκB, intercellular adhesion molecule-1 (ICAM-1) and vascular cell adhesion molecule-1 (VCAM-1).

Proteasome Inhibitors

Proteasomes belong to proteolytic enzymes called threonine proteases. Proteasome inhibitors were first synthesized as tools to probe the function and proteolytic activity specificity of the proteasome [38, 39].

Most of the proteasome inhibitors address the chymotryptic activity of the 20S proteasome core via adduct formation with N-terminal threonine hydroxyl group as part of the catalytically active center.

Results of both preclinical and clinical studies suggest that transformed cells are more sensitive to proteasome inhibition than normal cells [40-42].

Similarly, MM cell lines were more sensitive to apoptosis induced by proteasome inhibitors than were peripheral blood mononuclear cells from healthy individuals [43]. The biologic basis for the enhanced susceptibility of cancer cells to proteasome inhibitors has not been fully elucidated.

Several hypotheses have been proposed. One from them is the loss of checkpoint mechanisms for DNA repair by cancer cells. Other hypotheses are a greater sensitivity of rapidly proliferating tumor cells to proteasome inhibitors and more efficient uptake and slower inactivation of proteasome inhibitors by tumor cells [44-46]. Thus, the possibility that proteasome inhibitors could be drug candidates appeared as a new hope for cancer therapy.

Several classes of proteasome inhibitors were developed and several proteasome inhibitors are shown in Figure 3. There are six major classes of proteasome inhibitors: peptide aldehydes, peptide semicarbazones, peptide vinyl sulfones, peptide boronates, peptide epoxyketones (epoxomycin and eponomycin) and β-lactones (lactacystin and its derivatives), based on the pharmacophore that reacts with the threonine residue in the active site of the proteasome. In leukemia, three classes of proteasome inhibitors entered clinical trials (peptide boronates /bortezomib/, β-lactones /NPI-0052/ and epoxomycin derivatives /PR-171/). Toxicity profiles of other three classes of proteasome inhibitors (peptide aldehydes, peptide semicarbazones and peptide vinyl sulfones) prevent their use in clinical trials.

Resistance to apoptosis and enhanced proliferation is characteristic feature of cancer cells. Proteasome inhibitors induce cell cycle arrest by interfering with timely degradation of cyclins and cyclin-dependent kinases inhibitors.

Proteasome inhibitors function as apoptosis inducers by inhibition of transcription factor NF-κB and by endoplasmic reticulum stress and subse-quent generation of reactive oxygen species. Proteasome inhibitors stabilize proapoptotic proteins, such as p53, Bax, Bik and Bim while reduce levels of some antiapoptotic proteins, such as Bcl2, XIAP, or c-FLIP.

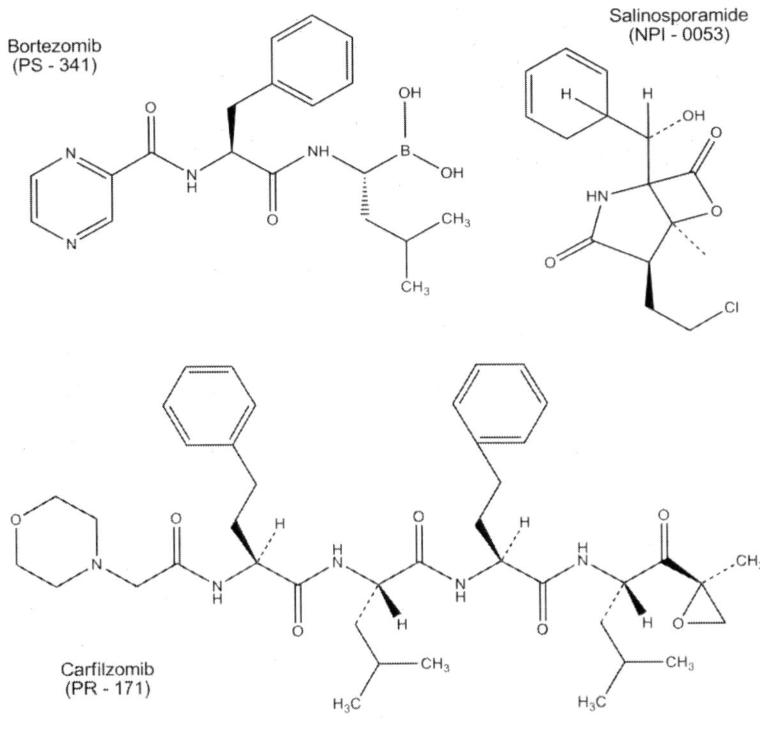

Figure 3. Chemical structures of several selected proteasome inhibitors.

The first developed proteasome inhibitors were peptide aldehydes, which mimic a protein substrate [47-49]. The peptide aldehydes form a reversible covalent hemiacetal intermediate between the aldehyde group of the inhibitor and the hydroxyl group of the amino terminal threonine. MG115 (N-benzo-yloxycarbonyl(Z)-1-L-leucinyl-L-leucinyl-L-norvalinal), MG132 (N-benzo-yloxycarbonyl (Z)-Leu-Leu-leucinal) and PSI (N-benzyloxycarbonyl (Z) - Ile-Glu(O-t-Bu)-Ala-leucinal) are members of this group of proteasome inhibitors. However, many peptide aldehydes, for example MG132 and others, cause significant neurotoxicity and therefore they were not used in clinical trials.

Bortezomib

Boronate inhibitors of the proteasome are more potent than structurally similar peptide aldehydes [50]. Bortezomib (VELCADE, formerly known as PS-341, pyrazinylcarbonyl-Phe-Leu-boronate) inhibits proteasome by binding reversibly to the chymotrypsin-like site in the 20S core of the proteasome [51]. Bortezomib is the first proteasome inhibitor approved by the US Food and Drug Administration for the treatment of relapsed or relapsed and refractory multiple myeloma (MM) and some forms of non-Hodgkin's lymphoma, mantle cell lymphoma [52-60]. Cellular mechanisms responsible for the clinical efficacy of bortezomib include inhibition of tumor cell adhesion to stroma and disruption cytokine-dependent survival pathways, in part through suppression of the transcription nuclear factor-κB (NF-κB) activity, inhibition of angiogenesis, induction of aggresome (aggregates of ubiquitin-conjugated proteins) formation, endoplasmic reticulum stress, and the unfolded protein response [61-67].

NF-κB as a Therapeutic Target in Multiple Myeloma

Proteasome inhibitors and several other anti-multiple myeloma agents, such as dexamethasone, thalidomide and its immunomodulatory derivatives (IMiDs), and arsenic trioxide As_2O_3, inhibit NF-κB activity as part of their diverse actions (Figure 4).

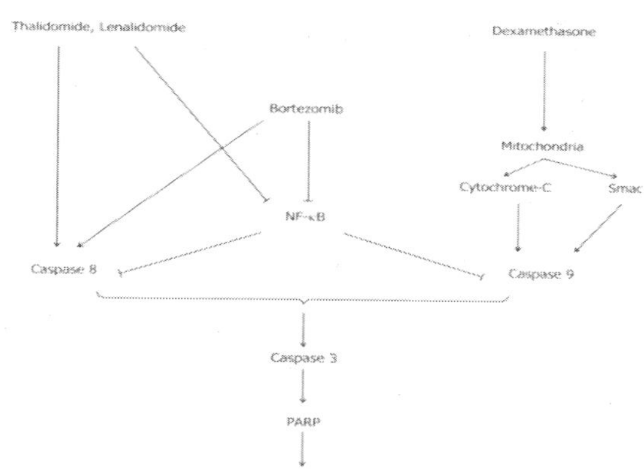

Figure 4. The role of NF-κB in the effects of anti-MM drugs. Apoptosis dependent on caspases is induced by anti-MM drugs (bortezomib, thalidomide, lenalidomide) that inhibit NF-κB activity.

The Role of the Myeloma's Microenvironment in Pathophysiology of Multiple Myeloma

Adhesion of tumor cells to extracellular matrix proteins and bone marrow stromal cells (BMSCs) plays a major role in the MM pathogenesis [68]. The most important factors for the development of osteoclasts are macrophage colony-stimulating factor (*M-CSF*) and receptor activator of nuclear factor – kappa B ligand (RANKL). M-CSF expands the pool of osteoclast precursors and subsequently RANKL stimulates osteoclast precursors to develop into mature osteoclasts (Figure 5). Myeloma cells induce RANKL expression and downregulatethe expression of osteoprotegerin (OPG), a soluble RANKL decoy receptor.

RANKL is responsible for osteoclast-mediated bone resorption in a broad range of conditions and plays a key role in establishment and propagation of skeletal disease in MM. The candidates for the stimulation of osteoclast activity are interleukin (IL)-6, macrophage inflammatory protein-1 alpha (MIP-1α), RANKL, and interleukin-1 beta (IL-1β) (Figure 6).

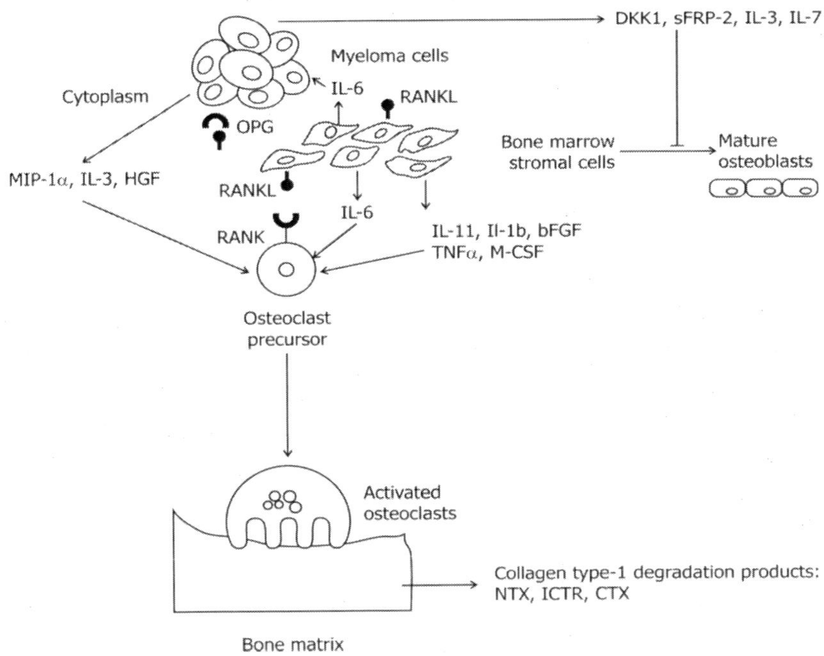

Figure 5. The role of the myeloma´s microenvironment in pathophysiology of multiple myeloma (MM) bone disease. MM is characterized by extensive bones loss and osteolytic lesions. MM cells bind to bone marrow stromal cells through the interaction of VCAM-1 and integrin α4b1. Myeloma cells produce RANKL and cause bone marrow stromal cells to overexpress RANKL and IL-6. Binding of RANKL to RANK on the surface of osteoclast precursors induces NF-κB activation, which leads to osteoclast differentiation and bone resorption. IL-6 acts as a growth factor for myeloma cells. RANKL and IL-6 induce differentiation of osteoclast precursors into mature osteoclasts. OPG is the soluble RANKL antagonist. Myeloma cells inhibit OPG. MM cells secrete factors that alter the biology of bone remodeling. Wnt signaling is essential for maintenance of osteoblast and osteoclast homeostasis. Production of Wnt signaling inhibitors dickopf-1 (DKK1) and sFRP2 contributes to osteolytic lesions through the direct inhibition of osteoblast differentiation. Myeloma cells express MIP-1α, which recruits osteoclast precursors and enhances osteoclast activity. The resulting enhanced bone resorption releases collagen type-1 degradation products, cytokines and growth factors that in turn promote myeloma cell proliferation and survival.

Adhesion of MM cells to extracellular matrix proteins confers cell adhesion-mediated drug resistance and binding of MM cells to BMSCs triggers transcription and secretion of cytokines, primarily NF-κB-dependent secretion of IL-6 [69-71].

This in turn triggers the proliferation of MM cells, promotes both tumor cells survival and upregulation of anti-apoptotic molecules [72, 73]. IL-6 mediates autocrine and paracrine growth of MM cells within the BM milieu. It also confers to tumor cells further resistance to conventional therapy and induces vascular endothelial growth factor (VEGF) expression and secretion [68]. The important role of BM microenvironment in MM pathogenesis is now well established [11, 12, 74, 75].

The balanced homeostasis between the cellular, the extracellular, and the liquid compartments within the BM is disrupted. The results of this disruption are immune suppression, cytopenias and lytic bone lesions.

All these effects are caused by the impact of tumor cells on the BM and other cells within the BM milieu. Tumor cell growth, survival, migration, and drug resistance are promoted by these effects. The therapeutic success of proteasome inhibitors, thalidomide and lenalidomide in relapsed refractory disease is associated with targeting interactions between MM cells and BM cells (Figure 6), including tumor angiogenesis and or cytokines or growth factors in the BM microenvironment (also called "niches").

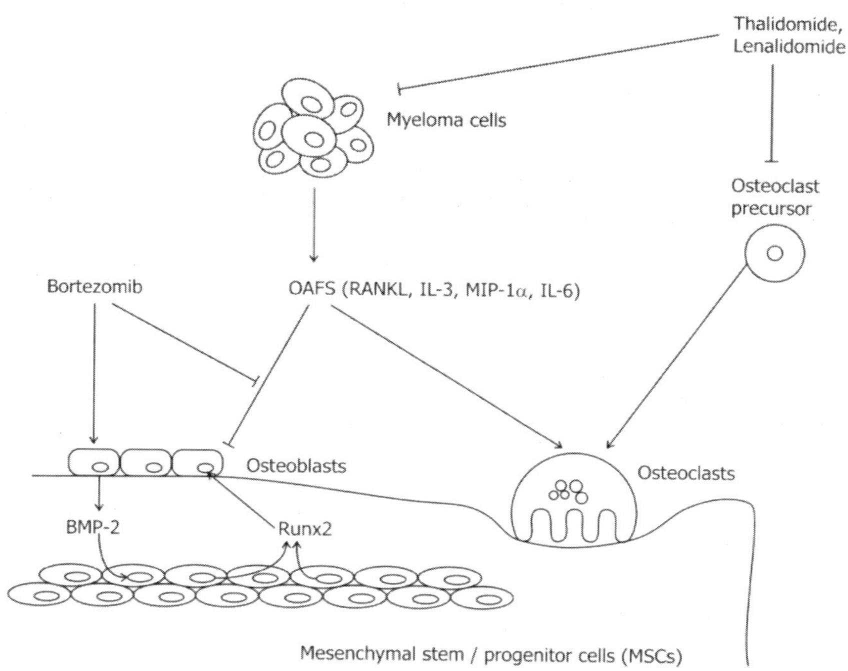

Figure 6. The sites of bortezomib, thalidomide and lenalidomide action in the pathophysiology of MM bone disease. Bortezomib directly inhibits osteoclast formation and function. Bortezomib enhances new bone formation and inhibits DKK1 expression and induces osteoblast differentiation. Bortezomib also increases the number of Runx2/Cbfa1-positive osteoblasts of responding MM patients, but not in those who did not respond. Bortezomib reduces serum receptor activator of nuclear NF-κB ligand (RANKL) levels. Thus, bortezomib prevents NF-κB activation, which leads to the prevention of bone resorption. Thalidomide and lenalidomide inhibit osteoclast development by affecting the lineage commitment of osteoclast precursors. These drugs, aside from their antiangiogenic effects, also activate apoptosis of MM cells.

Bortezomib in Preclinical Studies on Human Myeloma Cell Lines and Primary Patient Multiple Myeloma Cells

In these studies bortezomib inhibited the proliferation in human myeloma cell lines, which was both sensitive and refractory to conventional chemo-therapeutic agents (melphalan, doxorubicin, mitoxantrone and dexamethasone).

Bortezomib induced caspase-dependent apoptosis of myeloma cell lines and primary patient MM cells [71]. MM cell lines were up to 40 times more sensitive to the proapoptotic effects of bortezomib than were peripheral blood mononuclear cells from healthy individuals [71]. Bortezomib also inhibited NF-κB activation in tumor necrosis factor (TNF)-α-treated MM cells by blocking the degradation of the inhibitor protein IκBα and overcame the resistance to apoptosis in MM cells conferred by IL-6 [71, 76, 77].

Proapoptotic regulators upregulation and antiapoptotic proteins down-regulation were observed [76, 78]. Bortezomib stabilizes proapoptotic proteins, such as p53, Bax, Bik and Bim while reduce levels of some anti-apoptotic proteins, such as Bcl-2. Bortezomib responses are also linked to the upregulation of the proapoptotic Bcl-2 protein family member Noxa [79] and this effect is independent of constitutive activity of the phosphoinositide 3-kinase/AKT (protein kinase B) and NF-κB pathways. Bortezomib induces Noxa and the cleavage of antiapoptotic protein Mcl-1. The myeloid cell leukemia-1 (*Mcl-1*) protein is an antiapoptotic member of the Bcl-2 family.

Noxa induction allows the displacement of the direct apoptosis activator Bim, which is able to activate Bax/Bak by a “hit and run” mechanism, triggering mitochondrial dysfunction and apoptosis (Figure 7).

Bortezomib-mediated proteasome inhibition affect multiple signaling pathways, including cell cycle, growth arrest, stress response, microenvironment and apoptosis. Disruption of multiple cellular signaling by bortezomib initiates and maintains an active cell death pathway and causes apoptosis as we show in Figure 8.

Binding of MM cells to BMSCs and abrogation of the NF-κB-dependent transcription and secretion of IL-6 in BMSCs were also inhibited by borte-zomib [73]. Molecular mechanisms of the antimyeloma activity of bortezomib were studied by analysis of gene expression profiles of bortezomib-treated MM cells in comparison with nontreated MM cells. Bortezomib also induced the phosphorylation of c-Jun NH_2-terminal kinase (JNK), activating caspase-8 and, subsequently, caspase-3. The activated caspase-3 cleaved DNA protein kinase catalytic subunit and ATM/ATR proteins, and ultimately resulted in impaired DNA repair in MM cells [80]. DNA damage induced by activated caspase-3 was also observed. Subsequent phosphorylation of p53 and the degradation of Mdm2 (the product of expression of murine double minute oncogene that represses p53 transcriptional activity by p53 poly-ubiquitination and degradation, the human analogue HDM2) are in a time and dose-dependent on the level of bortezomib which is comparable with the serum level of bortezomib used in clinical practice [80].

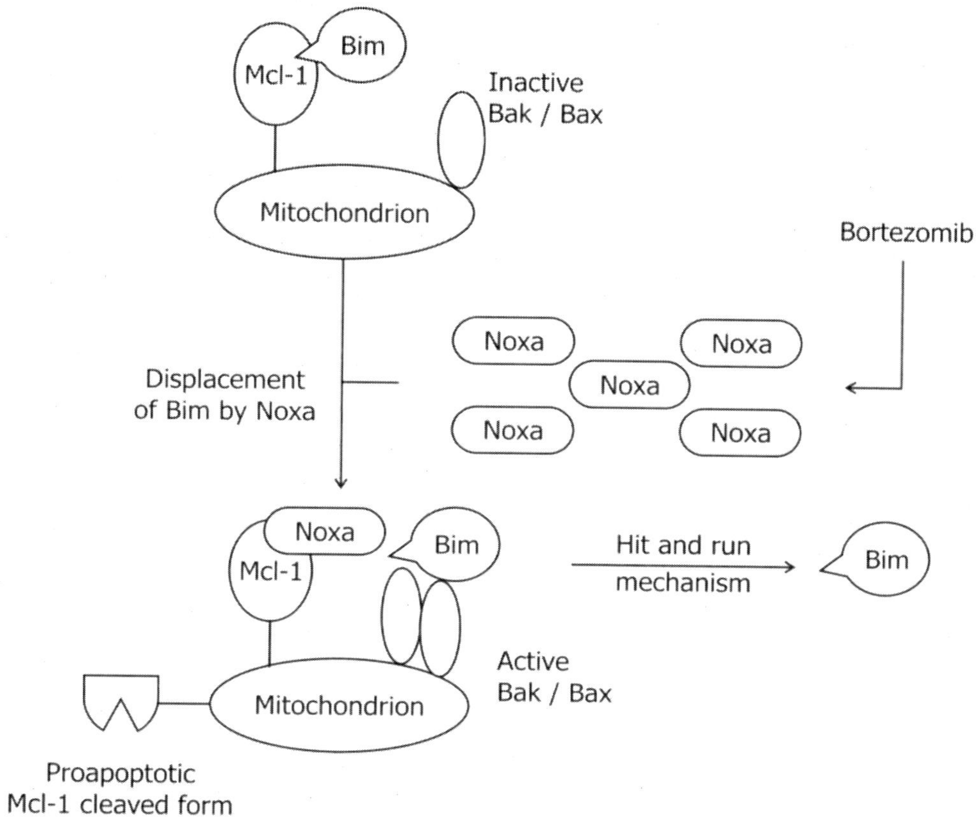

Figure 7. Effect of bortezomibe treatment on the interplay between antiapoptotic and proapoptotic members of the Bcl-2 family in myeloma cells. Myeloma cell death is totally dependent on Mcl-1/Bim complex disruption. Noxa induced by bortezomib is involved in the displacement of Bim from Mcl-1 binding. Released Bim triggers Bax/ Bak activation and through this it induces apoptosis.

Bortezomib increases osteoblast number, function, and gene expression [81-83] through targeting of a multipotent population of mesenchymal stem progenitor cells (MSCs). Bortezomib induces MSCs to preferentially undergo osteoblastic differentiation, in part by modulation of the bone-specifying transcription factor runt-related transcription factor 2 (Runx-2) [84].

Bortezomib promotes bone formation in myelomatous and nonmyelomatous bones by simultaneously inhibiting osteoclastogenesis and stimulating osteoblastogenesis. As clinical and experimental studies indicate that bone disease is both a consequence and necessity of MM progression our results suggest and that bortezomib's effects on bone remodeling contribute to the antimyeloma efficacy of this drug [85]. Three other studies [86-88] showed an inhibitory effect of bortezomib on osteoclastic bone resorption in MM patients with a significant reduction in serum dickkopf-1 (DKK1) and RANKL levels.

DKK1 is an inhibitor of the Wnt signaling pathway (wingless in *Drosophila*) that is important in the growth, development, and function of osteoblasts [89].

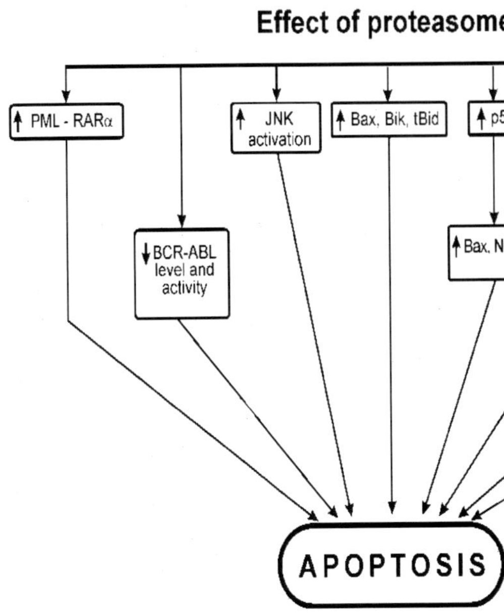

Figure 8. Molecular targets of proteasome inhibitors in the process of apoptosis induction.

Bortezomib in Relapsed and/or Refractory Multiple Myeloma - Clinical Studies

Based on preclinical studies and promising phase 1 trial, two pivotal phase 2 studies, SUMMIT [90] and CREST [91] were performed in relapsed and/or refractory MM patients. Patients were treated with bortezomib 1.3 mg/m^2 on days 1,4,8, and 11 every 3 weeks. Dexamethasone was allowed in patients with suboptimal responses to bortezomib alone.

The overall response rate was 35%, including 10% complete or near complete responses with an overall survival of 17 months. The randomized CREST study [91], comparing two dosages of bortezomib (1.3 versus 1,0 mg/m^2) showed that a reduced dose was able to produce responses in up to one third of patients and it was accompanied with a lower toxicity.

The addition of dexamethasone in patients with suboptimal responses to bortezomib alone resulted again in an improvement in the response degree [92].

A subsequent randomized phase 3 trial “the Assessment of Proteasome Inhibition for Extending Remissions” (APEX) including 669 patients with relapsed MM has shown that bortezomib is more effective than high dose dexamethasone as demonstrated by a significant improvement in response rate (43% vs. 18%), median time to progression (6.2 vs. 3.4 months) and 1-year survival rate (80% vs. 67%, respectively) [93]. In the updated APEX analysis (median follow-up: 22 months), survival was assessed in both arms (single-agent bortezomib versus high-dose dexamethasone), and efficacy updated for the bortezomib arm. Median survival was 29.8 months for bortezomib versus 23.7 months for dexamethasone, a 6-month benefit, despite substantial cross-over from dexamethasone to bortezomib.

Overall and complete response rates with bortezomib were 43% and 9%, respectively; among responding patients, 56% improved response with longer therapy beyond initial response, leading to continued improvement in overall quality of response. Higher response quality was associated with longer response duration; response duration was not associated with time to response. These data confirm the activity of borte-zomib and support extended treatment in relapsed multiple myeloma patients tolerating therapy [94].

Bortezomib therapy has become an important part of the standard of care for patients with relapsed multiple myeloma, and preliminary clinical evidence suggests that bortezomib retreatment in patients previously treated with the drug may prolong disease control. The retrospective study [94] was designed to clarify the utility of bortezomib as a repeat therapy. Records from 3 major cancer centers that had participated in the phase 2 (SUMMIT or CREST) or phase 3 (APEX) registration studies were used to identify patients who were subsequently retreated off protocol with bortezomib-based therapy. 22 patients who received bortezomib retreatment following a 60 or more day gap between bortezomib treatments were found. Twelve patients had intervening therapy between initial bortezomib treatment and bortezomib retreatment.

During retreatment, 14 of 22 patients received bortezomib in combination with another antineoplastic agent.

The overall response rate for bortezomib re-treatment was 50% (9% complete responses). The median length of retreatment was 5.1 months in responding patients and 2.4 months in nonresponding patients. Therapy was terminated due to unmanageable toxicity in 2 patients during retreatment, compared with 6 patients during initial treatment.

During retreatment, no patients required dose reduction due to peripheral neuropathy, compared to 4 patients during their initial treatment. Thus, borte-zomib retreatment appears to be safe and effective.

Favorable observed response rates with bortezomib retreatment suggest that it may be a viable option for relapsed or refractory multiple myeloma, even in patients previously exposed to bortezomib [95].

An important aspect of all these studies is the toxicity profile of bortezomib, particularly when used in combinations with other agents. The most common side effects of bortezomib were gastrointestinal symptoms, fatigue, and anorexia, although these were mostly grade 1-2 [96].

Thrombocytopenia grade 3-4, due to a reversible blockage in platelet release, was found in 30% of cases, while anemia and neutropenia are uncommon (<10%). The major dose-limiting adverse effect is painful peripheral neuropathy (37% with only 9% grade 3 and more) [97].

Unusual toxicities such as tumor lysis syndrome, severe pulmonary failure, toxic hepatitis or rhabdomyolysis have been also reported [96, 98, 99].

Thus, the toxicity profile of bortezomib is well defined and most complications are predictable and manageable.

Combinations of Bortezomib with Conventional Anti-Multiple Myeloma Agents

Bortezomib was combined in a phase 1 trial with liposomal doxorubicin in advanced MM patients [100]. The response rate among 22 evaluable patients was 73%, including 36% of complete response. An updated analysis [101] after extended follow-up showed the time to progression 9.3 months, the median time from start of therapy to start of subsequent therapy 24.2 months and median overall survival 38.3 months.

The phase 3 international study compared the efficacy and safety of a combination of pegylated liposomal doxorubicin (PLD) plus bortezomib with bortezomib monotherapy in patients with relapsed or refractory multiple myeloma [102]. 646 patients were randomly assigned to receive either intravenous bortezomib 1.3 mg/m^2) on days 1, 4, 8, and 11 of an every 21-days cycle, or the same bortezomib regimen with PLD 30 mg/m^2) on day 4. Median time to progression was increased from 6.5 months for bortezomib to 9.3 months with the PLD + bortezomib combination. The 15-month survival rate for PLD + bortezomib was 76% compared with 65% for bortezomib alone.

The complete plus partial response rate was 41% for bortezomib and 44% for PLD + bortezomib, a difference that was not statistically significant. Median duration of response was increased from 7.0 to 10.2 months with PLD + bortezomib. Grade 3/4 adverse events was more frequent in the combination group (80% vs. 64%), with safety profiles consistent with the known toxicities of the two agents. An increased incidence in the combination group was seen of grade 3/4 neutropenia, thrombocytopenia, asthenia, fatigue, diarrhea, and hand-foot syndrome. PLD with bortezomib is superior to borte-zomib monotherapy for the treatment of patients with relapsed or refractory multiple myeloma. The combination therapy is associated with a higher incidence of grade 3/4 myelosuppression, constitutional symptoms, gastro-intestinal symptoms, and dermatologic toxicities.

Following the remarkably positive results of a large phase 3 trial comparing bortezomib and PLD with bortezomib monotherapy, the FDA approved the use of this combination in May 2007 for patients who have not previously received bortezomib and who have received at least one prior therapy. Bortezomib can sensitize MM cells to conventional chemotherapeutics to which a patient has previously become resistant [76, 103].

Bortezomib has shown activity in relapsed and or refractory MM, even in patients refractory to thalidomide or lenalidomide (immunomodulatory drug [IMiD]) treatment [104]. Combination therapies with bortezomib- thalidomide - dexamethasone [105], bortezomib-melphalan-prednisone-thalidomide [106] or with bortezomib - lenalidomide - dexamethasone [107, 108] were highly effective in advanced and refractory MM. These treatment strategies will hopefully further prolong the survival of patients with myeloma.

The Second-Generation Proteasome Inhibitors with More Potency and Fewer Side-Effects Studied in Multiple Myeloma

The good clinical results obtained with bortezomib have validated the proteasome as a therapeutic target in MM. Two second-generation proteasome inhibitors have entered phase 1 and phase 2 trials: NPI-0052 (salinosporamide A, Marizomib) and carfilzomib (Kyprolis, formerly PR-171) (see Figure 3).

Salinosporamide A (Marizomib) was discovered by William Fenical and Paul Jensen from Scripps Institution of Oceanography in La Jolla, CA.

In preliminary screening, a high percentage of the organic extracts of cultured *Salinospora* strains possessed antibiotic and anticancer activities, which suggests that these bacteria are an excellent resource for drug discovery. *Salinospora* strain CNB-392 was isolated from a heat-treated marine sediment sample collected in the Bahamas and cytotoxicity-guided fractionation of the crude extract led to the isolation of salinosporamide A. Salinosporamide A shares its fused γ-lactam-β-lactone bicyclic ring structure with clasto-lactacystin-β-lactone, also called omuralide.

Thus, Salinosporamide A is a natural product derived from the fermentation of the marine gram-positive actinomycete *Salinospora tropica* and is a highly cytotoxic proteasome inhibitor [109-119].

Preclinical studies in MM models showed that NPI-0052 induces apoptosis of MM cells, including cells resistant to conventional anti-MM therapies as well as cells isolated from patients who had developed resistance to bortezomib-based therapies [111]. NPI-0052 is distinct from bortezomib in terms of chemical structure (Figure 3) and effects on individual proteolytic activities of the proteasome activities. While bortezomib inhibits exclusively the chymotrypsin-like activity of the 20S proteasome, NPI-0052 inhibits all three protease activities in the proteasome (Figure 9): the chymotrypsin-like, trypsin-like, and caspase-like activities [111]. Another important difference is that NPI-0052 is orally bioavailable, while bortezomib is not amenable to oral administration. Schematic representation of the mechanism of action of salino-sporamide A is shown in Figure 9. Inhibition of all three proteolytic activities of the 20S proteasome in leukemia cells by NPI-0052 results in activation of caspase-8. This leads to proapoptotic protein Bid cleavage and to the considerable decrease of mitochondrial transmembrane potential [115].

Mitochondrial membrane permeabilization, release of cytochrome c and activation of caspase-9 follow. Apoptosis proceeds then by activation of effector caspase-3 and consequent DNA fragmentation and increased levels of intracellular reactive oxygen species were detected [115].

Salinosporamide A potentiated the apoptosis induced by tumor necrosis factor α (TNF), bortezomib, and thalidomide, and this correlated with down-regulation of gene products that mediate cell proliferation (cyclin D1, cyclo-oxygenase-2 [COX-2], and c-Myc), cell survival (Bcl-2, Bcl-xL, cFLIP, TRAF 1, IAP1, IAP2, and surviving), invasion (matrix metalloproteinase-9 [MMP-9] and ICAM-1), and angiogenesis (vascular endothelial growth factor [VEGF]) [116]. Salinosporamide A also suppressed TNF-induced tumor cell invasion and receptor activator of NF-κB ligand (RANKL)-induced osteoclastogenesis.

It was also found that salinosporamidee A suppressed both constitutive and inducible NF-κB activation. Compared with bortezomib, MG-132, N-acetyl-leucyl-leucyl-norleucinal (ALLN), and lactacystin, salinosporamide A was found to be the most potent suppressor of NF-κB activation. Further studies showed that salinosporamide A inhibited TNF-induced inhibitory subunit of NF-κB α (IκBα) degradation, nuclear translocation of p65, and NF-κB-dependent reporter gene expression but had no effect on IκBα kinase activation, IκBα phosphorylation, or IκBα ubiquitination [117].

Thus, overall, results indicate that salinosporamide A enhances apoptosis, suppresses osteoclastogenesis, and inhibits invasion through suppression of the NF-κB pathway.

Combination of NPI-0052 and bortezomib induces synergistic anti-MM activity (Figure 10) [114]. These studies therefore provide the rationale for clinical protocols evaluating NPI-0052, alone and together with bortezomib, to improve patient outcome in MM.

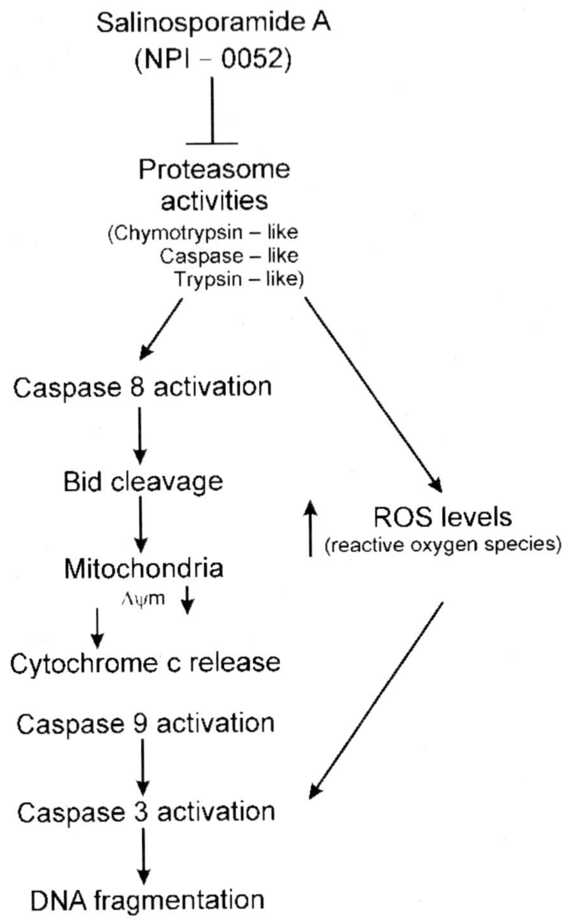

Figure 9. Schema of the mechanism of inhibition of all three proteasome proteolytic activities (the chymotrypsin-like, caspase-like, and trypsin-like activities) by salino-sporamide A (NPI-0052). NPI-0052 induces caspase-8, which initiates Bid cleavage and drops of mitochondrial membrane potential (Δψm). Mitochondrial perturbations lead to the release of cytochrome c from the mitochondria, which then activates the mitochondrial – mediated proapoptotic pathway (activation of caspases-9 and -3 and consequent DNA fragmentation). Parallel pathway of cell death induction by NPI-0052 is connected with reactive oxygen species generation.

Another new proteasome inhibitor of next generation is PR-171 (carfilzomib, Kyprolis; Onyx Pharmaceuticals, Inc., South San Francisco, CA) (Figure 3). PR-171 is tetrapeptide epoxyketone-based irreversible proteasome inhibitor that exhibits a high level of selectivity for a single active site in the proteasome, as well as minimal cross reactivity to other protease classes [120-130]. Carfilzomib binds β5 catalytic subunit of the 20S proteasome core particle and LMP7 subunit of the immunoproteasome. In models of MM, carfilzomib potently irreversibly bound and specifically inhibited the chymotrypsin-like proteasome and immunoproteasome activities, resulting in accumulation of ubiquitinated substrates. Carfilzomib induced a dose- and time-dependent inhibition of proliferation, ultimately leading to apoptosis.

Programmed cell death was associated with activation JNK, mitochondrial membrane depolarization, release of cytochrome c, and activation of both intrinsic and extrinsic caspase pathways.

This agent also inhibited proliferation and activated apoptosis in patient-derived MM cells, as well as neoplastic cells from patients with other hematologic malignancies. Importantly, carfilzomib showed increased efficacy compared to bortezomib (Figure 11), and was active against bortezomib-resistant MM cell lines, and samples from patients with clinical bortezomib resistance [121].

Carfilzomib had an acceptable tolerability profile in patients with relapsed, or relapsed and refractory MM in Phase I and Phase II clinical studies [122]. There was a low incidence of grade 3 or higher peripheral neuropathy.

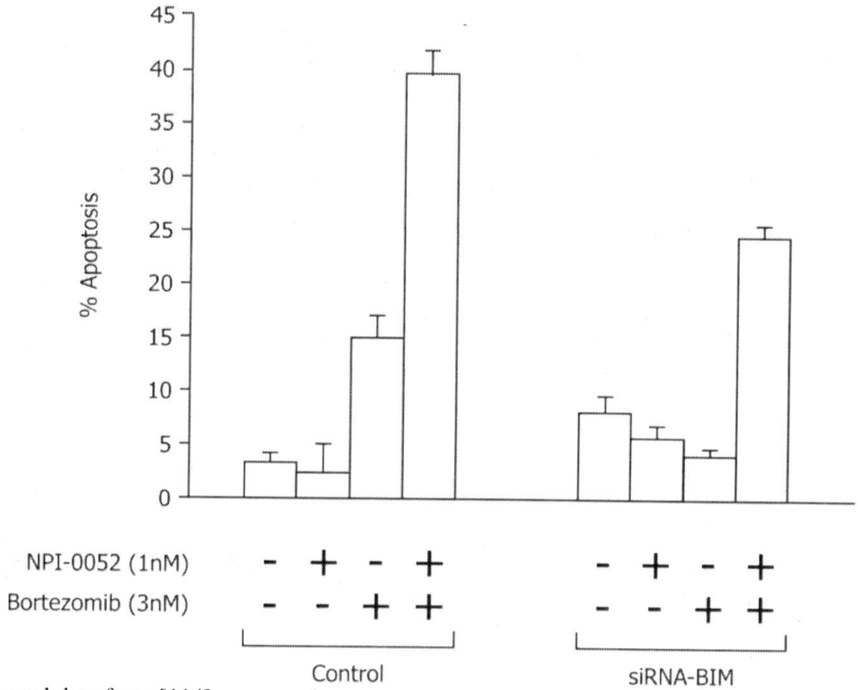

Experimental data from [114] were used.

Figure 10. The role of Bim, a proapoptotic relative of Bcl-2, in apoptosis induced by the second generation proteasome inhibitor NPI-0052 in comparison with bortezomib. MM.1S dexamethasone sensitive cells were transfected with Bim siRNA for 48 hours, followed by 12 hours of treatment with indicated proteasome inhibitor/s and analysis for apoptosis by annexinV/propidium iodide staining.

Carfilzomib was approved on July 20, 2012 by the FDA for use in patients with MM who have received at least two prior therapies, including the treatment with bortezomib and an immunomodulatory therapy and have demonstrated disease progression on or within 60 days of completion of the last therapy [126]. Results from a recent Phase 1 and 2 trials indicate that the combination of Kyprolis, Revlimid, and dexamethasone is effective in relapsed multiple myeloma patients [127, 128]. Specifically, the results show that 77% of patients responded to the treatment. The investigators point out the responses seen in the trial were rapid (median time to response was one month) and robust (median duration of response was 22 months). According to the investigators, the results are particularly encouraging because one-quarter of the patients were refractory (resistant) to bortezomib and almost half were refractory to lenalidomide. The researchers also note that the side effect profile of the combination was similar to that observed in previous trials. Most of the severe side effects were blood-related.

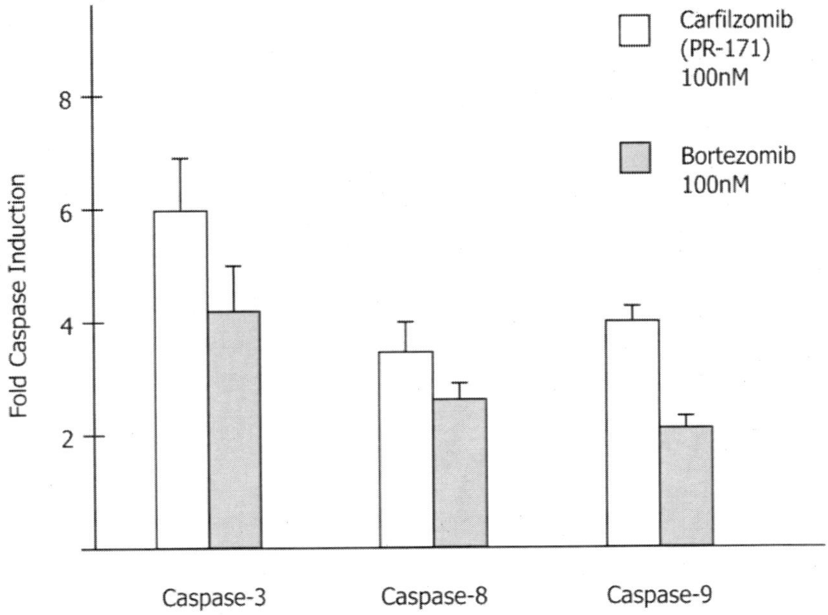

Experimental data from [121] were used.

Figure 11. Caspase induction by the second generation proteasome inhibitor carfilzomib (PR-171) in comparison with bortezomib in ANBL-6 MM cells. Cells were exposed to a 1-hour pulse of 100 nM carfilzomib or bortezomib and allowed to recover for 8 hours. Cellular lysates (30μg per reaction) were then incubated with 40μM fluorogenic substrate specific for caspase-3, caspase-8, and caspase-9 activity.

Twenty percent of the patients left the trial due to side effects - a dis-continuation rate the investigators describe as "moderate." Dr. Sara Bringhen from the University of Torino in Italy reported results from a Phase 2 study evaluating Kyprolis, cyclophosphamide, and dexamethasone as initial therapy for older, newly diagnosed multiple myeloma [129, 130]. After initial therapy, patients received further Kyprolis maintenance therapy.

Overall 96% of study participants responded, with 64% reaching a complete or near complete response, 12% a very good partial response, and 20% a partial response. The two-year progression-free survival rate was 76%, and the overall survival rate was 87%.

A poster presented at ASH (ASH 2013 Annual Meeting Abstract 3179) by Stewart´s group summarized the final results of a Phase 1/2 study of Kyprolis plus cyclophosphamide, thalidomide, and dexamethasone- a combination therapy known as "CYCLONE" - in newly diagnosed myeloma patients.

According to the researchers, the combination is highly efficacious. After four treatment cycles, 91% of patients responded, with 76% achieving at least a very good partial response. The two-year progression-free survival was 77%, and the two-year overall survival was 98%.

MM cells are characterized by high protein synthesis resulting in chronic endoplasmic reticulum (ER) stress, which is adaptively managed by the unfolded protein response. Inositol-requiring enzyme 1α (IRE1α) is activated to splice X-box binding protein 1 (XBP1) mRNA, thereby increasing XBP1s protein, which in turn regulates genes responsible for protein folding and degradation during the unfolded protein response. PI resistance mechanisms in MM remain controversial. Response of MM to the proteasome inhibitor bortezomib is correlated with the unfolded protein response regulator XBP1s protein [131,

132]. Leung-Hagesteijn et al. [133] reported the existence of a progenitor organization in primary MM that recapitulates maturation stages between B cells and plasma cells and that contributes to clinical PI resistance. Xbp1s^{-} tumor B cells and pre-plasmablasts with low level of Xbp1s survive therapeutic PI, preventing cure, while maturation arrest of MM before the plasmablast stage enables progressive disease on PI treatment.

Mechanistically, suppression of Xbp1s in MM is shown to induce bortezo-mib resistance via de-commitment to plasma cell maturation and immunoglobulin production, diminishing endoplasmic reticulum (ER) front-loading and cytotoxic susceptibility to PI-induced inhibition of ER-associated degradation.

These results reveal the tumor progenitor structure in MM and highlight its role in therapeutic failure.

The Third-Generation of Orally Active Proteasome Inhibitors

The novel orally active proteasome inhibitor CEP-18770 /[(1R)-1-[[(2 S,3 R)-3-hydroxy-2- [(6-phenylpyridine-2-carbonyl)amino]- 1-oxobutyl]amino] - 3-methylbutyl] boronic acid, Delanzomib/ was also studied in preclinical trials [134, 135]. CEP-18770 potently induces apoptotic cell death in MM cell lines and in primary purified CD138-positive cultures from untreated and bortezo-mib-treated MM patients [136].

In vitro, CEP-18770 has a strong antiangiogenic activity and potently represses RANKL-induced osteoclastogenesis. CEP-18770 exhibits a favorable cytotoxicity profile toward normal human epithelial cells, bone marrow progenitors, and bone marrow-derived stromal cells.

Thus, Delanzomib has a favorable tumor selectivity profile for the treatment of MM and other malignancies responsive to proteasome inhibition.

CEP-18770 combined with melphalan or bortezomib induces synergistic inhibition of MM cell viability in vitro. In MM xenograft models, the addition of CEP-18770 intravenously to melphalan completely prevented the growth of both melphalan-sensitive and melphalan-resistant tumours. The combination of CEP-18770 and bortezomib induced complete regression of bortezomib-sensitive tumours and markedly delayed progression of bortezomib-resistant tumours compared to treatment with either agent alone. Single agent CEP-18770 orally also showed marked anti-MM effects in these xenograft models. These studies provide strong preclinical rationale for further development of this novel PI in the treatment of MM as a monotherapy as well as combined with either melphalan or bortezomib [137, 138].

MLN9708 rapidly hydrolyzes to the biologically active form, MLN2238 (ixazomib). Ixazomib is an investigational oral proteasome inhibitor that, compared with bortezomib, has improved pharmacokinetics, pharmacodynamics, and antitumor activity in preclinical studies.

The in vivo activity of MLN2238 was evaluated in a variety of mouse models of hematologic malignancies, including tumor xenograft models derived from a human lymphoma cell line and primary human lymphoma tissue, and genetically engineered mouse models of plasma cell malignancies [139]. Treatment of MM cells with MLN2238 predominantly inhibits chymotrypsin-like activity of the proteasome and induces accumulation of ubiquitinated proteins. MLN2238 inhibits growth and induces apoptosis in MM cells resistant to conventional and bortezomib therapies without affecting the viability of normal cells [140]. In animal tumor model studies, MLN2238 is well tolerated and inhibits tumor growth with significantly reduced tumor recurrence. A head-to-head analysis of MLN2238 versus bortezomib showed a significantly longer survival time in mice treated with MLN2238 than mice receiving bortezomib. Immununostaining of MM tumors from MLN2238-treated mice showed growth inhibition, apoptosis, and a decrease in associated angiogenesis. Mechanistic studies showed that MLN2238-triggered apoptosis is associated with activation of caspase-3, caspase-8, and caspase-9; increase in p53, p21, NOXA, PUMA, and E2F; induction of endoplasmic reticulum (ER) stress response proteins Bip, phospho-eIF2-α, and CHOP; and inhibition of nuclear factor kappa B. Finally, combining MLN2238 with lenalidomide, histone deacetylase inhibitor suberoylanilide hydroxamic acid, or dexamethasone triggers synergistic anti-MM activity.

In December 2013 at the American Society of Hematology or ASH Annual Meeting, there was an abstract 535 presented by Dr. Paul Richardson of the Dana-Farber Cancer Institute and colleagues looking at the safety, tolerability, and efficacy of the combination of ixazomib, lenalidomide, and dexamethasone in patients with newly diagnosed multiple myeloma. They found that 93% of the patients had at least a partial response including 67% of the patients achieving a very good partial response. Because there were some dose interruptions due to toxicity such as rash and peripheral neuropathy, investigators continue to refine the dosing schedule to mitigate these adverse effects as they move on to phase 3 studies.

MLN9708 in combination with the existing drugs panobinostat and dexamethasone will be studied among patients with relapsed or refractory multiple myeloma. This study will also look at the response and clinical benefit of the treatment and the progression-free survival and overall survival of study participants. The further randomized phase I/II trial studies the side effects and best dose of pomalidomide and ixazomib when given together with dexamethasone and to see how well pomalidomide and dexamethasone with or without ixazomib works in treating patients with refractory multiple myeloma.

Biological therapies, such as pomalidomide and dexamethasone, may stimulate the immune system in different ways and stop tumor cells from growing. Ixazomib may stop the growth of tumor cells by blocking some of the enzymes needed for cell growth.

It is not yet known whether pomalidomide and dexamethasone are more effective with or without ixazomib in treating multiple myeloma.

Oprozomib (ONX 0912) is an oral, irreversible, tripeptide epoxyketone that exerts its activity via inhibition of chymotrypsin-like activity of the proteasome [141]. Biochemically, it is the oral analogue of carfilzomib, and demonstrates similar antiangiogenic and proapoptotic activity in vitro and in vivo [141].

A synergistic effect with bortezomib and with a combination of lenalidomide and dexamethasone was also seen in preclinical studies, and hypothesized to be secondary to differential effects on proapoptotic signaling pathways. The primary advantage with oprozomib is the ease of administration via the oral route. The strong preclinical data for equipotent efficacy to carfilzomib has laid the groundwork for clinical trials. Oprozomib is being evaluated as a single agent and in combination with low dose dexamethasone in relapsed and refractory MM.

The novel orally active PI K-7174 (*N,N´*-bis-(E)-[5-(3,4,5-trimethoxy-phenyl)-4-pentenyl]homopiperazine) exerts anti-MM activity by down-regulating the expression of class

I HDAC (HDAC1, -2, -3) [142]. K-7174 has the clinical utility in overcoming bortezomib resistance as a single agent or in combination with HDAC inhibitors [142].

Conclusion and Perspectives

The heterogeneity of MM biology and prognosis has become apparent over the last decade. The prognosis and treatment of an individual with MM depends on many patient-specific factors, including age, overall state of health, and comorbidities.

A more personalized approach to treatment is likely to become standard as increasingly robust molecularly based prognostic information becomes available. Insights into the role of the tumor microenvironment have provided new targets for the novel therapies. Pharmacogenomics analysis promises a new era of therapy tailored to the individual MM patient.

The first clinical trials evaluating the therapeutic potential of proteasome inhibition began before about 10 years. Since then, remarkable progress has been made [143, 144]. The role of bortezomib in the treatment of MM has evolved since the drug was introduced to the market.

Bortezomib-based combinations in newly diagnosed patients have resulted in high overall and complete response rates. Additionally, there does not seem to be a negative impact on stem cell harvest or engraftment in patients who received bortezomib as part of their induction regime [145].

A new next generation proteasome inhibitors (NPI-0052 and PR-171) have been evaluated in phase 1 and phase 2 trials of patients with relapsed and or refractory MM. As with bortezomib, next generation proteasome inhibitors trigger apoptosis in MM cells but are distinct from bortezomib in their chemical structure, effects on proteasome activities, and mechanism of action. The cellular response to next generation proteasome inhibitors occurs much earlier than that of bortezomib. Orally administered next generation proteasome inhibitors are cytotoxic to myeloma cells, with reduced toxicity against normal cells, compared with bortezomib. Because of the different kinetics and cellular responses, bortezomib and next generation proteasome inhibitors can be used in combination with synergistic apoptotic activity.

Survival outcomes are very poor when a patient with MM develops relapsed and/or refractory disease and treatment becomes more challenging. Significant progress has been made in the management of myeloma over the past 10 years with the development of new therapies including lenalidomide and bortezomib. Carfilzomib is a selective proteasome inhibitor with significant activity in relapsed and/or refractory MM at the FDA-approved dose and schedule. Carfilzomib has demonstrated robust and durable antitumor activity with evidence of a dose-response relationship in this patient population with a well-tolerated side-effect profile characterized by low rates of peripheral neuropathy. Data from clinical trials evaluating efficacy and safety of carfilzomib alone and in combination with other agents in various stages of disease will help define the MM treatment paradigm. Clinical trials continue to focus on single-agent, combination, consolidation, and maintenance treatment in the up-front and relapsed setting. Combination regimens are associated with higher response rates, and ongoing trials are concentrating on combinations with IMiDs (lenalidomide and pomalidomide), HDAC inhibitors (panobinostat and vorinostat), and cytotoxic therapies

(PLD, melphalan, and cyclophosphamide). These drug combinations have the potential to offer additional treatment options and further improve OS.

As carfilzomib data continue to evolve and demonstrate promise, the results of ongoing phase II and multiple phase III trials will help to further define the role of carfilzomib in MM therapy and will help establish the best dose, schedule, and supportive care in these patients.

When used with appropriate consideration, carfilzomib may help to provide patients with an improved overall survival and quality of life.

Bortezomib resistance can be overcome also by a novel small molecule 19S regulatory particle inhibitor b-AP15. This drug is simultaneously an inhibitor of deubiquitylating enzymes USP14 and UCHL5 [146, 147]. These enzymes are more highly expressed in MM cells than in normal plasma cells. Anti-MM activity of b-AP15 is associated with growth arrest as well as with induction of caspase-dependent apoptosis and activation of unfolded protein response. Combining b-AP15 with dexamethasone, lenalidomide, or HDAC inhibitors induces synergistic anti-MM activity. Preclinical data with b-AP15 provide the framework for clinical evaluation to improve patient outcome in MM.

The proteasome inhibitors and immunomodulatory agents represent the corner-stone of treatment of MM patients with combination regimens incorporating these drugs demonstrating encouraging rates and duration of response, including the newer agents, carfilzomib and pomalidomide.

In addition, novel drug classes have shown promising activity in refractory or relapsed MM patients, including the orally-administered proteasome inhibitors ixazomib and oprozomib; monoclonal antibodies such as the anti-CS1 mono-clonal antibody elotuzumab and anti-CD38 monoclonal antibody daratumumab; and histone deacetylase inhibitors such as panobinostat and rocilinostat [148, 149].

Acknowledgments

This work was supported by research project (Ministry of Health, Czech Republic) for conceptual development of research organization (00023736; Institute of Hematology and Blood Transfusion, Prague).

References

[1] Rajkumar, S. V. Multiple myeloma: 2013 update on diagnosis, risk-stratification, and management. *Am. J. Hematol.* 2013, 88, 226-235.

[2] Berenson, J. R.; Hilger, J. D.; Yellin, O.; Dichmann, R.; Patel-Donnelly, R., et al. Replacement of bortezomib with carfilzomib for multiple mye-loma patients progressing from bortezomib combination therapy. *Leukemia* accepted article preview 16 January 2014; doi: 10.1038/leu.2014.27.

[3] Palumbo, A.; Cavallo, F. Have drug combinations supplanted stem cell transplantation in myeloma? *Hematology* 2012, 335-341.

[4] Kyle, R.; Rajkumar, S. V. Multiple myeloma. *N. Engl. J. Med.* 2004, 351, 1860-1873.

[5] Chng, W. J.; Glebov, O.; Bergsagel, P. L.; Kuehl, W. M. Genetic events in the pathogenesis of multiple myeloma. *Best Pract. Res. Clin. Haematol.* 2007, 20, 571-596.

[6] Tonon, G. Molecular pathogenesis of multiple myeloma. *Hematol. Oncol. Clin. N. Am.* 2007, 21, 985-1006.

[7] Keats, J. J.; Fonseca, R.; Chesi, M.; Schop, R.; Baker, A.; Chng, W. J., et al. Promiscuous mutations activate the noncanonical NF-κB pathway in multiple myeloma. *Cancer Cell* 2007, 12, 131-144.

[8] Chapman, M. A.; Lawrence, M. S.; Keats, J. J.; Cibulskis, K.; Sougnez, C., et al. Initial genome sequencing and analysis of multiple myeloma. *Nature* 2011, 471, 467-472.

[9] Morgan, G. J.; Johnson, D. C.; Weinhold, N.; Goldschmidt, H.; Landgren, O.; Lynch, H. T., et al. Inherited genetic susceptibility to multiple myeloma. *Leukemia* 2014, 28, 518-524.

[10] Melchor, L.; Brioli, A.; Wardell, CP.; Murison, A.; Potter, N. E.; Kaiser, M. F., et al. *Leukemia* 2014 Jan. 13. doi: 10.1038/leu.2014.13.

[11] Podar, K.; Richardson, P. G.; Hideshima, T.; Chauhan, D.; Anderson, K. C. The malignant clone and the bone marrow environment. *Best Pract. Res. Clin. Haematol.* 2007, 20, 597-612.

[12] Mitsiades, C. S.; McMillin, D. V.; Klippel, S.; Hideshima, T.; Chauhan, D.; Richardson, P. G., et al. The role of the bone marrow microenvironment in the pathophysiology of myeloma and its significance in the development of more effective therapies. *Hematol. Oncol. Clin. N. Am.* 2007, 21, 1007-1034.

[13] Richardson, P. G.; Barlogie, B.; Berenson, J.; Singhal, S.; Jagannath, S.; Irwin, D., et al. Clinical factors predictive of outcome with bortezomib in patients with relapsed, refractory multiple myeloma. *Blood* 2008, 106, 2977-2981.

[14] Barlogie, B.; Shaughnessy, J.; Tricot, G.; Jacobson, J.; Zangari, M.; Anaissie, E., et al. Treatment of multiple myeloma. *Blood* 2004, 103, 20-32.

[15] Mitsiades, C. S.; Hayden, P. J.; Anderson, K. C.; Richardson, P. G. From the bench to the bedside: emerging new treatments in multiple myeloma. *Best Pract. Res. Clin. Haematol.* 2007, 20, 797-816.

[16] Kastritis, E.; Mitsiades, C. S.; Dimopoulos, M. A.; Richardson, P. G. Management of relapsed and relapsed refractory myeloma. *Hematol. Oncol. Clin. N. Am.* 2007, 21, 1007-1034.

[17] Schwartz, R. N. Current and emerging treatments for multiple myeloma. *J. Manag. Care Pharm.* 2008, 14, Suppl. S, S12-S18.

[18] Richardson, P. G.; Laubach, J.; Mitsiades, C. S.; Schlossman, R.; Hide-shima, T.; Redman, K., et al. Managing multiple myeloma: the emerging role of novel therapies and adapting combination treatment for higher risk settings. *Br. J. Haematol.* 2011, 154, 755-762.

[19] Jakubowiak, A. J.; Benson, D. M.; Bensinger, W.; Siegel, S. D. S.; Zimmerman, T. M.; Mohrbacher, A., et al. Phase I trial of anti-CS1 monoclonal antibody Elotuzumab in combination with bortezomib in the treatment of relapsed/refractory multiple myeloma. *J. Clin. Oncol.* 2012, 30, 1960-1965.

[20] Cavo, M.; Pantani, L.; Petrucci, M. T.; Patriarca, F.; Zamagni, E.; Donnarumma, D., et al. Bortezomib-thalidomide-dexamethasone is superior to thalidomide-dexamethasone as consolidation therapy after autologous hematopoietic stem cell transplantation in patients with newly diagnosed multiple myeloma. *Blood* 2012, 120, 9-19.

[21] Sonneveld, P.; Schmidt-Wolf, I. G. H.; van der Holt, B.; el Jarari, L.; Bertsch, U.; Salwender, H., et al. Bortezomib induction and maintenance treatment in patients with newly diagnosed multiple myeloma: results of the randomized phase III HOVON-65/GMMG-HD4 trial. *J. Clin. Oncol.* 2012, 30, 2946-2955.

[22] Richardson, P. G.; Mitsiades, C. S.; Laubach, J. P.; Hajek, R.; Spicka, I.; Dimopoulos, M. A., et al. Preclinical data and early clinical experience supporting the use of histone deacetylase inhibitors in multiple myeloma. *Leuk. Res.* 2013, 37, 829-837.

[23] Hajek, R.; Siegel, D.; Orlowski, R. Z.; Ludwig, H.; Palumbo, A.; Dimopoulos, M. The role of histone deacetylase inhibitors in patients with relapsed/refractory multiple myeloma. *Leuk. Lymphoma* 2014, 55, 11-18.

[24] Rosinol, L.; Bladé, J. Bortezomib and lenalidomide as front-line therapy for multiple myeloma. *Leuk. Lymphoma* 2014 Feb. 21 doi: 10.3109/104 28194.2014.896460.

[25] Genadieva-Stavric, S.; Cavallo, F.; Palumbo, A. New approaches to management of multiple myeloma. *Curr. Treat. Options Oncol.* 2014 Mar. 1 doi: 10.1007/s 11864-014-0276-6.

[26] Nooka, A. K.; Kaufman, J. L.; Mupiddi, S.;Langston, A.; Heffner, L. T.; Gleason, C., et al. Consolidation and maintenance therapy with lenalidomide, bortezomib and dexamethasone (RVD) in high-risk myeloma patients. *Leukemia* 2014, 28, 690-693.

[27] Ocio, E. M.; Richardson, P. G.; Rajkumar, S. V.; Palumbo, A.; Mateos, M. V.; Orlowski, R., et al. New drugs and novel mechanisms of action in multiple myeloma in 2013; a report from the International Myeloma Working Group (IMWG). *Leukemia* 2014, 28, 525-542.

[28] Hershko, A.; Ciechanover, A. The ubiquitin system. *Annu. Rev. Bio-chem.* 1998, 67, 425-479.

[29] Pickart, C. M. Mechanisms underlying ubiquitination. *Annu. Rev. Bio-chem.* 2001, 70, 503-533.

[30] Glickman, M. H.; Ciechanover, A. The ubiquitin-proteasome proteolytic pathway: destruction for the sake of construction. *Physiol. Rev.* 2002, 82, 373-428.

[31] Pickart, C. M.; Cohen, R. E. Proteasomes and their kin: proteases in the machine age. *Nat. Rev. Mol. Cell. Biol.* 2004, 5, 177-187.

[32] Hershko, A. Review: Nobel Lecture. The ubiquitin system for protein degradation and some of its roles in the control of the cell division cycle. *Cell Death Differ.* 2005, 12, 1191-1197.

[33] Ciechanover, A. Intracellular protein degradation from a vague idea through the lysosome and the ubiquitin-proteasome system and on to human diseases and drug targeting: Nobel Lecture, December 8, 2004. *Ann. N.Y. Acad. Sci.* 2007, 1116, 1-28.

[34] Rose, I. Review: Nobel Lecture. Ubiquitin at Fox Chase. *Cell Death Differ.* 2005, 12, 1162-1166.

[35] Wilkinson, K. D. Ubiquitin: A Nobel protein. *Cell* 2004, 119, 741-745.

[36] Koegl, M.; Hoppe, T.; Schlenker, S.; Ulrich, H. D.; Mayer, T. U.; Jentsch, S. A novel ubiquitination factor, E4, is involved in multiubiquitin chain assembly. *Cell* 1999, 96, 635-644.

[37] Staub, O.; Rotin, D. Role of ubiquitylation in cellular membrane trans-port. *Physiol. Rev.* 2006, 86, 669-707.

[38] Savory, P. J.; Rivett, A. J. Leupeptin-binding site(s) in the mammalian multicatalytic proteinase complex. *Biochem. J.* 1993, 289, 45-48.

[39] Vinitsky, A.; Cardozo, C.; Sepp-Lorenzino, L.; Michaud, C.; Orlowski, M. Inhibition of the proteolytic activity of the multicatalytic proteinase complex (proteasome) by substrate-related peptidyl aldehydes. *J. Biol. Chem.* 1994, 269, 29860-29866.

[40] Delic, J.; Masdehors, P.; Omura, S.; Cosset, J. M.; Dumont, J.; Binet, J. L. et al. The proteasome inhibitor lactacystin induces apoptosis and sensitizes chemo- and radio resistant human chronic lymphocytic leukemia lymphocytes to TNF-alpha-initiated apoptosis. *Br. J. Cancer* 1998, 77, 1103-1107.

[41] Masdehors, P.; Omura, S.; Merle-Beral, H.; Mentz, F.; Cosset, J. M.; Dumont, J., et al. Increased sensitivity of CLL-derived lymphocytes to apoptotic death activation by the proteasome-specific inhibitor lactacystin. *Br. J. Haematol.* 1999, 105, 752-757.

[42] Orlowski, R. Z.; Eswara, J. R.; Lafond-Walker, A.; Grever, M. R.; Orlowski, M.; Dang, C. V. Tumor growth inhibition induced in a murine model of human Burkitt's lymphoma by a proteasome inhibitor. *Cancer Res.* 1998, 58, 4342-4348.

[43] Hideshima, T.; Richardson, P. G.; Chauhan, D.; Palombella, V. I.; Elliott, P. J.; Adams, J., et al. The proteasome inhibitor PS-341 inhibits growth, induces apoptosis and overcomes drug resistance in human multiple myeloma cells. *Cancer Res.* 2001, 61, 3071-3076.

[44] Kisselev, A. F.; Goldberg, A. L. Proteasome inhibitors: from research tools to drug candidates. *Chem. Biol.* 2001, 8, 739-758.

[45] Voorhees, P. M.; Dees, E. C.; O'Neil, B.; Orlowski, R. Z. The proteasome as a target for cancer therapy. *Clin. Cancer Res.* 2003, 9, 6316-6325.

[46] Almond, J. B.; Cohen, G. M. The proteasome: a novel target for cancer chemotherapy. *Leukemia* 2002, 16, 433-443.

[47] Vinitsky, A.; Michaud, C.; Powers, J. C.; Orlowski, M. Inhibition of the chymotrypsin – like activity of the pituitary multicatalytic proteinase complex. *Biochemistry* 1992, 31, 9421-9428.

[48] Palombella, V. J., Rando, O. J., Goldberg, A. L., Maniatis, T. The ubiquitin-proteasome pathway is required for processing the NF-kappa B1 precursor protein and the activation of NF-kappa B. *Cell* 1994, 78, 773-785.

[49] Rock, K. L.; Gramm, C.; Rothstein, L.; Clark, K.; Stein, R.; Dick, L., et al. Inhibitors of the proteasome block the degradation of most cell proteins and the generation of peptides presented on MHC class I molecules. *Cell* 1994, 78, 761-771.

[50] Adams, J.; Behnke, M.; Chen, S.; Cruickshank, A. A.; Dick, L. R.; Grenier, L., et al. Potent and selective inhibitors of the proteasome: dipeptidyl boronic acids. *Bioorg. Med. Chem. Lett.* 1998, 8, 333-338.

[51] Adams, J.; Kauffman, M. Development of the proteasome inhibitor Velcade (Bortezomib). *Cancer Invest.* 2004, 22, 304-311.

[52] Adams, J. The proteasome: a suitable antineoplastic target. *Nat. Rev. Cancer* 2004, 4, 349-360.

[53] Kane, R. C.; Bross, P. F.; Farrell, A. T.; Pazdur, R. Velcade: US FDA approval for the treatment of multiple myeloma progressing on prior therapy. *Oncologist* 2003, 8, 508-513.

[54] Kane, R. C.; Farrell, A. T.; Sridhara, R.; Pazdur, R. United States Food and Drug Administration approval summary: bortezomib for the treatment of progressive multiple myeloma after one prior therapy. *Clin. Cancer Res.* 2006, 12, 2955-2960.

[55] Richardson, P. G.; Sonneveld, P.; Schuster, M. W.; Irwin, D.; Stadtmauer, E. A.; Facon, T., et al. Safety and efficacy of bortezomib in high-risk and elderly patients with relapsed multiple myeloma. *Br. J. Haematol.* 2007, 137, 429-435.

[56] Chauhan, D.; Hideshima, T.; Anderson, K. C. Targeting proteasomes as therapy in multiple myeloma. *Adv. Exp. Med. Biol.* 2008, 615, 251-260.

[57] Goy, A.; Younes, A.; McLaughlin, P.; Pro, B.; Romaguera, J. E.; Hagemeister, F., et al. Phase II study of proteasome inhibitor bortezomib in relapsed or refractory B-cell non-Hodgkin's lymphoma. *J. Clin. Oncol.* 2005, 23, 667-675.

[58] O'Connor, O. A.; Wright, J.; Moskowitz, C.; Muzzy, J.; MacGregor-Cortelli, B.; Stubblefield, M. Phase II clinical experience with the novel proteasome inhibitor bortezomib in patients with indolent non-Hodgkin's lymphoma and mantle cell lymphoma. *J. Clin. Oncol.* 2005, 23, 676-684.

[59] Suh, K. S.; Gay, A. Bortezomib in mantle cell lymphoma. *Future Oncol.* 2008, 4, 149-168.

[60] Hideshima, T.; Chauhan, D.; Richardson, P.; Mitsiades, C.; Mitsiades, N.; Hayashi, T., et al. NF-kappa B as a therapeutic target in multiple myeloma. *J. Biol. Chem.* 2002, 277, 16639-16647.

[61] Roccaro, A. M.; Vacca, A.; Ribatti, D. Bortezomib in the treatment of cancer. *Recent Patents Anticancer Drug Discov.* 2006, 1, 397-403.

[62] Roccaro, A. M.; Hideshima, T.; Raje, N.; Kumar, S.; Ishitsuka, K.; Yasui, H., et al. Bortezomib mediates antiangiogenesis in multiple myeloma via direct and indirect effects on endothelial cells. *Cancer Res.* 2006, 66,184-191.

[63] Hideshima, T.; Bradner, J. E.; Wong, J.; Chauhan, D.; Richardson, P.; Schreiber, S. L.; Anderson, K. C. Small-molecule inhibition of proteasome and aggresome function induces synergistic antitumor activity in multiple myeloma. *Proc. Natl. Acad. Sci. US* 2005, 102, 8567-8572.

[64] Nawrocki, S. T.; Carew, J. S.; Dunner, K. Jr.; Boise, L. H.; Chiao, P. J.; Huang, P., et al. Bortezomib inhibits PKR-like endoplasmic reticulum (ER) kinase and induces apoptosis via ER stress in human pancreatic cancer cells. *Cancer Res.* 2005, 65, 11510-11519.

[65] Nawrocki, S. T.; Carew, J. S.; Pino, M. S.; Highshaw, R. A.; Dunner, K. Jr.; Huang, P., et al. Bortezomib sensitizes pancreatic cancer cells to endoplasmic reticulum stress-mediated apoptosis. *Cancer Res.* 2005, 65, 11658-11666.

[66] Lee, A. H.; Iwakoshi, N. N.; Anderson, K. C.; Glimcher, L. H. Proteasome inhibitors disrupt the unfolded protein response in myeloma cells. *Proc. Natl. Acad. Sci. US* 2003, 100, 9946-9951.

[67] Obeng, E. A.; Carlson, L. M.; Gutman, D. M.; Harrington, W. J. Jr.; Lee, K. P.; Boise, H. Proteasome inhibitors induce a terminal unfolded protein response in multiple myeloma cells. *Blood* 2006, 107, 4907-4916.

[68] Gupta, D.; Treon, S. P.; Shima, Y.; Hideshima, T.; Podar, K.; Tai, Y. T., et al. Adherence of multiple myeloma cells to bone marrow stromal cells upregulates vascular endothelial growth factor secretion: therapeutic applications. *Leukemia* 2001, 15, 1950-1961.

[69] Chauhan, D.; Uchiyama, H.; Akbarali, Y.; Urashima, M.; Yamamoto, K.; Libermann, T. A., et al. Multiple myeloma cell adhesion – induced interleukin-6 expression in bone marrow stromal cells involves activation of NF-kappa B. *Blood* 1996, 87, 1104-1112.

[70] Chauhan, D.; Pandey, P.; Hideshima, T.; Treon, S.; Raje, N.; Davies, F. E., et al. SHP2 mediates the protective effect of interleukin-6 against dexamethasone – induced apoptosis in multiple myeloma cells. *J. Biol. Chem.* 2000, 275, 27845-27850.

[71] Dankbar, B.; Padro, T.; Leo, R.; Feldmann, B.; Kropff, M.; Mesters, R. M., et al. Vascular endothelial growth factor and interleukin-6 in paracrine tumor-stromal cell interactions in multiple myeloma. *Blood* 2000, 95, 2630-2636.

[72] Ogata, A.; Chauhan, D.; Teoh, G.; Treon, S P.; Urashima, M.; Schlossman, R. L.; Anderson, K. C. IL-6 triggers cell growth via the Ras-dependent mitogen-activated protein kinase cascade. *J. Immunol.* 1997, 159, 2212-2221.

[73] Lichtenstein, A.; Tu, Y.; Fady, C.; Vescio, R.; Berenson, J. Interleukin-6 inhibits apoptosis of malignant plasma cells. *Cell Immunol.* 1995, 162, 248-255.

[74] Hideshima, T.; Chauhan, D.; Richardson, P.; Anderson, K. C. Identification and validation of novel therapeutic targets for multiple myeloma. *J. Clin. Oncol.* 2005, 23, 6345-6350.

[75] Hughes, V. Neighbourhood watch. *Nature* 2011, 480, S48-S49.

[76] Mitsiades, N.; Mitsiades, C. S.; Richardson, P. G.; Poulaki, V.; Tai, Y. T.; Chauhan, D., et al. The proteasome inhibitor PS-341 markedly enhances sensitivity of multiple myeloma cells to conventional chemo-therapeutic agents: therapeutic applications. *Blood* 2003, 101, 2377-2380.

[77] Hideshima, T.; Chauhan, D.; Schlassman, R.; Richardson, P.; Anderson, R. C. The role of tumor necrosis factor alpha in the pathophysiology of human multiple myeloma: therapeutic applications. *Oncogene* 2001, 20, 4519-4527.

[78] Mitsiades, N.; Mitsiades, C. S.; Poulaki, V.; Chauhan, D.; Fanourakis, G.; Gu, X., et al. Molecular sequelae of proteasome inhibition in human multiple myeloma cells. *Proc. Natl. Acad. Sci. US* 2002, 99, 14374-14379.

[79] Gomez-Bougie, P.; Wuilléme-Toumi, S.; Ménoret, E.; Trichet, V.; Robillard, N.; Philippe, M., et al. Noxa up-regulation and Mcl-1 cleavage are associated to apoptosis induction by bortezomib in multiple myeloma. *Cancer Res.* 2007, 67, 5418-5424.

[80] Hideshima, T.; Mitsiades, C. S.; Akiyama, M.; Hayashi, T.; Chauhan, D.; Richardson, P., et al. Molecular mechanisms mediating antimyeloma activity of proteasome inhibitor PS-341. *Blood* 2003, 101, 1530-1534.

[81] Zangari, M.; Esseltine, D.; Lee, C. K.; Barlogie, B.; Elice, F.; Burns, M. J., et al. Response to bortezomib is associated to osteoblastic activation in patients with multiple myeloma. *Br. J. Haematol.* 2005, 131, 71-73.

[82] Oyajobi, B. O.; Garrett, I. R.; Gupta, A.; Flores, A.; Esparza, J.; Muñoz, S., et al. Stimulation of new bone formation by the proteasome inhibitor, bortezomib: implications for myeloma bone disease. *Br. J. Haematol.* 2007, 139, 434-438.

[83] Giuliani, N.; Morandi, F.; Tagliaferri, S.; Lazzaretti, M.; Bonomini, S.; Crugnola, M., et al. The proteasome inhibitor bortezomib affects osteoblast differentiation in vitro and in vivo in multiple myeloma patients. *Blood* 2007, 110, 334-338.

[84] Mukherjee, S.; Raje, N.; Schoonmaker, J. A.; Liu, J. C.; Hideshima, T.; Wein, M. N., et al. Pharmacologic targeting of a stem/progenitor population in vivo is associated with enhanced bone regeneration in mice. *J. Clin. Invest.* 2008, 118, 491-504.

[85] Yaccoby, S.; Wezeman, M. J.; Zangari, M.; Walker, R.; Cottler-Fox, M.; Gaddy, D., et al. Inhibitory effects of osteoblasts and increased bone formation on myeloma in

novel culture systems and a myelomatous mouse model. *Haematologica* 2006, 91, 192-199.

[86] Terpos, E.; Heath, D. J.; Rahemtulla, A.; Zervas, K.; Chantry, A.; Anagnostopoulos, A., et al. Bortezomib reduces serum dickkopf-1 and receptor activator of nuclear factor-kappaB ligand concentrations and normalises indices of bone remodelling in patients with relapsed multiple myeloma. *Br. J. Haematol.* 2006, 135, 688-692.

[87] Uy, G. L.; Trivedi, R.; Peles, S.; Fisher, N. M.; Zhang, Q. J.; Tomasson, M. H.; Dipersio, J. F.; Vij, R. Bortezomib inhibits osteoclast activity in patients with multiple myeloma. *Clin. Lymphoma Myeloma* 2007, 7, 587-589.

[88] Boissy, P.; Andersen, T. L.; Lund, T.; Kupisiewicz, K.; Plesner, T.; Delaissé, J. M. Pulse treatment with the proteasome inhibitor bortezomib inhibits osteoclast resorptive activity in clinically relevant conditions. *Leuk. Res.* 2008, 32, 1661-1668.

[89] Westendorf, J. J.; Kahler, R. A.; Schroeder, T. M. Wnt signaling in osteoblasts and bone diseases. *Gene* 2004, 341, 19-39.

[90] Richardson, P. G.; Barlogie, B.; Berenson, J.; Singhal, S.; Jagannath, S.; Irwin, D., et al. A phase 2 study of bortezomib in relapsed, refractory myeloma. *N. Engl. J. Med.* 2003, 348, 2609-2617.

[91] Jagannath, S.; Barlogie, B.; Berenson, J.; Siegel, D.; Irwin, D.; Richardson, P. G., et al. A phase 2 study of two doses of bortezomib in relapsed or refractory myeloma. *Br. J. Haematol.* 2004, 127, 165-172.

[92] Jagannath, S.; Richardson, P. G.; Barlogie, B.; Berenson, J.; Singhal, S.; Irwin, D., et al. Bortezomib in combination with dexamethasone for the treatment of patients with relapsed and or refractory multiple myeloma with less than optimal response to bortezomib alone. *Haematologica* 2006, 91, 929-934.

[93] Richardson, P. G.; Barlogie, B.; Berenson, J.; Singhal, S.; Jagannath, S.; Irwin, D., et al. Clinical factors predictive of outcome with bortezomib in patients with relapsed refractory multiple myeloma. The SUMMIT Investigators. *Blood* 2005, 106, 2977-2981.

[94] Richardson, P. G.; Sonneveld, P.; Schuster, M.; Irwin, D.; Stadtmauer, E.; Facon, T., et al. Extended follow-up of a phase 3 trial in relapsed multiple myeloma: final time-to-event results of the APEX trial. *Blood* 2007, 110, 3557-3560.

[95] Wolf, J.; Richardson, P. G.; Schuster, M.; LeBlanc, A.; Walters, I. B.; Battleman, D. S. Utility of bortezomib retreatment in relapsed or refract-tory multiple myeloma patients: a multicenter case series. *Clin. Adv. Hematol. Oncol.* 2008, 6, 755-760.

[96] San Miguel, J.; Bladé, J.; Boccadoro, M.; Cavenagh, J.; Glasmacher, A.; Jagannath, S., et al. A practical update on the use of bortezomib in the management of multiple myeloma. *Oncologist* 2006, 11, 51-61.

[97] Richardson, P. G.; Briemberg, H.; Jagannath, S.; Wen, P. Y.; Barlogie, B.; Berenson, J., et al. Frequency, characteristics, and reversibility of peripheral neuropathy during treatment of advanced multiple myeloma with bortezomib. *J. Clin. Oncol.* 2006, 24, 3113-3120.

[98] Rosiñol, L.; Montoto, S.; Cibeira, M. T.; Bladé, J. Bortezomib-induced severe hepatitis in multiple myeloma: a case report. *Arch. Intern. Med.* 2005, 165, 464-465.

[99] Cibeira, M. T.; Mercadal, S.; Arenillas, L.; Muntañola, A.; Salamero, O.; Bladé, J. Bortezomib-induced rhabdomyolysis in multiple myeloma. *Acta Haematol.* 2006, 116, 203-206.

[100] Orlowski, R. Z.; Voorhees, P. M.; Garcia, R. A.; Hall, M. D.; Kudrik, F. J.; Allred, T., et al. Phase 1 trial of the proteasome inhibitor bortezomib and pegylated liposomal doxorubicin in patients with advanced hematologic malignancies. *Blood* 2005, 105, 3058-3065.

[101] Biehn, S. E.; Moore, D. T.; Voorhees, P. M.; Garcia, R. A.; Lehman, M. J.; Dees, E. C.; Orlowski, R. Z. Extended follow-up of outcome measures in multiple myeloma patients treated on a phase I study with bortezomib and pegylated liposomal doxorubicin. *Ann. Hematol.* 2007, 86, 211-216.

[102] Orlowski, R. Z.; Nagler, A.; Sonneveld, P.; Bladé, J.; Hajek, R.; Spencer, A., et al. Randomized phase III study of pegylated liposomal doxorubicin plus bortezomib compared with bortezomib alone in relapsed or refractory multiple myeloma: combination therapy improves time to progression. *J. Clin. Oncol.* 2007, 25, 3892-3901.

[103] Ma, M. H.; Yang, H. H.; Parker, K.; Manyak, S.; Friedman, J. M.; Altamirano, C., et al. The proteasome inhibitor PS-341 markedly enhances sensitivity of multiple myeloma tumor cells to chemotherapeutic agents. *Clin. Cancer Res.* 2003, 9, 1136-1144.

[104] Sonneveld, P.; Hajek, R.; Nagler, A.; Spencer, A.; Bladé, J.; Robak, T., et al. Combined pegylated liposomal doxorubicin and bortezomib is highly effective in patients with recurrent or refractory multiple myeloma who received prior thalidomide/lenalidomide therapy. *Cancer* 2008, 112, 1529-1537.

[105] Pineda-Roman, M.; Zangari, M.; van Rhee, F.; Anaissie, E.; Szymonifka, J.; Hoering, A., et al. VTD combination therapy with bortezomib-thalidomide-dexamethasone is highly effective in advanced and refractory multiple myeloma. *Leukemia* 2008, 22, 1419-1427.

[106] Palumbo, A.; Ambrosini, M. T.; Benevolo, G.; Pregno, P.; Pescosta, N.; Callea, V., et al. Bortezomib, melphalan, prednisone, and thalidomide for relapsed multiple myeloma. *Blood* 2007, 109, 2767-2772.

[107] Fonseca, R.; Rajkumar, S. V. Consolidation therapy with bortezomib/ lenalidomide/ dexamethasone versus bortezomib/dexamethasone after a dexamethasone-based induction regimen in patients with multiple myeloma: a randomized phase III trial. *Clin. Lymphoma Myeloma* 2008, 8, 315-317.

[108] Richardson, P. G.; Xie, W.; Jagannath, S.; Jakubowiak, A.; Lonial, S.; Raje, N. S., et al. A phase 2 trial of lenalidomide, bortezomib, and dexamethasone in patient with relapsed and relapsed/refractory myeloma. *Blood* 2014, 123, 1461-1469.

[109] Feling, R. H.; Buchanan, G. O.; Mincer, T. J.; Kauffman, C. A.; Jensen, P. R.; Fenical, W. Salinosporamide A: a highly cytotoxic proteasome inhibitor from a novel microbial source, a marine bacterium of the new genus salinospora. *Angew. Chem. Int. Ed. Engl.* 2003, 42, 355-357.

[110] Macherla, V. R.; Mitchell, S. S.; Manam, R. R.; Reed, K. A.; Chao, T. H.; Nicholson, B., et al. Structure-activity relationship studies of salino-sporamide A (NPI-0052), a novel marine derived proteasome inhibitor. *J. Med.. Chem.* 2005, 48, 3684-3687.

[111] Chauhan, D.; Catley, L.; Li, G.; Podar, K.; Hideshima, T.; Velankar, M., et al. A novel orally active proteasome inhibitor induces apoptosis in multiple myeloma cells with mechanisms distinct from Bortezomib. *Cancer Cell* 2005, 8, 407-419.

[112] Chauhan, D.; Hideshima, T.; Anderson, K. C. A novel proteasome inhibitor NPI-0052 as an anticancer therapy. *Br. J. Cancer* 2006, 95, 961-965.

[113] Williamson, M. J.; Blank, J. L.; Bruzzese, F. J.; Cao, Y.; Daniels, J. S.; Dick, L. R., et al. Comparison of biochemical and biological effects of ML858 (salinosporamide A) and bortezomib. *Mol. Cancer Ther.* 2006, 5, 3052-3061.

[114] Chauhan, D.; Singh, A.; Brahmandam, M.; Podar, K.; Hideshima, T.; Richardson, P., et al. Combination of proteasome inhibitors bortezomib and NPI-0052 trigger in vivo synergistic cytotoxicity in multiple myeloma. *Blood* 2008, 111, 1654-1664.

[115] Miller, C. P.; Ban, K.; Dujka, M. E.; McConkey, D. J.; Munsell, M.; Palladino, M.; Chandra, J. NPI-0052, a novel proteasome inhibitor, induces caspase-8 and ROS-dependent apoptosis alone and in combination with HDAC inhibitors in leukemia cells. *Blood* 2007, 110, 267-277.

[116] Ahn, K. S.; Sethi, G.; Chao, T. H.; Neuteboom, S. T. C.; Chatuverdi, M. M.; Palladino, M. A., et al. Salinosporamide A (NPI-0052) potentiates apoptosis, suppresses osteoclastogenesis, and inhibit invasion through down-modulation of NF-κB-regulated gene products. *Blood* 2007, 110, 2286-2295.

[117] Potts, B. C.; Albitar, M. X.; Anderson, K. C.; Baritaki, S.; Berkers, C.; Bonavida, B., et al. Marizomib, a proteasome inhibitor for all seasons: preclinical profile and a framework for clinical trials. *Curr. Cancer Drug Targets* 2011, 11, 254-284.

[118] Lawasut, P.; Chauhan, D.; Laubach, J.; Hayes, C.; Fabre, C.; Maglio, M., et al. New proteasome inhibitors in myeloma. *Curr. Hematol. Malig. Rep.* 2012, 7, 258-266.

[119] Allegra, A.; Alonci, A.; Gerace, D.; Russo, S.; Innao, V.; Calabro, L.; Musolino, C. New orally aktive proteasome inhibitors in multiple myeloma. *Leuk. Res.* 2014, 38, 1-9.

[120] Demo, S. D., Kirk, C. J.; Aujay, M. A.; Buchholz, T. J.; Dajee, M.; Ho, M. N., et al. Antitumor activity of PR-171, a novel irreversible inhibitor of the proteasome. *Cancer Res.* 2007, 67, 6383-6391.

[121] Kuhn, D. J.; Chen, Q.; Voorhees, P. M.; Strader, J. S.; Shenk, K. D.; Sun, C. M., et al. Potent activity of carfilzomib, a novel, irreversible inhibitor of the ubiquitin-proteasome pathway, against preclinical models of multiple myeloma. *Blood* 2007, 110, 3281-3290.

[122] McCormack, P. L. Carfilzomib: in relapsed, or relapsed and refractory, multiple myeloma. *Drugs* 2012, 72, 2023-2032.

[123] Reece, D. E. Carfilzomib in multiple myeloma: gold, silver, or bronze? *Blood* 2012, 120, 2776-2777.

[124] Siegel, D. S.; Martin, T.; Wang, M.; Vij, R.; Jakubowiak, A. J.; Lonial, S., et al. A phase 2 study of single-agent carfilzomib (PX-171-003-A1) in patients with relapsed and refractory multiple myeloma. *Blood* 2012, 120, 2817-2825.

[125] Siegel, D. S. From clinical trials to clinical practice: single-agent carfilzomib averse events and the management in patients with relapsed and/or refractory multiple myeloma. *Ther. Adv. Hematol.* 2013, 4, 354-365.

[126] Herndon, T. M.; Deisseroth, A.; Kaminskas, E.; Kane, R. C.; Koti, K. M.; Rothmann, M. D., et al. US Food and Drug Administration approval: carfilzomib for the treatment of multiple myeloma. *Clin. Cancer Res.* 2013, 19, 4559.

[127] Niesvizky, R.; Martin, T. G.,3rd; Bensinger, W. I.; Alsina, M.; Siegel D. S.; Kunkel, L. A., et al. Phase 1b dose-escalation study (PX-171-006) of carfilzomib, lenalidomide, and low-dose dexamethasone in relapsed or progressive multiple myeloma. *Clinical Cancer Research* 2013a, 19, 2248–2256.
[128] Niesvizky, R.; Wang, M.; Martin, T.; Bensinger, W.; Alsina, M.; Siegel, D.; Kavalerchik, E. Final results from the phase 1b/2 study (PX-171-006) of carfilzomib (CFZ) in combination with lenalidomide and low-dose dexamethasone (CRD) for patients with relapsed or progressive multiple myeloma [Abstract S577]. *Haematologica* 2013b, 98(suppl. 1).
[129] Bringhen, S.; Federica, C.; Petrucci, M.; Gay, F.; Federico, V.; Conti-cello, C., et al. Carfilzomib, cyclophosphamide and dexamethasone (CCD) for newly diagnosed multiple myeloma (MM) patients: Initial results of a multicenter, open label phase II study [Abstract S578] *Haematologica* 2013, 98(suppl. 1).
[130] Palumbo, A.; Bringhen, S.; Petrucci, M.; Oliva, S.; Finsinger, P.; Conticello, C., et al. A phase II trial of carfilzomib, cyclophosphamide and dexamethasone (CCd) for newly diagnosed multiple myeloma patients [Abstract P-145]. *Clinical Lymphoma, Myeloma, and Leukemia* 2013, 13(suppl. 1).
[131] Ling, S. C.; Lau, E. K.; Al-Shabeeb, A.; Nikolic, A.; Catalano, A., Iland, H., et al. Response of myeloma to the proteasome inhibitor bortezomib is correlated with the unfolded protein response regulator XBP-1. *Haematologica* 2012, 97, 64-72.
[132] Gambella, M.; Rocci, A.; Passera, R.; Gay, F.; Omede, P.; Crippa, C., et al. High XBP1 expression is a marker of better outcome in multiple myeloma patiens treated with bortezomib. *Haematologica* 2014, 99, e14-e16.
[133] Leung-Hagesteijn, C.; Erdmann, N.; Cheung, G.; Keats, J. J.; Stewart, A. K.; Reece, D E., et al. Xbp1s-negative tumor B cells and pre-plasma-blasts mediate therapeutic proteasome inhibitor resistance in multiple myeloma. *Cancer Cell* 2013, 24, 289-304.
[134] Orlowski, R. Z.; Kuhn, D. J. Proteasome inhibitors in cancer therapy: lessons from the first decade. *Clin. Cancer Res.* 2008, 14, 1649-1657.
[135] Dorsey, B. D.; Iqbal, M.; Chatterjee, S.; Menta, E.; Bernardini, R.; Bernareggi, A., et al. Discovery of a potent, selective, and orally active proteasome inhibitor for the treatment of cancer. *J. Med. Chem.* 2008, 51, 1068-1072.
[136] Piva, R.; Ruggeri, B.; Williams, M.; Costa, G.; Tamagno, I.; Ferrero, D., et al. CEP-18770: A novel, orally active proteasome inhibitor with a tumor-selective pharmacologic profile competitive with bortezomib. *Blood* 2008, 111, 2765-2775.
[137] Sanchez, E.; Li, M.; Steinberg, J. A.; Wang, C.; Shen, J.; Bonavida, B., et al. The proteasome inhibitor CEP-18770 enhances the anti-myeloma activity of bortezomib and melphalan. *Br. J. Haematol.* 2010, 148, 569-581.
[138] Sanchez, E.; Li, M.; Li, J.; Wang, C.; Chen, H.; Jones-Bolin, S., et al. CEP-18770 (delanzomib) in combination with dexamethasone and lenalidomide inhibits the growth of multiple myeloma. *Leuk. Res.* 2012, 36, 1422-1427.
[139] Chauhan, D.; Tian, Z.; Zhou, B.; Kuhn, D.; Orlowski, R.; Raje, N., et al. In vitro and in vivo selective antitumor activity of a novel orally bio-available proteasome inhibitor MLN9708 against multiple myeloma cells. *Clin. Cancer Res.* 2011, 17, 5311-5321.
[140] Lee, E. C.; Fitzgerald, M.; Bannerman, B.; Donelan, J.; Bano, K.; Terkelsen, J., et al. Antitumor activity of the investigational proteasome inhibitor MLN9708 in mouse models of B-cell and plasma cell malignancies. *Clin. Cancer Res.* 2011, 17, 7313-7323.

[141] Chauhan, D.; Singh, A. V.; Aujay, M.; Kirk, C. J.; Bandi, M.; Ciccarelli, B., et al. A novel orally active proteasome inhibitor ONX 0912 triggers in vitro and in vivo cytotoxicity in multiple myeloma. *Blood* 2010, 116, 4906-4915.

[142] Manochakian, R.; Miller, K. C.; Chanan-Khan, A. A. Clinical impact of bortezomib in frontline regimens for patients with multiple myeloma. *Oncologist* 2007, 12, 978-990.

[143] Moreau, P.; Richardson, P. G.; Cavo, M.; Orlowski, R. Z.; San Miguel, J. F.; Palumbo, A.; Harousseau, J. L. Proteasome inhibitors in multiple myeloma, 10 years later. *Blood* 2012, 120, 947-959.

[144] Kubiczkova, L.; Pour, L.; Sedlarikova, L.; Hajek, R.; Sevcikova, S. Proteasome inhibitors-molecular basis and current perspectives in multiple myeloma. *J. Cell. Mol. Med.* 2014, DOI: 10.1111/jcmm.12279.

[145] Kapoor, P.; Ramakrishnan, V.; Rajkumar, S. V. Bortezomib combination therapy in multiple myeloma. *Sem. Hematol.* 2012, 49, 228-242.

[146] Feng, X.; Holmlund, T.; Zheng, C.; Fadeel, B. Proapoptotic effects of the novel proteasome inhibitor b-AP15 on multiple myeloma cells and natural killer cells. *Exp. Hematol.* 2014, 42, 172-182.

[147] Tian, Z.; D´Arcy, P.; Wang, X.; Ray, A., Tai, Y. T.; Hu, Y., et al. A novel small molecule inhibitor of deubiquitylating enzyme USP14 and UCHL5 induces apoptosis in multiple myeloma and overcomes bortezomib resistance. *Blood* 2014, 123, 706-716.

[148] Laubach, J. P.; Voorhees, P. M.; Hassoun, H.; Jakubowiak, A.; Lonial, S.; Richardson, P. G. Current strategies for treatment of relapsed/ refractory multiple myeloma. *Expert Rev. Hematol.* 2014, 7, 97-111.

[149] Ocio, E. M.; Mitsiades, C. S.; Orlowski, R. Z.; Anderson, K. C. Future agents and treatment directions in multiple myeloma. *Expert Rev. Hematol.* 2014, 7, 127-141.

In: Multiple Myeloma: Risk Factors, Diagnosis and Treatments ISBN: 978-1-63321-514-6
Editor: Steve Holt

Chapter 3

Cereblon as the Cellular Target Responsible for the Anti-Multiple Myeloma Activity of Immunomodulatory Drugs (Thalidomide, Lenalidomide and Pomalidomide)

Radka Bokorova, Jaroslav Polak, Martin Vostry, Arnost Kostecka and Ota Fuchs*

Institute of Hematology and Blood Transfusion, Prague, Czech Republic

Abstract

Cereblon (CRBN) was named according to its putative role in cerebral development, especially in memory and learning. A nonsense mutation in CRBN causes autosomal recessive nonsyndromic mental retardation. CRBN is a member and substrate receptor of the cullin 4 ring E3 ubiquitin ligase complex (CRL4). CRL4 consists of Cullin 4, RING finger protein (Roc1), and DNA damage binding protein 1 (DDB1). CRBN binds to its substrate proteins and it leads to ubiquitination of these substrates by the CRL4.

CRBN is a primary target of thalidomide teratogenicity. The binding of immunomodulatory drugs (IMiDs) to CRBN is associated with cytotoxicity of IMiDs and is used to treat multiple myeloma (MM), myelodysplastic syndromes (MDS) and lymphomas. The *CRBN* gene consists of 1329 base pairs, 11 exons, and encodes a protein of 443 amino acids. Exons 10-11 code for the binding site of IMiDs and exons 5-7 for the binding site of DDB1. CRBN plays a key role in mediating the antiproliferative and immunomodulatory activities of IMiDs in MM cells and T cells, respectively. Two target proteins, the zinc finger-containing transcription factors Ikaros (IKZF1) and Aiolos (IKZF3) have been recently revealed by analysis of MM cell lines treated with

* Corresponding author: Ota Fuchs, PhD; U Nemocnice 1, 128 20 Prague 2, Czech Republic; e-mail Ota.Fuchs@uhkt.cz, telephone +420221977313, fax +420221977370.

lenalidomide. IMiDs induce the CRBN-dependent proteasomal degradation of IKZF1 and IKZF3. Both these factors are required for the viability of MM cell lines. IKZF1 bind and activate interferon regulatory factor 4 gene (*IRF4*) promoter and *MYC* expression in B cells. IKZF1/3 are known repressors of the interleukin 2 gene (*IL-2*) promoter in T cells. CRBN directly interacts with the α-subunit of 5′-adenosine monophosphate-activated protein kinase (AMPK) and reduces the enzymatic activity of AMPK by suppressing phosphorylation of its catalytic subunit. This AMPK inhibition activates MdmX (murine double minute X, also known as MDM4) and the mammalian target of rapamycin (mTOR) pathway.

Keywords: Multiple myeloma; cereblon; cullin 4 E3 ubiquitin ligase; Ikaros transcription factors family; immunomodulatory drugs; 5′-adenosine monophosphate-activated protein kinase

Introduction

MM cells stably transduced with CRBN shRNA (short hairpin RNA that target gene encoding CRBN) had reduced CRBN mRNA and CRBN protein expression and were less sensitive than parental cells to antiproliferative effects by IMiDs [1]. In addition, MM cells with resistance to IMiDs had reduced CRBN mRNA and CRBN protein expression [1-9]. This indicates the importance of CRBN expression for IMiDs function. Reduced CRBN expression in T cells treated by CRBN siRNA (small interfering RNA) abrogates the T cell costimulatory activity of the IMiDs compounds. This finding supports again the crucial role of CRBN on IMiDs function. Quantification of only variants with CRBN binding site is therapeutically relevant as there are also variants lacking the exon 10 [5, 6]. The interaction of IMiDs and CRBN inhibits the function of the cullin 4 ring E3 ubiquitin ligase complex (CRL4) which may prevent ubiquitination of CRBN. On the other hand, this interaction induces the ubiquitination of specific target proteins which may differ in various hematological diseases. Ubiquitin-mediated proteolysis is a central mechanism by which regulatory proteins and their consequent signaling events are controlled. Cullins encode the structural components for one of the most abundant E3 ubiquitin ligase families in eukaryotes [10-13].

Two target proteins, the zinc finger-containing transcription factors Ikaros (IKZF1) and Aiolos (IKZF3) have been recently revealed by analysis of MM cell lines treated with lenalidomide. IMiDs induce the CRBN-dependent proteasomal degradation of IKZF1 and IKZF3 by the RING finger E3 ubiquitin ligase complex (CRL4) [14-18]. Both these factors IKZF1 and IKZF 3 are required for the viability of MM cell lines. IKZF1 binds and activates interferon regulatory factor 4 gene (*IRF4*) promoter and *MYC* expression in B cells. IKZF1/3 are known repressors of the interleukin 2 gene (*IL-2*) promoter in T cells. Thus, a decrease in IKZF1/3 explains how IMiDs can both activate the immune system and degrade B cell function. After direct binding of IMiDs to cereblon, CRL4 tags Ikaros and Aiolos with ubiquitin, thereby targeting them for proteolysis. Ikaros and Aiolos are transcriptional regulators of B and T cell development. Aiolos is required for normal plasma cell development. Both these transcription factors are essential for MM. The toxic effects on MM cells resulting from the loss of these two transcription factors are reversed by deletion of critical CRBN-binding regions of Ikaros before treatment by IMiDs. Transcription factor

IRF4 was shown to be essential for MM cells proliferation. IRF4 stimulates the expression of *Myc,* which is normally down regulated in the mature plasma cells, but is upregulated in MM. Thus, a decrease in Ikaros explains how IMiDs can both activate the immune system and degrade B cell function. More selective and effective therapeutics and biomarkers for drug response can be developed on the base of analysis of the CRBN-Ikaros/Aiolos-IRF4/Myc signaling pathway.

Cereblon and Its Role in Memory and Learning

CRBN gene encodes a protein related to the Lon protease protein family. In rodents and other mammals this gene product is found in the cytoplasm localized with a calcium channel membrane protein, and is thought to play a role in brain development. *CRBN* gene is located at chromosome site 3p26.2 (Chromosome: 3; Gen Bank Accession NC_000003.12; 3149633…3179717).

Genetic linkage analysis revealed that mutations in this gene are associated with autosomal recessive nonsyndromic mental retardation [19].

Higgins et al. [19] used a private genealogic database to reconstruct the relationships among 32 individuals from 5 nuclear families in a single pedigree in which 10 members had nonsyndromic mental retardation. Standard IQ ranged from 50 to 70, consistent with mild mental retardation. IQ scores were lower in males than females. Developmental milestones were mildly delayed. There were no dysmorphic or autistic features. The kindred was consanguineous, and the evidence clearly indicated autosomal recessive inheritance. Several branches traced back to a founder couple who arrived in America in 1849 from a town in the Rhineland-Palatinate region of Germany. Higgins et al. [20] identified in this family by single-strand conformational polymorphism analysis and direct DNA sequencing a homozygous nonsense mutation in the *CRBN* gene (On line Mendelian Inheritance in Man/OMIM/609262.0001) that segregated with the phenotype. This nonsense mutation (R419X) led to truncation of the C-terminal 24 amino acids and resulted in mental retardation.

Although this mutation has been linked to mild mental retardation, the mechanism by which the mutation affects CRBN function is unknown. Xu et al. [21] used biochemical and mass spectrometric approaches to explore the function of this mutant. They showed that the protein retains its ability to assemble into a Cullin-RING E3 ligase complex and catalyzes the ubiquitination of CRBN-target proteins. However, they found that this mutant exhibits markedly increased levels of autoubiquitination and is more readily degraded by the proteasome than the wild type protein. They also showed that the level of the mutant protein can be restored by a treatment of cells with a clinically utilized proteasome inhibitor, suggesting that this agent may be useful for the treatment of mental retardation associated with the CRBN R419X mutation. These data demonstrate that enhanced autoubiquitination and degradation account for the defect in CRBN activity that leads to mental retardation.

Animal studies show that CRBN is a cytosolic protein with abundant expression in the hippocampus (HPC) and neocortex (CTX). Its diverse functions include the developmental regulation of ion channels at the neuronal synapse, the mediation of developmental programs by ubiquitination, and a target for herpes simplex type I virus in HPC neurons. To test the hypothesis that anomalous CRBN expression leads to HPC-mediated memory and learning deficits, germ-line CRBN knock-out mice (CRBN(-/-)) was generated [22]. Rajadhyaksha et al. [22] also inactivated cereblon in forebrain neurons in conditional knock-out mice in which *CRBN* exons 3 and 4 are deleted by cre recombinase under the direction of the Ca^{2+}/calmodulin-dependent protein kinase II alpha promoter (CamKII(cre/+), CRBN(-/-)). Cre recombinase is a Type I topoisomerase from bacteriophage P1 that catalyzes the site-specific recombination of DNA between *LoxP* sites. Cre-*L*ox recombination is widely used to carry out deletions, insertions, translocations and inversions at specific sites in the DNA of cells. CRBN mRNA levels were negligible in the HPC, CTX, and cerebellum (CRBM) of the CRBN(-/-) mice.

In contrast, CRBN mRNA levels were reduced 3- to 4-fold in the HPC, CTX but not in the CRBM in CamKII(cre/+), CRBN(-/-) mice as compared to wild type (CamKII(cre/+), CRBN(+/+)). Contextual fear conditioning showed a significant decrease in the percentage of freezing time in CamKII(cre/+), CRBN(-/-) and CRBN(-/-) mice while motor function, exploratory motivation, and anxiety-related behaviors were normal.

These findings suggest that CamKII(cre/+), CRBN(-/-) mice exhibit selective HPC-dependent deficits in associative learning and supports the use of these mice as in vivo models to study the functional consequences of CRBN aberrations on memory and learning in humans.

CRBN was identified as a binding protein for large-conductance calcium-activated potassium channel (BK_{Ca}) alpha subunit KCNT1 in rat and mouse brain [23-25]. CRBN may play an important role in assembly and surface expression of functional BK_{Ca} channels by direct interaction with cytosolic C-terminus of its α-subunit. The mutation in CRBN may cause autosomal recessive nonsyndromic mental retardation by disrupting the developmental regulation of BK_{Ca} in brain regions that are critical for memory and learning.

Cereblon as a Negative Modulator of the Adenosine Monophosphate-Activated Protein Kinase (AMPK)

AMPK plays a key role in sensing intracellular ATP levels and acts as a crucial component in maintaining the energy balance within cells. AMPK is activated when the intracellular AMP-to-ATP ratio rises in response to cellular stress or pharmacological inducers [26-33]. AMPK promotes catabolic path-ways to generate more ATP and inhibits anabolic pathways. Once activated, AMPK phosphorylates several downstream substrates, the overall effect of which is to switch off ATP-consuming pathways (e.g., fatty acid synthesis and cholesterol synthesis) and to switch on ATP-generating pathways (e.g., fatty acid oxidation and glycolysis) [26-33].

AMPK is a highly evolutionarily conserved serine/threonine protein kinase made up of a heterotrimer of catalytic α subunit and two regulatory subunits (β and γ) [34-36]. In mammals, each subunit is encoded by multiple genes (α1, α2, β1, β2, γ1, γ2, γ3). So, 12 combinations of these genes in AMPK structure are possible. The catalytic α subunit is composed of three functional domains, including an NH_2-terminal protein kinase catalytic domain, a central auto-inhibitory region (AID), and a COOH-terminal regulatory subunits (β and γ)-binding domain [37]. The β-subunits contain conserved C-terminal domains that are sufficient on their own to form a complex with α and γ subunits [38].

Three-dimensional structural studies revealed that hydrophobic contacts between the kinase domain and the AID have a predominant role in the allosteric control by AMP [39, 40]. Upon binding of AMP, conformational change between low and high activity forms of AMPK removes the effect of the AID on kinase activation and also on threonine residue 172 (Thr-172) dephosphorylation. The key step in AMPK activation is its phosphorylation on Thr-172 within the catalytic domain, by upstream kinases. The combination of the allosteric and phosphorylation effects causes sharp increase in kinase activity.

AMPK is phosphorylated and activated by an upstream protein kinase, AMPK kinase (AMPKK), (Figure 1). The main upstream AMPKK is the tumor suppressor LKB1 (liver kinase B1), which phosphorylates AMPK at Thr-172 [41]. In addition to LKB1, there are another AMPKK, the Ca^{2+}/ calmodulin-dependent protein kinases (CaMKKα and CaMKKβ) and trans-forming growth factor-β-activated kinase (TAK1) [30].

CaMKKα and CaMKKβ phosphorylate AMPK in an AMP-independent manner. However, the normal physiological conditions under which TAK1 phosphorylates AMPK are currently unclear.

Lee et al. [42, 43] demonstrated that CRBN directly interacts with the α-subunit of AMPK and reduces the enzymatic activity of AMPK by suppressing phosphorylation of its catalytic subunit. The interaction between AMPKα1 and CRBN functioned as an endogenous negative regulator and reduced the level of the γ-subunit in the AMPK complex. The activation of endogenous AMPK was greatly enhanced by knockdown of endogenous CRBN. Therefore, it is possible that at least some CRBN may be present in the endogenous AMPK complex as a binding partner and limits the activation of AMPK.

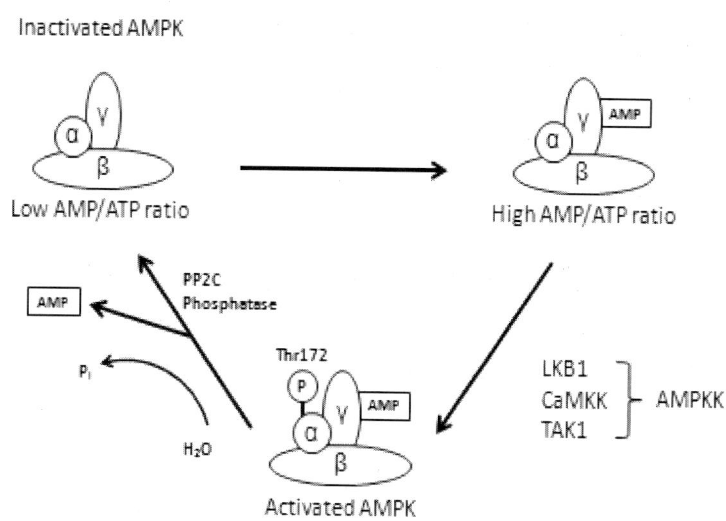

Figure 1. Regulation of AMP-activated protein kinase (AMPK). AMPK contains free subunits (α, β and γ). The Ser/Thr kinase activity of AMPK is controlled by α subunit, containing a threonine residue (Thr172), whose phosphorylation is required for AMPK activation. AMPK is activated when the intracellular AMP-to-ATP ratio rises.

In the absence of CRBN, Thr-172 could be better protected from dephosphorylation than in its presence. CRBN interacts with the AMPKα1 subunit via separate binding sites in the N-terminal and C-terminal regions. The stability of the AMPK complex could be also regulated by cereblon. Dissociation of the γ- subunit caused by cereblon may have implications for the suppression of AMPK enzymatic activity and lack of phosphorylation of downstream targets.

The AMP-binding γ-subunit could induce a conformational change in the kinase domain of the α-subunit that protects AMPK from Thr-172 dephosphorylation [44]. This AMPK inhibition activates MdmX (murine double minute X, also known as MDM4) [45] and the mammalian target of rapamycin (mTOR) pathway [46]. AMPK is expressed and activated in MM cells. The inhibition of AMPK induces growth arrest and reduction of cell viability [47]. Induction of apoptosis was determined by annexin-V and propidium iodide staining. The AMPK activators 5-aminoimidazole-4-carboxamide riboside (AICAr) and a small molecule compound 5-(3-(4-(2-(4-fluorophenyl)ethoxy) phenyl)propyl)furan-2-carboxylic acid (D942) inhibit cell growth in MM cell lines [48]. AICAr also induces an S-phase cell cycle arrest in all four tested MM cell lines and it leads to phosphorylation and thus activation of AMPK.

Activation of AMPK inhibits basal extracellular signal-regulated kinase (ERK), mTOR and P70S6 kinase (P70S6K) as well as AKT phosphorylation, and blocks IL-6, and IGF-1. AMPK activation inhibits MM cell growth despite stimulation with IL-6, and IGF-1 and represents a potential new target in the therapy of MM.

Immunomodulatory Drugs

At present, IMiDs include thalidomide, lenalidomide and pomalidomide (Figure 2). Both, pomalidomide (Pomalyst®, initially known as CC-4047, Actimid) and lenalidomide (Revlimid®, initially known as CC-5013), are a synthetic derivative of thalidomide (Thalomid®, Immunoprin, Talidex, Talizer). Pomalidomide [4-Amino-2-(2,6-dioxopiperidin-3-yl) isoindole-1,3-dione] is a potent second-generation IMiD [49-53]. Pomalidomide has direct antiproliferative, pro-apoptotic, and antiangiogenic effects, as well as modulatory effects on bone resorption and on the immune system. Lenalidomide [3-(4-amino-1-oxo1,3-dihydro-2H-isoindol-2-yl)piperidine-2,6-dione] is 4-amino-glutarimide analog of thalidomide with potent immunomodulatory, antiangiogenic and direct neoplastic cell inhibitory activity [54-61]. Chemical structure of the IMiD drugs is shown in Figure 2.

Thalidomide [(*RS*)-2-(2,6-dioxopiperidin-3-yl)-1*H*-isoindole-1,3(2*H*)-dione] was synthesized in Germany in 1954, from α-phtaloylisoglutamine, to be used as a non-barbiturate sedative and antimetic drug (Contergan). In 1957, after a short period of preclinical studies, thalidomide was approved for first trimester gestational sickness in humans. The appearance of malformations such as phocomelia in the newborn banned its use three years later.

Thalidomide was responsible for birth defects in more than 10,000 children [62, 63]. The US Food and Drug Administration (FDA) approved thalidomide in 1998 for the treatment of erythema nodosum leprosum [64]. Thalidomide exhibits potent antiangiogenic and immunomodulatory effects, and is currently used around the world to treat a range of conditions, mainly multiple myeloma. However, long-term use of thalidomide has detrimental side effects, such as peripheral neuropathy [65, 66].

Lenalidomide was developed in order to avoid thalidomide side effects (sedation and neuropathy), and to increase efficacy [67, 68]. Lenalidomide shares a number of structural and biological properties with thalidomide but is safer and more potent than thalidomide.

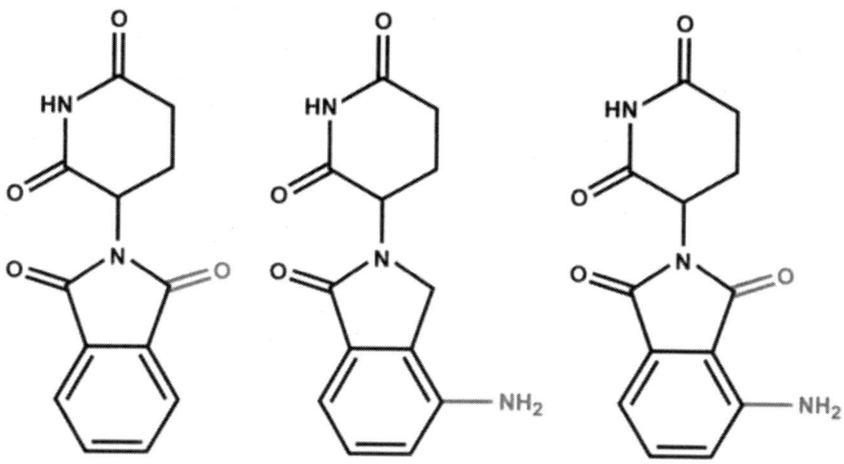

Figure 2. Chemical structures of immunomodulatory drugs (IMiDs) including thalidomide, lenalidomide and pomalidomide. Lenalidomide and pomalidomide are synthetic compounds derived by modifying the chemical structure of thalidomide.

Mechanism of Immunomodulatory Drugs Action in the Treatment of Multiple Myeloma

IMiDs target both MM cells and their microenvironment, while also modulating the immune system (Figure 3). The exact molecular mechanisms of the antitumor effects of IMiDs remain uncertain.

IMiDs affect various molecular and cellular elements within the tumor microenvironment. IMiDs change the concentration of various cytokines that support tumor cell growth [49, 60, 69-72]. IMiDs disrupt bone marrow stromal support for malignant MM cells, although the exact mechanisms of these actions remain unclear. IMiDs decrease the expression of adhesion molecules that facilitate the interaction between MM cells and bone marrow stromal cells (BMSCs) [73].

Importantly, the downregulation of MM cells adherence to BMSCs can overcome the cellular adhesion-mediated drug resistance by malignant MM cells. This effect of IMiDs is further increased by their ability to downregulateTNFα [60, 70, 74, 75].

Surprisingly, in contrast to the inhibitory effect of lenalidomide in BMSCs, lenalidomide was totally ineffective in inhibiting TNFα mRNA expression in MM cells [76].

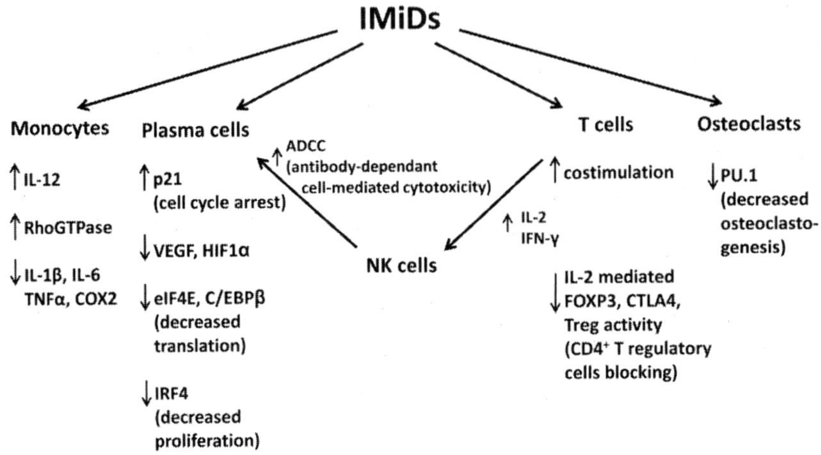

Figure 3. Various mechanisms of action of immunomodulatory drugs (IMiDs). IMiDs have multiple effects including immunomodulatory activity, anti-angiogenic activity, intervention of cell surface adhesion molecules, cell cycle arrest, inhibition of cell migration and metastasis, anti-proliferation activity and anti-inflammatory activity and pro-apoptotic activity.

Immunomodulatory Activities of IMiDs

IMiDs are a potent co-stimulator of primary human T cells, synergizing with stimulation via T-cell receptor complex to increase IL-2-mediated T-cell proliferation and interferon gamma (IFN-γ) production [77]. Secretion of IL-2 and IFN-γ increases the number of natural killer (NK) cells, improves their function and mediates lysis of MM cells (Figure 3).

NKT cells are a heterogeneous group of T-cells that recognize lipids and glycolipids presented by CD1d molecules. NKT cells activated in presence of lenalidomide have greater ability to secrete IFN-γ. Lenalidomide enhances antigen-specific expansion of NKT cells [78]. Regulatory T-cells (Tregs) are a component of the immune system that suppresses immune response of other cells. Tregs were elevated in MM patients. IMiDs strongly inhibit Tregs proliferation via decreased FOXP3 mRNA expression [79].

Anti-Angiogenic Properties of IMiDs

All IMiDs have anti-angiogenic activity. Thalidomide has predominant anti-angiogenic activity while lenalidomide and pomalidomide have far greater immune enhancing effects [60]. It appears that anti-angiogenesis occurs via the modulation of chemotactic factors involved in endothelial cells migration including TNFα, vascular endothelial growth factor (VEGF) and basic fibro-blast growth factor (bFGF) from BMSCs rather than a direct inhibition of endothelial cells proliferation [80, 81].

Inhibition of VEGF and bFGF production by IMiDs is likely to have multiple other biological effects beyond that of anti-angiogenesis including inhibition of IL-6 production by BMSCs. VEGF and bFGF up-regulate IL-6 and other pro-inflammatory cytokines [82].

Inhibition of Cell Cycle and Induction of Apoptosis by IMiDs

IMiDs induce cell cycle arrest via upregulation of tumor suppressor genes (cyclin dependent kinase inhibitors $p15^{INK4b}$, $p16^{INK4a}$, $p21^{Cip1,Waf1}$, $p27^{Kip1}$; early response transcription factors /Erg1, Erg2 and Erg3/) and apoptosis by caspase activation [83, 84].

The inhibition of the transcription factor NF-κB activity by IMiDs results in reduced expression of anti-apoptotic proteins including cellular inhibitor of apoptosis protein 2 (cIAP2) [85] and FLIP [Fas-associated protein with death protein (FADD)-like interleukin-1β-converting enzyme (FLICE) inhibitor protein] [86]. These anti-apoptotic proteins inhibit caspase-8 that is on the other hand stimulated by IMiDs [84].

Disruption of Bone Marrow Stromal Support for Malignant MM Cells

IMiDs down-regulate the expression of adhesion molecules [leukocyte function-associated antigen 1 (LFA-1, CD11a), intercellular adhesion molecule 1 (ICAM-1, CD54), vascular cell adhesion molecule 1 (VCAM-1, CD106) and very late antigen 4 (VLA-4)] that facilitate the interaction between MM cells and BMSCs [73].

As we described, IMiDs inhibit NF-κB, a transcription factor that has important growth and anti-apoptotic roles and which is connected with the upregulation of intracellular adhesion molecules and many cytokines [87].

Effect of IMiDs on Myeloma Cell Proliferation

The direct anti-MM effect of IMiDs was shown to occur through the induction of grow arrest of MM cells in G1 phase of cell cycle [81]. This effect is associated with a decrease in interferon regulatory factor 4 (IRF4), a transcription factor that is critical for MM cell growth and survival (Figure 3) [88, 89].

Raje et al. [90] showed strong synergism of anti-MM activity of rapamycin (Rapamune), a specific mTOR inhibitor, combined with lenalidomide. Importantly, this combination is able to overcome drug resistance when tested against MM cell lines resistant to conventional chemotherapy. Moreover, the combination, but not rapamycin alone, is able to overcome the growth advantage conferred on MM cells by interleukin-6 (IL-6), insulin-like growth factor-1 (IGF-1), or adherence to bone marrow stromal cells (BMSCs). Combining rapamycin and lenalidomide induces apoptosis of MM cells. Differential signaling cascades including the mitogen-activated protein kinase (MAPK) and the phosphatidylinositol 3'-kinase/Akt kinase (PI3K/Akt) path-ways [91-94] are targeted by these drugs individually and in combination, suggesting the molecular mechanism by which they interfere with MM growth and survival. These studies, therefore, provide the framework for clinical evaluation of mTOR inhibitors combined with IMiDs to improve patient outcome in MM. IMiDs down-regulate CCAAT/enhancer-binding protein-β (C/EBPβ) resulting in abrogation of cell proliferation

[95]. Overexpression of C/EBPβ rescues MM cells from IMiD compounds-induced inhibition of proliferation, indicating that C/EBPβ is critical in mediating antiproliferative effects. IMiD compounds-induced decrease of C/EBPβ protein leads to impaired transcription of interferon regulatory factor 4 (IRF4). Downregulation of IRF4 by lenalidomide was confirmed by longitudinal studies of bone marrow samples from 23 patients obtained before and during lenalidomide treatment using $CD138^{+}/IRF4^{+}$ double labeling. In contrast to down-regulation of C/EBPβ protein, IMiD compounds do not alter C/EBPβ mRNA levels or protein stability, suggesting translational regulation of C/EBPβ. Expression of the C/EBPβ protein is under the initiation factor of translation 4E (IF4E) control in MM cells.

However, this control by IF4E was not observed in IMiD compounds-resistant MM cells. Targeting translation by inhibiting IF4E-binding protein 1 phosphorylation overcomes resistance. So, this pathway is critical and may be a target to overcome drug resistance. MM cell lines and primary MM cells strongly expressed C/EBPβ, whereas normal B cells and plasma cells have little or no detectable levels of C/EBPβ [96]. Silencing of C/EBPβ leads to down-regulation of transcription factors such as IRF4, XBP1, and BLIMP1 accompanied by a strong inhibition of proliferation.

Further, silencing of C/EBPβ leads to a complete down-regulation of antiapoptotic B-cell lymphoma 2 (BCL2) expression. In chromatin immuno-precipitation assays, C/EBPβ directly binds to the promoter region of IRF4, BLIMP1, and BCL2.

C/EBPβ is involved in the regulatory network of transcription factors that are critical for plasma cell differentiation and survival. Targeting C/EBPβ may provide a novel therapeutic strategy in the treatment of multiple myeloma.

Exposure of plasma cells to lenalidomide activates the Wnt/β-catenin pathway and its downstream targets such as cyclin D1 and MYC [97]. The accumulation of β-catenin during treatment with lenalidomide may be the cause of drug resistance [97]. N-cadherin-based interaction between MM cells and osteoblasts blocks MM cell growth. Therefore the high levels of N-cadherin expression in osteoblasts confer strong proliferation block on MM cells. Since β-catenin associates with N-cadherin at the cell membrane, N-cadherin adhesion is disrupted, β-catenin is released and translocates to the nucleus where it regulates the transcription of target genes with effect on cell proliferation [98]. Resistance of myeloma to lenalidomide is an emerging clinical problem.

Though it is associated in part with activation of Wnt/β-catenin signaling, the mediators remain undefined. Wnt/β-catenin inhibition by N-(2-Methyl-4-nitrophenyl)-2,5-dichlorobenzenesulfonamide (FH535), a sulfonamide based and cell-permeable compound that suppresses both Wnt/β-catenin and peroxisome proliferator-activated receptor (PPAR) signaling, enhances the activity of lenalidomide.

Cereblon as the Direct Target Protein of IMiDs

Ito et al. [100-102] developed a new affinity bead technology for isolating ligand-binding proteins. Polymer-coated beads were constructed that allow single-step purification of ligand target molecules.

These beads include styrene-glycidyl-methacrylate (SG) beads and ferrite-glycidyl-methacrylate (FG) beads. FG beads were used for the purification of thalidomide-binding proteins from various cell extracts. Thalidomide-modified beads were incubated with cell extracts and then washed with buffer.

Bound proteins were eluted with free thalidomide and analyzed by gel electrophoresis. Only two specific protein bands were detected (55 kDa and 127 kDa). These proteins were identified as CRBN and DDB1.

As we described in Abstract and Introduction, both CRBN and DDB1 are subunits of the cullin 4 ring E3 ubiquitin ligase complex (CRL4). Auto-ubiquitination of CRBN was inhibited by thalidomide *in vitro*, suggesting that thalidomide is an inhibitor of E3 ubiquitin ligase.

Cereblon as a Primary Target for Thalidomide Teratogenicity

The zebrafish was adopted as a model animal for *in vivo* study of thalidomide teratogenicity [100-102]. Zebrafish have a protein zCrbn, which is 70% homologous to human CRBN and possesses thalidomide binding activity. Thalidomide exposure induces fin and ear (otic vesicle) defects in zebrafish. A reduction in the size of otic vesicle was observed in zebrafish following thalidomide exposure. Zebrafish fins and tetrapod limbs are homologous with respect to early patterning and gene expression, although skeletal structures in adult fish and tetrapods are quite different. Shortening of the pectoral fins along the proximodistal axis and the inhibition of fibroblast growth factor 8 (*Fgf8*) gene expression were found in thalidomide-treated zebrafish embryos. Finally, chicks were employed for the investigation of the conserved role of CRBN. Down-regulation of Fgf8 and Fgf10 cause multiple birth defects and limb deformities.

The Role of Ikaros Family Proteins in IMiDs and CRBN Mechanism

Using distinct but complementary proteomic techniques and systems, three groups have recently simultaneously reported that IMiDs induce the CRBN-dependent proteasomal degradation of IKZF1 (Ikaros) and IKZF3 (Aiolos) [14-16]. Schema is shown in Figure 4.

IKZF1, a zinc finger transcription factor initially discovered as a regulator of the T cell receptor, is required for hematopoiesis, particularly lymphocyte development and plasma cell maturation. Mutations that cause loss of function of IKZF1 and IKZF3 are associated with acute lymphoblastic leukemia, consistent with a tumor suppressor function.

On the other hand, IKZF1 and IKZF3 are required for the viability of many MM cell lines. IKZF1 and IKZF3 are also involved in the complex process of chromatin remodeling, and the nature of their interactions is poorly understood.

IKZF1 binds and activates the *IRF4* gene promoter and loss of IKZF1 leads to decreased *IRF4* and *MYC* expression.

However, lenalidomide can also inhibit MM cell lines with high basal levels of IRF4 unchanged by drug treatment, suggesting that other IKZF1/3 targets can play a role in the therapeutic response to IMiDs.

IKZF1/3 are known repressors of *IL-2* gene promoter. The degradation of IKZF1/3 in response to IMiDs explains enhanced T cell IL-2 production.

Hence, many of the effects of IMiDs can be explained by a unified mechanism: IMiDs re-target the cullin 4 ring E3 ubiquitin ligase activity toward IKZF1/3 in a change-of-function effect (Figure 4).

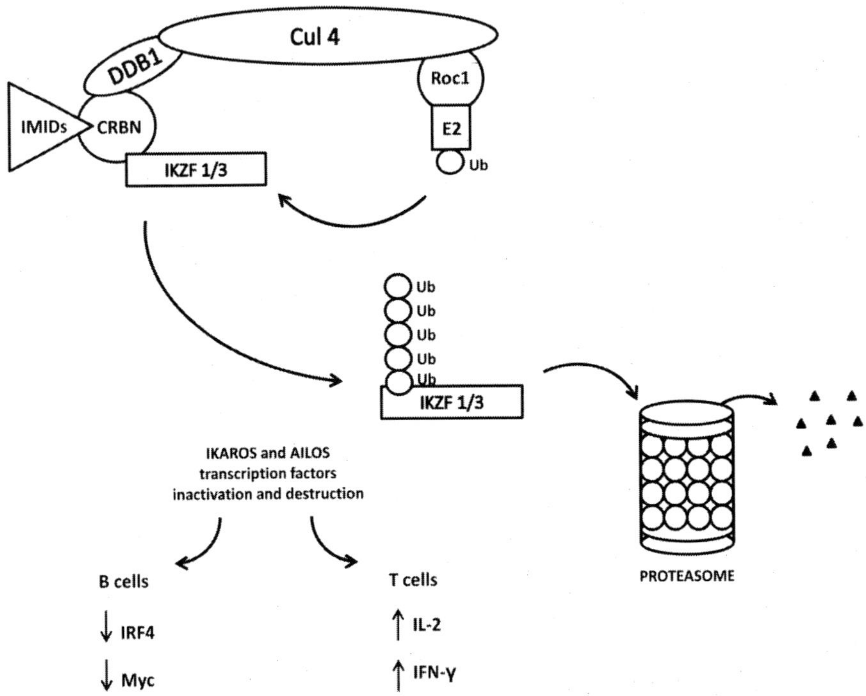

Figure 4. Schematic model of CRBN-directed cullin 4 ring E3 ubiquitin ligase complex (CRL4) action after binding of IMiDs to CRBN. CRBN forms an E3 ubiquitin ligase complex with three other proteins-damaged DNA binding protein 1 (DDB1), cullin 4 (CUL4), and regulator of cullins 1 (Roc1). IMiDs binding to CRBN results in the selective ubiquitination and proteasomal degradation of Ikaros family zinc finger transcription factors IKZF1 and IKZF3. This degradation decreases interferon regulatory factor 4 (IRF4) in plasma cells and increases IL-2 expression in T cells.

Measurement of Cereblon mRNA and Cereblon Protein Levels as Biomarkers for IMiDs Response

The measurement of CRBN mRNA by quantitative RT-PCR typically uses commercial assays, such as predesigned TaqMan assays, where primers and probe are optimized with respect to known gene splicing information.

For CRBN mRNA, the current "best coverage assay" detects the exon 8-exon 9 junction and exon 10 as a measure of gene expression [6]. This assay (Hs00372271_m1; Applied

Biosystems, Life Technologies Corp.) measures all CRBN mRNA variants that are translated to functional protein with exception of the variants with removed exon 10 (part of IMIDs binding region). The presence of multiple CRBN mRNA splice variants complicates the transcript measurement by Affymetrix array.

Currently available commercial antibodies are neither sensitive nor specific for reliable detection of CRBN protein levels. Gandhi et al. [6] characterized a monoclonal antibody CRBN65 and compared its properties with the commonly used, currently available commercial antibodies against CRBN. This antibody is the most sensitive and specific and can detect as little as 200 pg of CRBN protein via Western blot [6].

Appropriate antibodies and validated assays for cereblon protein detection and *CRBN* gene expression that account for the known gene splicing information are needed for CRBN measurements in the clinic.

While it has been shown that CRBN and IRF4 levels correlate with lenalidomide responsiveness in MM patients, previous *in vitro* investigations using cytogenetically discrete human myeloma cell lines have not been able to replicate this phenomenon [1, 103, 104]. The implications of this apparent discordance are two-fold. First, these results show that it is important to investigate *CRBN* and *IRF4* gene expression in both $CD138^-$ and $CD138^+$ myeloma cells. Second, because there are multiple isoforms of CRBN, it may be important to study expression levels of each one in the context of both *in vivo* and *in vitro* settings [6].

Conclusion and Perspectives

The studies showing IMiDs induced the CRBN-dependent proteasomal degradation of IKZF1 and IKZF3 [14-16] have greatly advanced our under-standing of the mechanism of action of IMiDs in MM. The small-molecule drug lenalidomide modulates the activity of the CRBN-CRL4 E3 ubiquitin ligase complex to increase ubiquitination of two transcription factors, IKZF1 and IKZF3. It does so by specific binding to one component of the system, cereblon. These studies may have wider implications for the targeting of E3 ubiquitin ligases in drug discovery for other diseases.

There are very few approved and experimental drugs that modulate the ubiquitin system like lenalidomide in this case. Other small molecules could develop to alter the specificity of ubiquitylation complexes with the aim of inducing the specific degradation of previously "undruggable" oncoproteins such as Ras and Myc in many different types of cancer.

Nevertheless, there are still gaps in our understanding of the mechanism of action of IMiDs in MM. For example, the proteasomal inhibitor bortezomib (Velcade™, PS-341) is used for the treatment of MM. Bortezomib is used efficiently also in combination with lenalidomide. There is an apparent paradox, because inhibition of proteasomal destruction of IKZF1 and IKZF3 by bortezomib contradicts the proposed mechanism.

Lu et al. [15] hypothesize that since the proteasomal inhibition by bortezomib is incomplete with therapeutic dosing, this might allow sufficient destruction of IKZF1 and IKZF3 while retaining other therapeutic effect of bortezomib. Alternatively, they hypothesize that IKZF1 and IKZF3 once poly-ubiquitylated, may be inactive or act as dominant-negatives.

Future dissection of CRBN direct down-stream substrates and CRBN indirect down-stream factors will help to identify mechanisms of IMiD action and find new biomarkers for prediction of IMiD response and IMiD resistance as well as developing a new therapies to treat the patients with MM.

It is also possible to speculate whether or not anti-myeloma activity of IMiDs is associated with the interaction between CRBN and AMPK or KCNT 1.

Both AMPK and KCNT1 are potential substrates of the CRBN-CRL4 E3 ubiquitin ligase complex, but they may not be associated with downstream signaling that leads to anti-myeloma activity of IMiDs.

Acknowledgments

This work was supported by the research grant NT/13836 from the Internal Grant Agency of the Ministry of Health of the Czech Republic.

References

[1] Lopez-Girona, A.; Mendy, D.; Ito, T.; Miller, K.; Gandhi, A. K.; Kang, J., et al. Cereblon is a direct protein target for immunomodulatory and antiproliferative activities of lenalidomide and pomalidomide. *Leukemia* 2012, 26, 2326-2335.

[2] Zhu, Y. X.; Braggio, E.; Shi, C. X.; Bruins, L. A.; Schmidt, J. E.; Van Wier, S., et al. Cereblon expression is required for the antimyeloma activity of lenalidomide and pomalidomide. *Blood* 2011, 118, 4771-4779.

[3] Broyl, A.; Kuiper, R.; van Duin, M.; van der Holt, B.; El Jarari, L.; Bertsch, U., et al. High cereblon expression is associated with better survival in patients with newly diagnosed multiple myeloma treated with thalidomide maintenance. *Blood* 2013, 121, 624-627.

[4] Heintel, D.; Rocci, A.; Ludwig, H.; Bolomsky, A.; Caltagirone, S.; Schreder, M., et al. High expression of cereblon (*CRBN*) is associated with improved clinical response in patients with multiple myeloma treated with lenalidomide and dexamethasone. *Br. J. Haematol.* 2013, 161, 748-751.

[5] Lodé, L.; Amiot, M.; Maiga, S.; Touzeau, C.; Menard, A.; Magrangeas, F., et al. Cereblon expression in multiple myeloma: not ready for prime time. *Br. J. Haematol.* 2013, 163, 282-284.

[6] Gandhi, A. K.; Mendy, D.; Waldman, M.; Chen, G.; Rychak, E.; Miller, K., et al. Measuring cereblon as a biomarker of response or resistance to lenalidomide and pomalidomide requires use of standardized reagents and understanding of gene complexity. *Br. J. Haematol.* 2014, 164, 233-244.

[7] Schuster, S. R.; Kortuem, K. M.; Zhu, Y. X.; Braggio, E.; Shi, C. X.; Bruins, L. A., et al. The clinical significance of cereblon expression in multiple myeloma. *Leuk. Res.* 2014, 38, 23-28.

[8] Pearse, R. N. IMiDs: Not for the CRBN weak. *Leuk. Res.* 2014, 38, 21-22.

[9] Zhu, Y. X.; Kortuem, K. M.; Stewart, A. K. Molecular mechanism of action of immune–modulatory drugs thalidomide, lenalidomide and pomalidomide in multiple myeloma. *Leuk. Lymphoma* 2013, 54, 683-687.

[10] Angers, S.; Li, T.; Yi, X.; MacCoss, M. J.; Moon, R. T.; Zheng, N. Molecular architecture and assembly of the DDB1-CUL4A ubiquitin ligase machinery. *Nature* 2006, 443, 590-593.

[11] Jackson, S.; Xiong, Y. CRL4s: the CUL4-RING E3 ubiquitin ligases. *Trends Biochem. Sci.* 2009, 34, 562-570.

[12] Zhao, Y.; Sun, Y. Cullin-RING ligases as attractive anti-cancer targets. *Curr. Pharm. Des.* 2013, 19, 3215-3225.

[13] Sharma, P.; Nag, A. CUL4A ubiquitin ligase: a promising drug target for cancer and other human diseases. *Open Biol.* 2014, 4, 130217.

[14] Krönke, J.; Udeshi, N. D.; Narla, A., et al. Lenalidomide causes selective degradation of IKZF1 and IKZF3 in multiple myeloma cells. *Science* 2014, 343, 301-305.

[15] Lu, G.; Middleton, R. E.; Sun, H., et al. The myeloma drug lenalidomide promotes the cereblon-dependent destruction of Ikaros proteins. *Science* 2014, 343, 305-309.

[16] Gandhi, A. K.; Kang, J.; Havens, C. G., et al. Immunomodulatory agents lenalidomide and pomalidomide co-stimulate T cells by inducing degradation of T cell repressors Ikaros and Aiolos via modulation of the E3 ubiquitin ligase complex $CRL4^{CRBN}$. *Br. J. Haematol.* 2014, 164, 811-821.

[17] Stewart, A. K. How thalidomide works against cancer. *Science* 2014, 343, 256-257.

[18] Licht, J. D.; Shortt, J.; Johnstone, R., From anecdote to targeted therapy: the curious case of thalidomide in multiple myeloma. *Cancer Cell* 2014, 25, 9-11.

[19] Higgins, J. J.; Rosen, D. R.; Loveless, J. M.; Clyman, J. C.; Grau, M. J. A gene for nonsyndromic mental retardation maps to chromosome 3p25-pter. *Neurology* 2000, 55, 335-340.

[20] Higgins, J. J.; Pucilowska, J.; Lombardi, R. Q.; Rooney, J. P. A mutation in a novel ATP-dependent Lon protease gene in a kindred with mild mental retardation. *Neurology* 2004, 63, 1927-1931.

[21] Xu, G.; Jiang, X.; Jaffrey, S. R. A mental retardation-linked nonsense mutation in cereblon is rescued by proteasome inhibition. *J. Biol. Chem.* 2013, 288, 29573-29585.

[22] Rajadhyaksha A. M.; Ra, S.; Kishinevsky, S.; Lee, A. S.; Romanienko, P.; DuBoff, M., et al. Behavioral characterization of cereblon forebrain-specific conditional null mice: a model for human non-syndromic intellectual disability. *Behav. Brain Res.* 2012, 226, 428-434.

[23] Jo, S.; Lee, K. H.; Song, S.; Jung, Y. K., Park, C. S. Identification and functional characterization of cereblon as a binding protein for larged-conductance calcium-activated potassium channel in rat brain. *J. Neuro-chem.* 2005, 94, 1212-1224.

[24] Higgins, J. J.; Tal, A. L.; Sun, X.; Hauck, S. C.; Hao, J.; Kosofsky, B. E.; Rajadhyaksha, A. M. Temporal and spatial mouse brain expression of cereblon, an ionic channel regulator involved in human intelligence. *J. Neurogenet.* 2010, 24, 18-26.

[25] Chang, X. B.; Stewart, A. K. What is the functional role of the thalidomide binding protein cereblon? *Int. J. Biochem. Mol. Biol.* 2011, 2, 287-294.

[26] Hardie, D. G.; Carling, D. The AMP-activated protein kinase: fuel gauge of the mammalian cell. *Eur. J. Biochem.* 1997, 246, 259-273.

[27] Hardie, D. G.; Carling, D.; Carlson, M. The AMP-activated SNF1 protein kinase subfamily: metabolic sensors of the eukaryotic cell? *Annu. Rev. Biochem.* 1998, 67, 821-855.

[28] Hardie, D. G.; Scott, J. W.; Pan, D. A.; Hudson, E. R. Management of cellular energy by the AMP-activated protein kinase system. *FEBS Lett.* 2003, 546, 113-120.

[29] Carling, D. The AMP-activated protein kinase cascade-a unifying system for energy control. *Trends Biochem. Sci.* 2004, 29, 18-24.

[30] Lage, R.; Diéguez, C.; Vidal-Puig, A.; López, M. AMPK: a metabolic gauge regulating whole-body energy homeostasis. *Trends Mol. Medicine* 2008, 14, 539-549.

[31] Mihaylova, M. M.; Shaw, R. J. The AMPK signalling pathway coordinates cell growth, autophagy and metabolism. *Nat. Cell Biol.* 2011, 13, 1016-1023.

[32] Gowans, G. J.; Hardie, D. G. AMPK: a cellular energy sensor primarily regulated by AMP. *Biochem. Soc. Trans.* 2014, 42, 71-75.

[33] Hardie, D. G.; Ashford, M. L. AMPK: Regulating energy balance at the cellular and whole body levels. *Physiology* 2014, 29, 99-107.

[34] Dyck, J. R.; Gao, G.; Widmer, J.; Stapleton, D.; Fernandez, C. S.; Kemp, B. E.; Witters, L. A. Regulation of 5´-AMP-activated protein kinase activity by the noncatalytic beta and gamma subunits. *J. Biol. Chem.* 1996, 271, 17798-17803.

[35] Tangeman, L.; Wyatt, C. N.; Brown, T. L. Knockdown of AMP-activated protein kinase alpha 1 and alpha 2 catalytic subunits. *J. RNAi Gene Silencing* 2012, 8, 470-478.

[36] Pang, T.; Xiong, B.; Li, J. Y.; Qiu, B. Y.; Jin, G. Z.; Shen, J. K.; Li, J. Conserved α-helix acts as auto inhibitory sequence in AMP-activated protein kinase α subunits. *J. Biol. Chem.* 2007, 282, 495-506.

[37] Crute, B. E.; Seefeld, K.; Gamble, J.; Kemp, B. E.; Witters, L. A. Functional domains of the alpha1 catalytic subunit of the AMP-activated protein kinase. *J. Biol. Chem.* 1998, 273, 35347-35354.

[38] Woods, A.; Cheung, P. C.; Smith, F. C.; Davison, M. D.; Scott, J.; Beri, R. K.; Carling, D. Characterization of AMP-activated protein kinase β subunit and γ subunit-assembly of the heterotrimeric complex *in vito. J. Biol. Chem.* 1996, 271, 10282-10290.

[39] Chen, L.; Jiao, Z. H.; Zheng, L. S.; Zhang, Y. Y.; Xie, S. T.; Wang, Z. X.; Wu, J. W. Structural insight into the autoinhibition mechanism of AMP-activated protein kinase. *Nature* 2009, 459, 1146-1149.

[40] Zhu, L.; Chen, L.; Zhou, X. M.; Zhang, Y. Y.; Zhang, Y. J.; Zhao, J., et al. Structural insights into the architecture and allostery of full-length AMP-activated protein kinase. *Structure* 2011, 19, 515-522.

[41] Alexander, A.; Walker, C. L. The role of LKB1 and AMPK in cellular responses to stress and damage. *FEBS Lett.* 2011, 585, 952-957.

[42] Lee, K. M.; Jo, S.; Kim, H.; Lee, J.; Park, C. S. Functional modulation of AMP-activated protein kinase by cereblon. *Biochim. Biophys. Acta* 2011, 1813, 448-455.

[43] Lee, K. M.; Yang, S. J; Kim, Y. D.; Choi, Y. D.; Nam, J. H.;Choi, C. S.; Choi, H. S.; Park, C. S. Disruption of the cereblon gene enhances hepatic AMPK activity and prevents high-fat diet-induced obesity and insulin resistance in mice. *Diabetes* 2013, 62, 1855-1864.

[44] Riek, U.; Scholz, R.; Konarev, P.; Rufer, A.; Suter, M.; Nazabal, A., et al. Structural properties of AMP-activated protein kinase: dimerization, molecular shape, and changes upon ligand binding. *J. Biol. Chem.* 2008, 283, 18331-18343.

[45] He, G.; Zhang, Y. W.; Lee, J. H.; Zeng, S. X.; Wang, Y. W.; Luo, Z., et al. AMP-activated protein kinase induces p53 by phosphorylating MDMX and inhibiting its activity. *Mol. Cell. Biol.* 2014, 34, 148-157.

[46] Xu, J.; Ji, J.; Yan, X. H. Cross-talk between AMPK and mTOR in regulating energy balance. *Crit. Rev. Food. Sci. Nutr.* 2012, 52, 373-381.
[47] Baumann, P.; Mandl-Weber, S.; Emmerich, B.; Straka, C.; Schmid-maier, R. Inhibition of adenosine monophosphate-activated protein kinase induces apoptosis in multiple myeloma cells. *Anticancer Drugs* 2007, 18, 405-410.
[48] Baumann, P.; Mandl-Weber, S.; Emmerich, B.; Straka, C.; Schmid-maier, R. Activation of adenosine monophosphate activated protein kinase inhibits growth of multiple myeloma cells. *Exp. Cell Res.* 2007, 313, 3592-3603.
[49] Lacy, M. Q.; McCurdy, A. R. Pomalidomide. *Blood* 2013, 122, 2305-2309.
[50] Richardson, P. G.; Mark, T. M.; Lacy, M. Q. Pomalidomide: New immunomodulatory agent with potent antiproliferative effects. *Crit. Rev. Oncol. Hematol.* 2013, 88, S36-S44.
[51] Chanan-Khan, A. A.; Swaika, A.; Paulus, A.; Kumar, S. K.; Mikhael, J. R.; Rajkumar, S. V., et al. Pomalidomide: the new immunomodulatory agent for the treatment of multiple myeloma. *Blood Cancer Journal* 2013, 3, e143.
[52] McCurdy, A. R.; Lacy, M. Q. Pomalidomide and its clinical potential for relapsed or refractory multiple myeloma: an update for the haematologist. *Ther. Adv. Hematol.* 2013, 4, 211-218.
[53] Mark, T. M.; Coleman, M.; Niesvizky, R. Preclinical and clinical results with pomalidomide in the treatment of relapsed/refractory multiple myeloma. *Leuk. Res.* 2014, 38, 517-524.
[54] Corral, L. G.; Haslett, P. A.; Muller, G. W.; Chen, R.; Wong, L. M., et al. Differential cytokine modulation and T cell activation by two distinct classes of thalidomide analogues that are potent inhibitors of TNF-alpha. *J. Immunol.* 1999, 163, 380-386.
[55] Davies, F. E.; Raje, N.; Hideshima, T.; Lentzsch, S.; Young, G., et al. Thalidomide and immunomodulatory derivatives augment natural killer cell cytotoxicity in multiple myeloma. *Blood* 2001, 98, 210-216.
[56] Richardson, P. G.; Schlossman, R. L.; Weller, E.; Hideshima, T.; Mitsiades, C.; Davies, F., et al. (2002) Immunomodulatory drug CC-5013 overcomes drug resistance and is well tolerated in patients with relapsed multiple myeloma. *Blood* 2002, 100, 3063-3067.
[57] Bartlett, J. B.; Dredge, K.; Dalgleish, A. G. The evolution of thalidomide and its IMID derivatives as anticancer agents. *Nature Rev. Cancer* 2004, 4, 314-322.
[58] Vallet, S.; Palumbo, A.; Raje, N.; Boccadoro, M.; Andersson, K. C. Thalidomide and lenalidomide: mechanism-based potential drug combinations. *Leuk. Lymphoma* 2008, 49, 1238-1245.
[59] Kotla, V.; Goel, S.; Nischal, S.; Heuck, C.; Vivek, K., et al. Mechanism of action of lenalidomide in haematological malignancies. *J. Hematol. Oncol.* 2009, 2, 36.
[60] Quach, H.; Ritchie, D.; Stewart, A. K.; Neeson, P.; Harrison, S., et al. Mechanism of action of immunomodulatory drugs (IMiDs) in multiple myeloma. *Leukemia* 2010, 24, 22-32.
[61] Cives, M.; Milano, A.; Dammacco, F.; Silvestris, F. Lenalidomide in multiple myeloma: current experimental and clinical data. *Eur. J. Haematol.* 2012, 88, 279-291.
[62] Smithells, R. W.; Newman, C. G. Recognition of thalidomide defects. *J. Med. Genet.* 1992, 29, 718-723.
[63] Vargesson, N. Thalidomide-induced limb defects: Resolving a 50-year-old puzzle. *Bioessays* 2009, 31, 1327-1336.

[64] Franks, M. E.; Macpherson, G. R.; Figg, W. D. Thalidomide. *Lancet* 2004, 363, 1802-1811.

[65] Delforge, M.; Bladé, J.; Dimopoulos, M. A.; Facon, T.; Kropff, M.; Ludwig, H., et al. Treatment-related peripheral neuropathy in multiple myeloma: the challenge continues. *Lancet Oncol.* 2010, 11, 1086-1095.

[66] Richardson, P. G.; Delforge, M.; Beksac, M.; Wen, P.; Jongen, J. L.; Sezer, O., et al. Management of treatment-emergent peripheral neuropathy in multiple myeloma. *Leukemia* 2012, 26, 595-608.

[67] Andhavarapu, S.; Roy, V. Immunomodulatory drugs in multiple myeloma. *Expert Rev. Hematol.* 2013, 6, 69-82.

[68] Saini, N.; Mahindra, A. Novel immunomodulatory compounds in multiple myeloma. *Expert Opin. Investig. Drugs* 2013, 22, 207-215.

[69] Davies, F.; Baz, R. Lenalidomide mode of action: linking bench and clinical fin dings. *Blood Rev.* 2010, 24 Suppl. 1, S13-S19.

[70] Quach, H.; Kalff, A.; Spencer, A. Lenalidomide in multiple myeloma: Current status and future potential. *Amer. J. Hematol.* 2012, 87, 1089-1095.

[71] Chan, A. C.; Neeson, P.; Leeansyah, E.; Tainton, K.; Quach, H.; Prince, H. M. Natural killer T cell defects in multiple myeloma and the impact of lenalidomide therapy. *Clin. Exper. Immunol.* 2013, 175, 49-58.

[72] Chang, X.; Zhu, Y.; Shi, C.; Stewart, A. K. Mechanism of immune-modulatory drugs´ action in the treatment of multiple myeloma. *Acta Biochim. Biophys. Sin.* 2014, 46, 240-253.

[73] Geitz, H.; Handt, S.; Zwingenberger, K. Thalidomide selectively modulates the, density of cell surface molecules involved in the adhesion cascade.- *Immunopharmacology* 1996, 31, 213-221.

[74] Muller, G. W.; Chen, R.; Huang, S. Y.; Corral, L. G.; Wong, L. M.; Patterson, R. T., et al. Amino-substituted thalidomide analogs: potent inhibitors of TNF-alpha production. *Bioorg. Med. Chem. Lett.* 1999, 9, 1625-1630.

[75] Hideshima, T.; Chauhan, D.; Schlossman, R.; Richardson, P.; Anderson, K. C. The role of tumor necrosis factor alpha in the pathophysiology of human multiple myeloma: therapeutic applications. *Oncogene* 2001, 20, 4519-4527.

[76] Maiga, S.; Gomez-Bougie, P.; Bonnaud, S.; Gratas, C.; Moreau, P.; Le Gouil, S., et al. Paradoxial effect of lenalidomide on cytokine/growth factor profiles in multiple myeloma. *Brit. J. Cancer* 2013, 108, 1801-1806.

[77] Haslett, P. A.; Colrral, L. G.; Albert, M.; Kaplan, G. Thalidomide costimulates primary human T lymphocytes, preferentially inducing proliferation, cytokine production, and cytotoxic responses in the CD8+ subset. *J. Exp. Med.* 1998, 187, 1885-1892.

[78] Chang, D. H.; Liu, D.; Klimek, V.; Hassoun, H.; Mazumder, A.; Nimer, S. D., et al. Enhancement of ligand-dependent activation of human natural killer T cells by lenalidomide.: therapeutic implications. *Blood* 2006, 108, 618-621.

[79] Galustian, C.; Meyer, B.; Labarte, M. C.; Dredge, K.; Klaschka, D.; Henry, J., et al. The anti-cancer agents lenalidomide and pomalidomide inhibits the proliferation and function of T regulatory cells. *Cancer Immunol. Immunother.*2009, 58, 1033-1045.

[80] Dredge, K.; Marriott, J. B.; Macdonald, C. D.; Man, H. W.; Chen, R.; Muller, C. W., et al. Novel thalidomide analogues display anti-angiogenic activity independently of immunomodulatory effects. *Br. J. Cancer* 2002, 87, 1166-1172.

[81] Dredge, K.; Horsfall, R.; Robinson, S. P.; Zhang, L. H.; Lu, L.; Tang, Y., et al. Orally administrated lenalidomide (CC-5013) is anti-angiogenic *in vivo* and inhibits endothelial cell migration and Akt phosphorylation *in vitro*. *Microvascular Res.* 2005, 69, 56-63.

[82] Dankbar, B.; Paadro, T.; Leo, R.; Feldman, B.; Kropff, M.; Mesters, R. M., et al. Vascular endothelial growth factor and interleukin-6 in paracrine tumor-stromal cell interactions in multiple myeloma. *Blood* 2000, 95, 2630-2636.

[83] Escoubet-Lozach, L.; Lin, I. L.; Jensen-Pergakes, K.; Brady, H. A.; Gandhi, A. K.; Schafer, P. H., et al. Pomalidomide and lenalidomide induce p21 WAF-1 expression in both lymphoma and multiple myeloma through a LSD1-mediated epigenetic mechanism. *Cancer Res.* 2009, 69, 7347-7356.

[84] Mitsiades, N.; Mitsiades, C. S.; Poulaki, V.; Chauhan, D.; Richardson, P. G.; Hideshima, T., et al. Apoptotic signaling induced by immuno-modulatory thalidomide analogs in human multiple myeloma cells: Therapeutic implications. *Blood* 2002, 99, 4525-4530.

[85] Chu, Z. L.; McKinsey, T. A.; Liu, L.; Gentry, J. J.; Malim, M. H.; Ballard, D. W. Suppression of tumor necrosis factor-induced cell death by inhibitor of apoptosis c-IAP2 is under NF-κB control. *Proc. Natl. Acad. Sci. US* 1997, 94, 10057-10062.

[86] Kreuz, S.; Siegmund, D.; Scheurich, P, Wajant, H. NF-κB inducers upregulate cFLIP, a cycloheximide-sensitive inhibitor of dech receptor signaling. *Mol. Cell. Biol.* 2001, 21, 3964-3973.

[87] Li, Z. W.; Chen, H.; Campbell, R. A.; Bonavida, B.; Berenson, J. R. NF-κB in the pathogenesis and treatment of multiple myeloma. *Curr. Opin. Hematol.* 2008, 15, 391-399.

[88] Lopez-Girona, A.; Heintel, D.; Zhang, L. H.; Mendy, D.; Gaidarova, S.; Brady, H., et al. Lenalidomide downregulates the cell survival factor, interferon regulatory factor-4 providing a potential mechanistic link for predicting response. *Br. J. Haematol.*, 2011, 154, 325-336.

[89] Shaffer, A. L.; Emre, N. C.; Lamy, L.; Ngo, V. N.; Wright, G.; Xiao, W., et al. IRF4 addiction in multiple myeloma. *Nature* 2008, 454, 226-231.

[90] Raje, N.; Kumar, S.; Hideshima, T.; Ishitsuka, K.; Chauhan, D; Mitsiades, C., et al. Combination of the mTOR inhibitor rapamycin and CC-5013 has synergistic activity in multiple myeloma. *Blood* 2004, 104, 4188-4193.

[91] Steinbrunn, T.; Stühmer, T.; Sayehli, C.; Chatterjee, M.; Einsele, H.; Bargou, R. C. Combined targeting of MEK/MAPK and PI3K/Akt signaling in multiple myeloma. *Br. J. Haematol.*, 2012, 159, 430-440.

[92] Yang, J.; He, J.; Wang, J.; Cao, Y.; Ling, J.; Qian, J.; Lu, Y.; Li, H.; Zheng, Y.; Lan, Y.; Hong, S.; Matthews, J.; Starbruck, M. W.; Navone, N. M.; Orlowski, R. Z.; Lin, J.; Kwak, L. W.; Yi, Q. Constitutive activation of p38 MAPK in tumor cells contributes to osteolytic bone lesions in multiple myeloma. *Leukemia*, 2012, 26, 2114-2123.

[93] Tu, Y.; Gardner, A.; Lichtenstein, A. The phosphatidylinositol 3-kinase/ AKT kinase pathway in multiple myeloma plasma cells: roles in cytokine-dependent survival and proliferative responses. *Cancer Res.* 2000, 60, 6763-6770.

[94] Younes, H.; Leleu, X.; Hatjiharissi, E.; Moreau, A. S.; Hideshima, T.; Richardson, P.; Anderson, K. C.; Ghobrial, I. M. Targeting the phospha-tidylinositol 3-kinase pathway in multiple myeloma *Clin. Cancer Res.* 2007, 13, 3771-3775.

[95] Li, S.; Pal, R.; Monaghan, S. A.; Schafer, P.; Ouyang, H.; Mapara, M., et al. IMiD immunomodulatory compounds block C/EBPβ translation through eIF4E down-regulation resulting in inhibition of MM. *Blood* 2011, 117, 5157-5165.

[96] Pal, R.; Janz, M.; Galson, D. L.; Gries, M.; Li, S; Jöhrens, K., et al. C/ EBPβ regulates transcription factors critical for proliferation and survival of multiple myeloma cells. *Blood* 2009, 114, 3890-3898.

[97] Bjorklund, C. C.; Ma, W.; Wang, Z. Q.; Davis, R. E.; Kuhn, D. J.; Kornblau, S. M., et al. Evidence of a role for activation of Wnt/β-catenin signaling in the resistance of plasma cells to lenalidomide. *J. Biol. Chem.* 2011, 13, 11009-11020.

[98] Sadler, N. M.; Harris, B. R.; Metzger, B. A.; Kirshner, J. N-cadherin impedes proliferation of the multiple myeloma cancer stem cells. *Am. J. Blood Res.* 2013, 3, 271-285.

[99] Bjorklund, C. C.; Baladandazuthapani, V.; Lin, H. Y.; Jones, R. J.; Kuiatse, I.; Wang, H., et al. Evidence of a role for CD44 and cell adhesion in mediating resistance to lenalidomide in multiple myeloma: therapeutic implications. *Leukemia* 2014, 28, 373-383.

[100] Ito, T.; Ando, H.; Suzuki, T.; Ogura, T.; Hotta, K.; Imamura, Y., et al. Identification of a primary target of thalidomide teratogenicity. *Science* 2010, 327, 1345-1350.

[101] Ito, T.; Ando, H.; Handa, H. Teratogenic effects of thalidomide: molecu-lar mechanisms. *Cell. Mol. Life Sci.* 2011, 68, 1569-1579.

[102] Ito, T.; Handa, H. Deciphering the mystery of thalidomide teratogeni-city. *Congenit. Anom.* 2012, 52, 1-7.

[103] Greenberg, A. J.; Walters, D. K.; Kumar, S. K.; Vincent Rajkumar, S.; Jelinek, D. F., et al. Responsiveness of cytogenetically discrete human myeloma cell lines to lenalidomide: lack of correlation with cereblon and interferon regulatory factor 4 expression levels. *Eur. J. Haematol.* 2013, 91, 504-513.

In: Multiple Myeloma: Risk Factors, Diagnosis and Treatments
Editor: Steve Holt
ISBN: 978-1-63321-514-6

Chapter 4

Review of Risk Factors, Diagnosis Criteria and Treatment in Multiple Myeloma

Elena Flores-Ballester * ***and Julio Garcia-Suárez***
Hospital Universitario Príncipe de Asturias,
Alcalá de Henares, Madrid, Spain

Abstract

Introduction: Multiple myeloma (MM) is a malignant disease characterized by uncontrolled plasma tumor cell proliferation, produced by extrinsic stromal cell support and intrinsic chromosomal abnormalities together with the presence of monoclonal protein in blood or urine or both. Typical clinical presentation at diagnosis includes anemia, skeletal lesions, renal impairment, and hypercalcemia. In recent years, the introduction of novel agents such as proteasome inhibitor bortezomib, thalidomide, lenalidomide, which are associated with high-dose therapy and autologous stem cell transplantation in young patients and standard chemotherapy in elderly patients, has changed the management of myeloma and extended overall survival (OS) times. In this chapter, we will review the risks factors, diagnosis and treatment of Multiple myeloma.

Risk factors: There are few risk factors that may affect someone's chance of getting multiple myeloma, for example age, other plasma cell diseases, sex, race, radiation, family history or obesity. A causal relationship between MGUS and MM and chronic antigenic stimulation has been suggested by the results of several studies. Hyperphosphorylated paratarg-7 carrier state was shown to be the first molecularly defined autosomal dominantly inherited risk factor for MGUS and MM.

Multiple myeloma diagnosis is based on a step by step diagnosis approach. *Screening test:* Full Blood Counts, Urea, creatinine, calcium, albumin, electrophoresis of serum and urine, quantification of non-isotypic immunoglobulins, X-ray of symptomatic areas. Test to establish diagnostic: Bone marrow aspirates and trephine biopsy with plasma cell phenotyping, skeletal survey, immunofixation of serum and urine. Tests to

* Email: elenafloresballester@gmail.com.

estimate tumour burden and prognosis: FISH analysis, quantification of Monoclonal protein in serum and urine, Albumin, b2-microglobulin. Tests to assess myeloma related organ impairment (ROTI): Full blood count, Serum urea and creatinine, creatinine clearance (measured or calculated), Calcium, Albumin, Plasma viscosity, Tissue biopsy (or fat pad aspirate) for amyloid (if suspected) Quantification of non-isotypic immunoglobulins, Skeletal survery. The diagnosis criteria proposed by International Multiple myeloma working Group, in 2003, distinguish between myeloma and MGUS principally. Other differential diagnoses in patient with Multiple myeloma are solitary plasmacytoma and other B-cell lymphoproliferative disorders.

Treatment: Therapy for multiple myeloma has advanced over the past 5 to 7 years, but with this progress, be uncertainty which is the optimal therapy, particularly in the newly diagnosed patient. A reasonable aim of multiple Myeloma treatment in younger "transplant eligible" patients is to initiate therapy with a target of durable complete remission, and the anticipated consequence of long-term disease control. To achieve this situation, recommended induction therapy with multiagent combination chemotherapies (usually selected from bortezomib, lenalidomide, thalidomide, cyclophosphamide, and corticosteriods) which when employed together elicit frequent, rapid, and good responses. The earliest reports say that there are a very good partial response rates combining various drugs in triplets or even using 4 drugs together. After that, consolidation with high-dose melphalan and autologous stem cell transplantation in the majority of patients, especially in those failing to achieve a complete response or at high risk for early relapse based on prognostic, genetically defined risk factors.

Introduction

Multiple myeloma (MM) is a malignant disease characterized by uncontrolled plasma tumor cell proliferation, produced by extrinsic stromal cell support and intrinsic chromosomal abnormalities together with the presence of monoclonal protein in blood or urine or both. Typical clinical presentation at diagnosis includes anemia, skeletal lesions, renal impairment, and hypercalcemia.

The median patient age at diagnosis is 70 years; only 37% of patients with newly diagnosed (ND) disease are aged 65 years, 26% are aged 65-74 years, and 37% are aged 75 years. The annual prevalence of MM in patients aged 65-74 years is 31 cases per 100 000 people, and it increases to 46 cases per 100 000 people in patients aged 75 years. Furthermore, the number of elderly patients with MM will probably increase because of the improved survival times.

In recent years, the introduction of novel agents such as proteasome inhibitor bortezomib, thalidomide, lenalidomide, which are associated with high-dose therapy and autologous stem cell transplantation in young patients and standard chemotherapy in elderly patients, has changed the management of myeloma and extended overall survival (OS) times. An estimate of the 5-year relative survival of patients with MM in the United States from 1990-1992 to 2002-2004 reported a significant survival increase from 29%-35%. More substantial increases were seen in patients aged 50 years (5-year relative survival from 45%-57%) and patients aged 50-59 years (5-year relative survival from 39%-48%). By contrast, increases were much less pronounced in patients aged 60-69 years (5-year relative survival from 31%-36%), and no improvement was seen in patients aged 70 years. Further research into the best treatment strategies for vulnerable elderly patients with MM is therefore required, including an improved definition of clinical vulnerability in the elderly. This review discusses the effect of age and vulnerability on outcomes in patients with MM, specifically focusing on the effect of these factors on treatment regimens in elderly patients.

In this chapter, we will review the risks factors, diagnosis and treatment of Multiple myeloma.

Risk Factors

Risk factors are anything that changes probabilities for some person ill. But risk factors don't tell us everything. People who have no risk factors can still get the disease. There are few risk factors that may affect someone's chance of getting multiple myeloma, for example:

- Age: The risk of multiple myeloma goes up with age. Less than 1% of cases are diagnosed in people younger than 35. Most people diagnosed with this cancer are at least 65 years old.
- Other plasma cell diseases: Many people with monoclonal gammopathy of undetermined significance (MGUS) or solitary plasmacytoma will eventually develop multiple myeloma.
- Sex: Men are slightly more likely to develop multiple myeloma than women
- Race: Multiple myeloma is more than twice as common among black Americans as white Americans. The reason is not known.
- Radiation: People who were exposed to radiation from an atomic bomb blast had a higher risk of multiple myeloma. Exposure to lower levels of radiation may also increase the risk of multiple myeloma. At most, this accounts for a very small number of cases.
- Family history: Multiple myeloma seems to run in some families. Someone who has a sibling or parent with myeloma is 4 times more likely to get it than would be expected. Still, most patients have no affected relatives, so this accounts for only a small number of cases.
- Obesity: A study by the American Cancer Society has found that being overweight or obese increases a person's risk of developing myeloma.

A causal relationship between MGUS and MM and chronic antigenic stimulation has been suggested by the results of several studies. Hyperphosphorylated paratarg-7 carrier state was shown to be the first molecularly defined autosomal dominantly inherited risk factor for MGUS and MM.

Diagnosis

Diagnosis and Diagnosis Criteria

For diagnosed a patient with suspected myeloma should include the screening tests indicated at the list, followed by further tests to confirm the diagnosis.

Screening test:

- Full Blood Counts, Erythrocyte Sedimentation Ratio, or plasma viscosity
- Urea, creatinine, calcium, albumin.
- Electrophoresis of serum and urine
- Quantification of non-isotypic immunoglobulins
- X-ray of symptomatic areas

Test to establish diagnostic:

- Bone marrow aspirate + trephine biopsy with plasma cell phenotyping
- Skeletal survey
- Immunofixation of serum and urine

Tests to estimate tumour burden and prognosis:

- FISH analysis
- Quantification of Monoclonal protein in serum and urine, Albumin, b2-microglobulin
- Skeletal survery

Tests to assess myeloma related organ impairment (ROTI)

- Full blood count
- Serum urea and creatinine, Creatinine clearance (measured or calculated), Calcium, Albumin, Plasma viscosity, Tissue biopsy (or fat pad aspirate) for amyloid (if suspected) Quantification of non-isotypic immunoglobulins.
- Skeletal survery

Special tests indicated in some patients:

- SFLC (Serum free light chain) assay in oligo-secretory, light chain only and non-secretory disease
- MRI (Magnetic resonance imaging)/CT (computerized tomography) scan

PET CT can be used in patients with initial diagnosis are extramedullary disease, for example plasmocytoma.

Quantification of SFLC levels and j/k ratio is an additional tool for the assessment of light chain production.

It is recommended that a diagnosis of myeloma be confirmed by the demonstration of an aberrant plasma cell phenotype and/or monoclonality. Plasma cell phenotyping may be performed by flow cytometry and/or immunohistochemistry

The Diagnosis criteria for symptomatic multiple myeloma adapted from International Myeloma Working Group, 2003 are these:

- M-protein in serum and/or urine (no specific concentration required for diagnosis. A small percentage of patients have no detectable M-protein in serum or urine, but do have myeloma-related organ impairment (ROTI) and increased bone marrow plasma cells (non-secretory myeloma).
- Myeloma-related organ or tissue impairment (including bone lesions) unohistochemistry on trephine sections

ROTI, Myeloma-related organ or tissue impairment, adapted from International Myeloma Working Group, 2003:

Clinical effects due to myeloma	Definition
Increased calcium levels	Upper limit of normal or >2.75mmol/l
Renal insufficiency	Creatinine >1.73mcmol/l
Anaemia	Haemoglobin 2g/dl below the lower limit of normal or haemoglobin< 10g/dl
Bone lesions	Lytic lesions or osteoporosis with compression fractures
Other	Symptomatic hyperviscosity, amyloidosis, recurrent bacterial infection (>2 episodes in 12 month)

Differential Diagnosis

The diagnosis criteria proposed by International Multiple Myeloma working Group, in 2003, distinguish between myeloma and MGUS principally. Other differential diagnoses in patient with Multiple Myeloma or M-proteins are solitary plasmacytoma and other B-cell lymphoproliferative disorders.

MGUS	Asymptomatic myeloma	Symptomatic myeloma
M-protein in serum‹30g/l	M-protein in serum≥ 30g/l and/or	M-protein in serum and/or urine*
Bone marrow clonal plasma cells 10% and low level of plasma cells infiltration in a terpherine biopsy (if done)	Bone marrow clonal plasma ≥10%	Bone morrow (clonal) plasma cells or biopsy proven plasmacytoma
No related organ or tissue impairment (no end organ damage including bone lesions)	No related organ or tissue impairment (no end organ damage including bone lesions) or symptoms	Myeloma-related organ or tissue impairment (including bone lesions)

*No specific concentration required for diagnosis. A small percentage of patients have no detectable M-protein in serum or urine but do have myeloma-related organ impairment (ROTI) and increased bone marrow plasma cells (non-secretory myeloma).

Treatment

Therapy for multiple myeloma has advanced over the past 5 to 7 years, but with this progress, be uncertainty which is the optimal therapy, particularly in the newly diagnosed patient.

A reasonable aim of Multiple Myeloma treatment in younger "transplant eligible" patients is to initiate therapy with a target of durable complete remission, and the anticipated consequence of long-term disease control. To achieve this situation, recommended induction therapy with multiagent combination chemotherapies (usually selected from bortezomib, lenalidomide, thalidomide, cyclophosphamide, and corticosteriods) which when employed together elicit frequent, rapid, and good responses. After that, consolidation with high-dose melphalan and autologous stem cell transplantation in the majority of patients, especially in those failing to achieve a complete response or at high risk for early relapse based on prognostic, genetically defined risk factors.

When Should Treatment Be Started?

The dates say that up to 25% of smoldering myeloma patients will not require active treatment for 10 to 15 years, although the majority will indeed progress during that time. There is still no evidence that early treatment will improve survival in asymptomatic and biochemically stable patients. The clinician should avoid treating asymptomatic and biochemically stable patients with active therapy, allowing current drug development efforts to mature to their maximal efficacy at a time when systemic treatment does become a necessity.

Choice Initial Drug Therapy

When we start treat one patient, we search a long-term remission. The earliest reports say that have been achieved complete and very good partial response (VGPR) rates can be substantially increased by combining these various drugs in triplets or even using 4 drugs together. Triplet therapies came from the combination of bortezomib, thalidomide, and dexamethasone (VTD), and the encouraging results have now been replicated using lenalidomide, bortezomib, and dexamethasone (RVD), liposomal doxorubicin, bortezomib, and dexamethasone (DVD), and cyclophosphamide, bortezomib, and dexamethasone (CVD) as examples. Preliminary results from ongoing phase 3 randomized trials show improved initial response rates and increased frequency of CR after induction therapy in patients randomized to bortezomib and dexamethasone versus VAD (vincristine, doxorubicin, dexamethasone) chemotherapy, and in patients randomized to bortezomib, thalidomide, and dexamethasone versus thalidomide and dexamethasone alone. These initial higher quality responses translate into a higher frequency of CR after transplantation and at least in preliminary reports improved PFS. Because durable CR and PFS appear to be valuable surrogates for long-term outcome and an important platform for better disease control, we therefore favor multiple drug, combination therapies be applied in younger patients able to tolerate potential toxicities and pursue high-dose therapy approaches.

Transplantation

Autologous stem cell transplantation (ASCT) has been shown in randomized trials to be of value to patients in helping achieve or consolidating and is thus used in the majority of our patients eligible and willing to undergo this procedure. New trials will address whether or not transplantation remains useful in the era of novel drugs; but until proven otherwise. Upper age limits vary widely from center to center and country to country, but in general the overall health of the patient rather than a specific chronologic age is probably most relevant. Earlier studies demonstrated an advantage to a second or tandem transplantation in patients who do not obtain at least a VGPR after the first procedure and may overcome the negative prognostic effect of del(17p13) and/or t(4;14) and that achievement of molecular remission resulted in long-term freedom from disease. However, because CR rates are now achieved more than 50% to 70% of the time with effective induction therapies combined with single ASCT and because responses may be further enhanced by post transplantation consolidation/maintenance therapies, there is less frequently the need to perform a second (or tandem) transplantation early in the disease course. The choice for maintenance therapies that can be used after transplantation will be discussed in the next section. The timing of ASCT is also an area of active research. Patients are usually more fit for intensive therapy early in the course of the disease, but prior studies using conventional chemotherapy as induction demonstrated that a delayed ASCT had no adverse impact on OS and is feasible as part of salvage therapy in first relapse. Randomized trials to better define populations served by this approach are planned, and a delayed transplantation may be considered in some patients doing well on induction drugs, obtaining an excellent response and who are not inclined to pursue the social and quality of life disruptions entailed by high-dose melphalan-based therapy. Allogeneic transplantation should infrequently be performed outside of clinical trials, as the risk of morbidity and early mortality of even nonmyeloablative transplantations is considerable and thus not acceptable for most patients in the current era of longer survival. In very young patients, particularly those who experience early relapse or with very high risk features at diagnosis, this therapeutic strategy may, however, offer some hope of long-term.

Consolidation and Maintenance Therapy After Transplantation

Three separate phase 3 studies found thalidomide maintenance to improve overall survival, despite these findings; thalidomide is not being routinely used for maintenance in many centers, presumably reflecting concerns about cumulative toxicity. Lenalidomide may offer the same advantages with less toxicity, and large randomized trials are now addressing its role in the post transplantation setting. It has become our practice to use maintenance routinely when patients have not achieved a CR after stem cell transplantation or when genetic risk markers suggest a very high risk of early relapse. There are insufficient data on bortezomib maintenance on which to form an opinion although trials are under way. Perhaps thalidomide or lenalidomide probably proves suitable. It is not known how long maintenance should be continued, but we generally use it indefinitely and taper dosing for tolerance. Anticoagulation is not a requirement in the maintenance setting, but is recommended.

Treatment Options for Unfit Patient

The prevalence of MM is expected to rise over time because of an aging population. Most patients with newly diagnosed multiple myeloma (MM) are aged > 65 years with 30% aged > 75 years. Many elderly patients are also vulnerable because of comorbidities that complicate the management of MM. Most elderly patients with MM are ineligible for autologous transplantation, and the standard treatment has, until recently, been melphalan plus prednisone. The introduction of novel agents, such as thalidomide, bortezomib, and lenalidomide, has improved outcomes; however, elderly patients with MM are more susceptible to side effects and are often unable to tolerate full drug doses. For these patients, lower-dose intensity regimens improve the safety profile and thus optimize treatment outcome. Appropriate screening for vulnerability and an assessment of cardiac, renal, hepatic, pulmonary, and neurologic functions, as well as age > 75 years, at the start of therapy allows treatment strategies to be individualized and drug doses to be tailored to improve tolerability and optimize efficacy.

No data are available that assess screening for vulnerability before choosing and starting therapy for MM, because of the underrepresentation in clinical trials of elderly adults and patients with comorbidities, it is reasonable to translate data on elderly general population to the MM population. We can, speculate that the continued poor prognosis of elderly patients with MM may be attributable, at least in part, to physical vulnerability and the effect that this has on patients' ability to tolerate complex treatment regimens. It is, therefore, important to consider the age, physical condition, and comorbidity status for all elderly patients with MM when planning treatment. There is a classification of levels of frailty and disability in elderly patients (table 1).

Table 1. Levels of frailty and disability in elderly patients and related description

Frailty grade Description	
Very fit	Active, energetic patients, who exercise regularly or occasionally
Moderately fit	Patients not regularly active beyond routinely walking
Vulnerable	Patients who can perform limited activities but yet do not need help from other people
Mildly frail	Patients who need help for household tasks (shopping, walking several blocks, managing their finances, and medications)
Moderately frail	Patients who need partial help for their personal care (dressing, bathing, toileting, eating)
Severely frail	Patients completely dependent on other people for their personal care

Table 2. Appropriate dose adjustments or use of modified treatment regimens according to elderly patients classifications

	GO-GO	MODERATE-GO	SLOW-GO
	NO RISK FACTORS: DOSE LEVEL 0	At least one risk factor. DOSE LEVEL -1	At least one risk factor plus occurrence of grade 3-4 nonhematologic AE: DOSE LEVEL -2
AGENT	DOSE LEVEL 0	DOSE LEVEL-1	DOSE LEVEL -2
Dexamethasone	40mg/d d 1,8,15,,22/4 weeks	20 mg d 1,8,15,22 /4 weeks	10 mg/d d1,8,15,22/4 weeks
Melphalan	0,25mg/Kg or 9 mg/m2 d 1-4/4-6 weeks	0,18mg/Kg or 7.5 mg/m2 d 1-4/4-6 weeks	0.13mg/kg or 5 mg/m2 d 1-4/4-6 weeks
Thalidomide	100 mg/ d	50 mg/d	50 mg qod
Lenalidomide	25mf/d d 1-21/4 weeks	15 mg/d d 1-21 /4 weeks	10 mg/d d 1-21/4 weeks
Bortezomib	1.3 mg/m2 twice weekly d 1,4,8,11/3 weeks	1.3 mg/m2 twice weekly d 1,4,8,11/3 weeks	1,0 mg/m2 twice weekly d 1,4,8,11/3 weeks
Prednisone	60 mg/m2 1-4 or 50 mg qod	30 mg/m2 1-4 or 25 mg qod	15 mg/m2 1-4 or 12.5 mg qod
Cyclophosphamide	100 mg/d d 1-21 /4 weeks or 300 mg/m2/d d 1,8,15/ 4 weeks	50 mg/d d 1-21 /4 weeks or 150 mg/m2/d d 1,8,15/ 4 weeks	50 mg/d d 1-21 /4 weeks or 75 mg/m2/d d 1,8,15/ 4 weeks

Risk Factors
Age over 75 Mild, moderate or severe frailty: Patients needing help for household tasks and personal care Comorbidities: Cardiac dysfunction Pulmonary dysfunction Hepatic dysfunction Renal dysfunction

Appropriate dose adjustments or use of modified treatment regimens according to elderly patients classifications, should be made to improve the tolerability of treatment. (Table 2) Well tolerated regimens will probably reduce the need for treatment interruptions and thereby should optimize treatment efficacy. Future trials should address the role of age, comorbidities, and geriatric assessment by stratifying patients with MM into treatment groups at different risk of mortality and, maybe, personalized therapy for elderly patients. To promote the enrollment of elderly adults in clinical trials it may be necessary to relax standard protocol eligibility criteria by focusing on developing therapeutics suitable for patients with comorbid conditions.

References

A. Keith Stewart, Paul G. Richardson, and Jesus F. San-Miguel Mayo Clinic Arizona, Scottsdale; Dana-Farber Cancer Institute, Boston, MA; and University Salamanca, Salamanca, Spain. *Blood. 2009 114: 5436-5443 doi:10.1182/blood-2009-07-204651.*

Prepublished online October 27, 2009; How I treat multiple myeloma in younger patients.

Antonio Palumbo, Sara Bringhen, Heinz Ludwig, Meletios A. Dimopoulos, Joan Blade´, Maria V. Mateos, Laura Rosinõl, Mario Boccadoro, Michele Cavo, Henk Lokhorst, Sonja Zweegman, Evangelos Terpos, Faith Davies, Christoph Driessen, Peter Gimsing, Martin Gramatzki, Roman Hájek, Hans E. Johnsen, Fernando Leal Da Costa, Orhan Sezer, Andrew Spencer, Meral Beksac, Gareth Morgan, Hermann Einsele, Jesus F. San Miguel, and Pieter Sonneveld Myeloma Unit, Division of Hematology. *Blood 2011 118: 4519-4529, doi: 10.1182/blood-2011-06-358812 Prepublished online August 12, 2011*; Personalized therapy in multiple myeloma according to patient age and vulnerability: a report of the European Myeloma Network (EMN).

Jennifer M. Bird, Roger G. Owen, Shirley D'Sa, John A. Snowden, Guy Pratt, John Ashcroft, Kwee Yong, Gordon Cook, Sylvia Feyler, Faith Davies, Gareth Morgan, Jamie Cavenagh, Eric Low and Judith Behrens on behalf of the Haemato-oncology Task Force of the British Committee for Standards in Haematology (BCSH) and UK Myeloma Forum. BJH-2011 Guidelines for the diagnosis and management of multiple myeloma 2011.

Antonio Palumbo, S. Vincent Rajkumar, Jesus F. San Miguel, Alessandra Larocca, Ruben Niesvizky, Gareth Morgan, Ola Landgren, Roman Hajek, Hermann Einsele, Kenneth C. Anderson, Meletios A. Dimopoulos, Paul G. Richardson, Michele Cavo, Andrew Spencer, A. Keith Stewart, Kazuyuki Shimizu, Sagar Lonial, Pieter Sonneveld, Brian G.M. Durie, Philippe Moreau, and Robert Z. Orlowski Published Ahead of Print on January 13, 2014 as 10.1200/JCO.2013.48.7934 The latest version is at http://jco.ascopubs.org/cgi/doi/10.1200/JCO.2013.48.7934 International Myeloma Working Group Consensus Statement for the Management, Treatment, and Supportive Care of Patients with Myeloma Not Eligible for Standard Autologous Stem-Cell Transplantation.

In: Multiple Myeloma: Risk Factors, Diagnosis and Treatments ISBN: 978-1-63321-514-6
Editor: Steve Holt

Chapter 5

Diagnosis and Management of Oral Manifestations of Multiple Myeloma

Annie Karoline de Oliveira Tanaka[1], Gustavo Zanna Ferreira[1], Fábio Luiz Coracin[2] and Paulo Sérgio da Silva Santos[1,*]

[1]Stomatology Department of Bauru School of Dentistry, University of São Paulo, Bauru, SP, Brazil

[2]Clinicas Hospital of University of São Paulo, SP, Brazil

Abstract

The oral manifestations arising from multiple myeloma (MM) are resultant effects of the moclonal proliferation of atypical plasmocytes derived from bone marrow, kappa and lambda light chains and osteoclast activating factors. The initial manifestation of the MM in maxillofacial complex involves 12-15% of cases, mainly the posterior region of the jaw, justified by the intense hematopoietic activity. The main signs and symptoms include facial pain, gingival bleeding, paresthesias, tooth mobility, ulceration, soft tissue edema, pathological fractures and deposition of amyloidosis in the tongue. The radiographic aspects vary from discreet localized bone resorption until generalized bone rarefaction, may present osteolytic areas in "punched-out". Other osteolytic lesions as osteoporosis, chronic osteomyelitis, bone metastasis, osteoradionecrosis, arteriovenous malformations, osteonecrosis associated with bisphosphonates should be included in the differential diagnosis due to clinical and radiographic similarity. For elucidation of the diagnosis, laboratory exams and biopsy are indicated. Atypical plasmocytes with hyperchromatic core in histopathological analysis and kappa and lambda chains in immunohistochemistry analysis lead to the diagnosis of multiple myeloma.

From the established diagnosis, treatment is given in conjunction with the oncohematologist. Oral care include: oral preparation prior to chemotherapy, with the removal of focus of infection, such as caries, periodontal disease and residual roots; prevention of osteonecrosis associated with bisphosphonates and prevention and

* Corresponding author: Paulo Sérgio da Silva Santos. Bauru School of Dentistry, University of São Paulo, Alameda Otávio Pinheiro Brizolla 9-75, Bauru, SP, Brazil – 17012-901. Phone: 55 (14) 3235-8000 (8552), cel.: 55 14 99670-0921, e-mail: paulosss@fob.usp.br.

treatment of oral complications resulting from chemotherapy, such as oral mucositis, xerostomia, and opportunistic infections. The knowledge of the oral manifestations of the MM can lead to early diagnosis and optimal management of patients during the various stages of treatment.

1. Incidence and Case Series

Among hematologic malignancies, up to 10% of them are represented by multiple myeloma and it represents 1% of all malignancies in humans. It occurs with an estimated incidence of 3-15 cases per 100,000 habitants each year. In general, it represents approximately 0.8% of new cancer cases and 0.9% of cancer deaths. Multiple myeloma affects individuals with mean age of 60 years, ranging from 50 to 80 years with a predilection for the black race and the men with a ratio male:female of 3:2 (Alvarez - Cordovés, 2013; Soares Pinto, 2007; Ozdemir, 2005; Witt, 1997). Oral manifestations, as the first sign of the disease, comprises 12-15% of all cases and the maxillofacial involvement relatively is very common (Lee, 1996; Ozdemir, 2005).

The lesions in the jaws represent 10-30% of the cases and they are more frequent site is the posterior region of the mandible (molar region, branch and angle) due to the high hematopoietic activity in this area. The involvement of the jaws usually occurs after the involvement of other bones of the body, as vertebrae, pelvic bones, rib, humerus, femur and, mainly, the skull (Silveira et al., 2005; Mozaffari, 2002; Second, 2008; Pinto, 2007). Another important site in the jaws involves the upper region of the premolar and molar teeth, hard and soft palate, soft tissues, although, nose and sinus bones may also be affected (Owotade, 2005; Ozdemir, 2005).

2. Clinical Diagnosis

The most common clinical manifestation of multiple myeloma is related to the uncontrolled proliferation of atypical and neoplasic plasma cells in the bone marrow. Thus, the erythrocytes, leukocytes and platelets are unable to perform their functions leading to anemia, increased the incidence of bacterial, viral and fungal infections and abnormal bleeding, respectively.

The hypercalcemia and renal dysfunction may also be present (Alvarez - Cordovés 2013).

The oral manifestations present as pain associated with facial swelling, expansion and pain in the jaws, gingival bleeding, toothache, paresthesia, tooth mobility, ulceration, soft tissue edema (Figure 1), pathological fractures and deposition of amyloid protein in the tongue (Gray et al., 1997, Owotade, 2005; Ozdemir, 2005).

For establishing the diagnosis of multiple myeloma, the clinical findings are insufficient and it needs to be associated with blood and biochemical exams, urine and radiographic. The diagnostic criteria for multiple myeloma include: evidence of multiple osteolytic lesions on skull presented in x-ray examination, identification of atypical plasma cells obtained by biopsy and abnormalities in the production of immunoglobulins.

The final diagnosis is based on the presence of at least one major criteria associated with one minor or three minor criteria, and must be included the criteria 1 and 2, as shown in the Table 1 (Pinto, 2007; Owotade, 2005; Alvarez – Cordovés 2013).

Table 1. Major and minor criteria to multiple myeloma diagnosis

Major Criteria
1. Plasmocytoma proven on histopathological examination
2. Bone marrow plasmacytosis ≥30%
3. Component M
• Serum IgG ≥3.5g/dl; IgA ≥2g/dl.
• Urine ≥1g/24 hours of Bence Jones proteins.
Minor Criteria
a. Bone marrow plasmacytosis between 10-30%
b. Presence of component M, but in lesser amounts than the major criteria #3.
c. Osteolytic lesions
d. Reduced normal serum immunoglobulins: IgM<50 mg/dl, IgA<100 mg/dl or IgG<600 mg/dl (<50% of the normal rates)

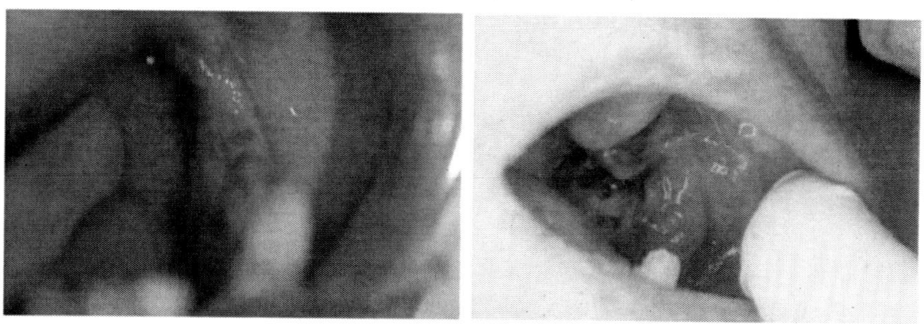

A B

Figure 1. A and B extramedular lesion multiple myeloma in the posterior mandible with soft tissue edema, central area ulcerated and erythematous borders.

3. Diagnostic Imaging

Imaging exams remain the primary method of diagnosis of the osteolytic lesions caused by multiple myeloma. The incidence suggests that up to 50% of bone destruction occur before any radiographic sign can be observed, and up to 75% of patients with multiple myeloma will have any radiographic findings of the disease (Angtuaco, 2004).

The radiographic features of multiple myeloma in the jaws is similar to the other bone sites and include: (1) normal findings, which did not detect bone resorption; (2) multiple radiolucent with "piecemeal" pattern due to the proliferation of plasma cells in the bone marrow (Figure 2); and (3) osteoporotic bone thinning and changes due to diffuse replacement of bone marrow by malignant plasma cells (Mozaffari, 2002).

The mandible is affected in about 15.6% of cases of multiple myeloma and, mainly, in the posterior region of the mandible (Witt et al., 1997).

Computed tomography and cone beam computed tomography findings include lesions in "piecemeal" pattern, osteolytic lesions leading to drilling and expansion of cortical with soft tissue masses, diffuse osteopenia, pathologic fractures and bone sclerosis (Figure 3) (Angtuaco, 2004; Elias, 2009; Santos 2012).

Magnetic resonance imaging is another useful tool that to determine the extent of injury and the relationship with the adjacent maxillary bone structures (Rodríguez - Caballero, 2011).

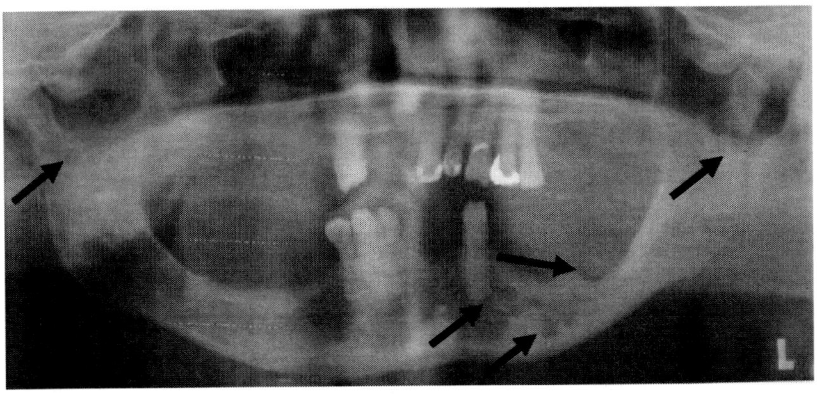

Figure 2. Panoramic radiography with multiple radiolucent with "piecemeal" in the mandible (arrows).

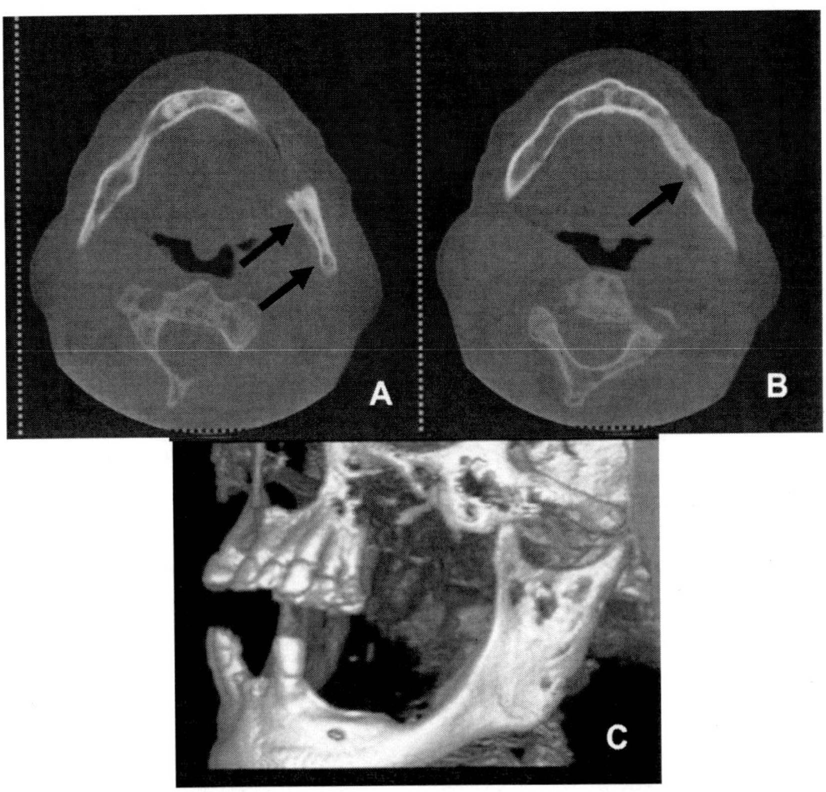

Figure 3. Cone Bean Computed Tomography, A and B axial reformatting, C 3D reformatting showing multiple osteolytic lesions with drilling cortical bone in "piecemeal" pattern in the mandible ramus (arrows).

4. Differential Diagnosis

The radiographic patterns of poorly defined osteolytic lesions with destruction of cortical bone are usually induced by rapid and aggressive growth and destructive lesions, such as malignant diseases of the central bone.

In addition, conditions such as chronic osteomyelitis, osteoradionecrosis and arteriovenous malformations can produce similar imaging aspects and should be included in the differential diagnosis. The presence of multiple lesions with disruption of cortical bone in the mandible and the skull bone are features of lesions such as Langerhans cell histiocytosis or metastatic malignant lesions (Mozaffari, 2002).

5. Histopathological and Immunohistochemistry Features

The histopathological features of plasmacytoma or multiple myeloma show a proliferation of atypical plasma cells forming monotone cell sheets.

These cells show individually varying degrees of differentiation with hyperchromatic nuclei, cellular and nuclear pleomorphism. The monoclonal nature of the malignant cells can differentiate them by immunohistochemistry were positive for immunoglobulin light chain (kappa or lambda). These features allow differentiating monoclonal plasmacytoma or multiple myeloma of other reactive inflammatory infiltrate present in plasma cell gingivitis (Jain, 2013; Sperandio, 2013). The malignant plasma cells usually show positivity for anti-CD138 antibody as an auxiliary diagnosis (Rodriguez - Caballero, 2011).

6. Management

The dental management of patients with multiple myeloma involving the maxillofacial complex comprises the treatment of adverse effects caused by antineoplastic therapy (Ozdemir, 2005). Concerning the chemotherapy and radiotherapy schedule, factors such as the type of drug/ radiation therapy, dose and frequency of treatment will interfere with oral manifestations of multiple myeloma patients due to the potential toxicity of the oral tissues.

Before the start of the antineoplastic therapy, the oral cavity should be prepared with the goal being to prevent the oral complications of this therapy. The removal of infection foci (tooth decay, periodontal disease and residual roots) should always be done before the onset of chemotherapy and/or radiotherapy. The schedule of the best time to invasive procedures, such as dental extractions, should be planned and considerer the counts values of the CBC and hemostasis tests should always be performed in conjunction with a hematologist.

Oral mucositis is the major oral complication in patients under cancer treatment and treatment approaches include the use of isotonic, anti-inflammatory and antimicrobial therapy topics and solutions with low-level laser (Santos, 2006). Low-level laser therapy may be used to improve erythema, ulcerative oral mucositis and pain associated with this condition and provide an improvement in the quality of food intake since these symptoms may lead to dysphagia. The use of topical anesthetics can also help control pain.

Another common complication of the treatment to multiple myeloma is the xerostomia. The concentration of chemotherapeutic agents in saliva results in mucosal exposure to the drug cytotoxicity. Furthermore, the xerostomia can be marked worse due to total or partial destruction of the glandular parenchyma if radiotherapy will be used in combination to chemotherapy. The main changes comprise the reduction in salivary flow, changes in the saliva constituents with changes of the oral microorganisms and reduced level of salivary immunoglobulin. The use of intraoral splint made to protect the parenchyma of the salivary gland during the use of ionizing radiation and the use of artificial saliva substitutes may be used in order to minimize the damage glandular structures and provide some comfort to patients, respectively (Ozdemir, 2005; Silva, 2006).

Opportunistic infections such as candidiasis and herpes (both herpes simplex or zoster) are other complications resulting of myelosuppression.

The use of antifungal therapy (e.g., Nystatin mouthwash 100.00 IU/ml) and antivirals (e.g., topical use of acyclovir) is recommended to control and prevent the spread of microorganisms to other organs.

The period of thrombocytopenia in the patients undergoing chemotherapy can lead to bleeding episodes that can be worse when there is accumulation of dental plaque leading to gingival inflammation and spontaneous bleeding. Thus, the oral hygiene comprehensive care including dental biofilm control, removal of gingival calculus and periodontal treatment becomes critical for prevention of bleeding episodes.

A recent described complication associated with the use of bisphosphonates is osteonecrosis of the jaws associated with the use of bisphosphonates that affects jawbones. Preventive strategies to avoid or reduce the risks should be adopted. Patients should receive a complete dental examination and be educated about optimal oral hygiene.

The dental abnormalities should be treated prior to initiating therapy with bisphosphonates and unnecessary invasive dental procedures should be avoided after the use. Dental health should be monitored at least annually and dental problems treated conservatively as possible.

The temporary suspension of the use of bisphosphonates should be considered if invasive dental procedures are necessary. Discontinuation of the drug occurs for 90 days before and after dental invasive procedures (e.g., tooth extraction, dental implants). Bisphosphonates need not be stopped for routine dental procedures, including endodontic treatment (Terpos et al., 2013).

The initial treatment of osteonecrosis associated with bisphosphonates depends on the stage of the disease including administration of antibiotics, antibacterial mouthwash solutions such as chlorhexidine gluconate 0.12%, pain control, surface bone debridement, bone resection (Salvatore et al., 2014).

After the development of osteonecrosis a review the benefits of therapy with bisphosphonates should be performed, considering the advantages and disadvantages of long-term therapy with these drugs (Terpos et al., 2013).

References

Alvarez-Cordovés, M. M., Mirpuri-Mirpuri, P. G., Pérez-Monje, A.: Diagnosis of multiple myeloma in primary care. Suspicion with an appropriate clinical history. *Semergen* 39:21, 2013.

Angtuaco, E. J., Fassas, A. B., Walker, R., Sethi, R., Barlogie, B. Multiple myeloma: clinical review and diagnostic imaging. *Radiology*. Apr.;231(1):11-23, 2004

Da Silva Santos, P. S., Klingbeil, M. F. G., Abrahão, A. C., Gallottini, M., and de Sousa, S. C. O. M. Multiple myeloma with primary manifestation in mandibular area. *Oral Surgery*, 5: 26–29, 2012. doi: 10. 1111/j.1752-248X.2011.01141.x.

Elias, H. G., Scott, J., Metheny, L., Quereshy, F. A. Multiple myeloma presenting as mandibular ill-defined radiolucent lesion with numb chin syndrome: a case report. *J. Oral Maxillofac. Surg*. Sep.;67(9), 2009: 1991-6 doi: 10.1016/j.joms.2009.04.016.

Gray, S. T., Antunovic, D. M., White, A. E. Non secretory multiple myeloma involving the maxilla: Report of a case with update of biology and new approaches to management. *Oral. Oncol.* 33:136, 1997.

Jain, S., Kaur, H., Kansal, G., Gupta, P. Multiple myeloma presenting as gingival hyperplasia. *J. Indian Soc. Periodontol.* 17(3):391-3, 2013.

Lee, S.-H., Huang, J.-J., Pan, W.-L., Chan, C.-P.: Gingival mass as the primary manifestation of multiple myeloma. *Oral Surg. Oral Med. Oral Pathol. Oral Radiol. Endod.* 82:75, 1996.

Mozaffari, E., Mupparapu, M., Otis, L.: Undiagnosed multiple myeloma causing extensive dental bleeding: Report of a case and review. *Oral Surg. Oral Med. Oral Pathol. Oral Radiol. Endod.* 94:448, 2002.

Ozdemir, R., Kayiran, O., Oruc, M., et al.: Plasmacytoma of the hard palate. *J. Craniofac. Surg*. 16:164, 2005.

Pinto, L. S. S., Campagnoli, E. B., Leon, J. E., et al.: Maxillary lesion presenting as a first sign of multiple myeloma: case report. *Med. Oral Patol. Oral Cir. Bucal* 12:344, 2007.

Rodriguez-Caballero, B., Sanchez-Santolino, S., Garcia-Montesinos-Perea, B., Garcia-Reija, M. F., Gomez-Roman, J., Saiz-Bustillo, R. Mandibulary solitary plasmocytoma of the jaw: a case report. *Med. Oral Patol. Oral Cir. Bucal*. 1; 16(5): 647-650, 2011.

Salvatore, L., Ruggiero, S. L., Dodson, T. B., Fantasia, J., Goodday, R., Aghaloo, T., Mehrotra, B., O'Ryan, F. Medication-Related Osteonecrosis of the Jaw—2014 Update. *American Association of Oral and Maxillofacial Surgeons,* 2014.

Santos, P. S., Fernandes, K. S.: Complicações bucais da quimioterapia. Prática Hospitalar, São Paulo - SP, v. 44, p. 29-31, 2006.

Segundo, A. V. L., Falcão, M. F. L., Filho, R. C. L., et al.: Multiple myeloma with primary manifestation in the mandible: a case report. *Med. Oral Patol. Oral Cir. Bucal* 13:232, 2008.

Silveira, E. J. D., Godoy, G. P., Freitas, T. M. C., et al.: Multiple myeloma: a clinic and epidemiologic analysis. *Rev. Odontol. UNESP* 34: 61, 2005.

Soares Pinto, L. S., Campagnoli, E. B., Leon, J. E., et al.: Maxillary lesion presenting as a first sign of multiple myeloma: case report. *Med. Oral Patol. Oral Cir. Bucal* 12:344, 2007.

Sperandio, F. F., Giudice, F. S. *Atlas de histopatologia oral básica*. São Paulo: Santos, P.272-273, 2013.

Terpos, E., Moulopoulos, L. A., Dimopoulos, M. A. Advances in imaging and the management of myeloma bone disease. *J. Clin. Oncol.* 10;29(14), 2011:1907-15. doi: 10.1200/JCO.2010.32.5449.

Witt, C., Borges, A. C., Klein, K., et al.: Radiographic manifestations of multiple myeloma in the mandible: a retrospective study of 77 patients. *J. Oral Maxillofac. Surg.* 55:450, 1997.

In: Multiple Myeloma: Risk Factors, Diagnosis and Treatments ISBN: 978-1-63321-514-6
Editor: Steve Holt

Chapter 6

New Drugs and New Strategies for the Treatment of Multiple Myeloma Patients

A. Reale, A. Melaccio, R. Ria and A. Vacca
Department of Biomedical Sciences and Human Oncology,
Section of Internal Medicine and Clinical Oncology,
University of Bari Medical School, Bari, Italy

Abstract

Multiple myeloma still remains an incurable disease with a high incidence rate in the elderly. Near the old active classes of drugs: alkylators (e.g., melphalan and cyclophosphamide), corticosteroids (e.g., prednisone and dexamethasone), and anthracyclines (e.g., doxorubicin), new drug formulations (e.g., liposomal doxorubicin) and new active classes of drugs such as proteasome inhibitors (e.g., bortezomib) and immunomodulatory drugs (e.g., thalidomide and lenalidomide) have been introduced in myeloma therapy. The high heterogeneity of this disease leads to large differences in clinical responses to treatments. High response rates and good quality responses with a long-term disease control can be observed with the introduction of new drugs. Changes in treatment strategies due to the introduction of novel drugs have been able to improve significantly the quality of responses. In fact, if in the past, Complete Remission (CR) in MM was rare to achieve, while the introduction of new treatments have increased the rate in younger patients as well as in non-transplant setting. CR represents a surrogated marker of long survival. It correlates with the long-term Progression-Free Survival (PFS) and Overall Survival (OS). Achieving CR and sustaining CR within a 3-year landmark from the treatment initiation is associated with highly superior survival. Actually, we agree that "The more profound the remission, the longer the duration of response".

Moreover, the interactions between tumor cells and their bone marrow microenvironment play a pivotal role in myeloma progression, inducing also drug resistance. This knowledge has improved treatment options leading to the approval of new drugs which target the malignant cell itself and also its microenvironment. These agents are in preclinical/early clinical evaluation and they appear to further improve disease control but their use is still not approved outside of clinical trials.

Keywords: Myeloma; bone marrow microenvironment; autologous stem cell transplantation; elderly patients; continuous treatments; relapsed/refractory; new drugs; new proteasome inhibitors; new immunomodulatory drugs; clinical trials

Introduction

Multiple myeloma (MM) is a disease that accounts for 10% of hematological malignancies. MM is a clonal B-cell malignancy characterized by the uncontrolled growth of malignant plasma cells in the bone marrow, resulting in an accumulation of monoclonal immunoglobulins (M-spike) in the blood and urine of the patient. Common symptoms at diagnosis include bone lesions, hypercalcemia, kidney failure, anemia and recurrent infections. Of outmost importance for the growth of the MM tumor is the interaction with the bone marrow (BM) microenvironment. The various bidirectional interactions between MM cells and the BM compartment stimulate survival, growth, drug resistance, migration and immune escape of MM cells. In addition, increased angiogenesis and bone lesions further contribute to MM development. The above interactions are mediated by secretion of multiple cytokines, including Interleukin-6 (IL-6), Insulin-like Growth Factor-1 (IGF-1), IL-1, Tumor Necrosis Factor-α (TNF-α), Vascular Endothelial Growth Factor (VEGF), that support paracrine interactions between MM cells and endothelial cells, Bone Marrow Stromal Cells (BMSC), osteoblasts, osteoclasts and immune cells. In addition, direct cell-cell and cell-matrix interactions by expression of adhesion molecules such as Integrin-α4β1 (VLA-4) and CD138 (syndecan-1) on MM cells stimulate the expression and secretion of growth factors into the BM microenvironment [1].

MM tumors evolve from a pre-malignant state (Monoclonal Gammopathy of Undetermined Significance or MGUS). MGUS evolves to symptomatic MM with a rate of 1% per year. The progression from MGUS to MM involves accumulating cytogenetic abnormalities, including the translocations t(4;14), t(11;14) and t(14;16 or 20). Progression of MGUS to MM is associated with additional aberrations including activating RAS mutations, deletion of 13q or 17p, MYC overexpression and mutations of TP53 [1].

MM primarily affects older individuals; the median age at diagnosis is 70 years [2]. It is still an incurable disease and it is characterized from the alternating of periods of remission and relapse which arise from the residual myeloma cells surviving after complete clinical response to treatment [3], and from the development of multiple drug resistance [4].

The treatment of MM is rapidly evolving. The introduction of high-dose therapy, followed by autologous stem cell transplantation (HDT-ASCT) up-front, and the use of novel agents as rescue therapy, has determined a benefit in young patients. Only a marginal change has been observed in patients older than 65 years. However, the availability of new treatment options has improved the management also for non-transplantation-eligible MM patients [2]. In particular the introduction of new treatment options for non-transplantation-eligible patients has altered the goals of therapy. Prolongation of disease-free survival and Overall Survival (OS) remains the ultimate goal, but achieving prolonged treatment-free intervals and good quality of life have also become important aims, especially for this subset of patients [2].

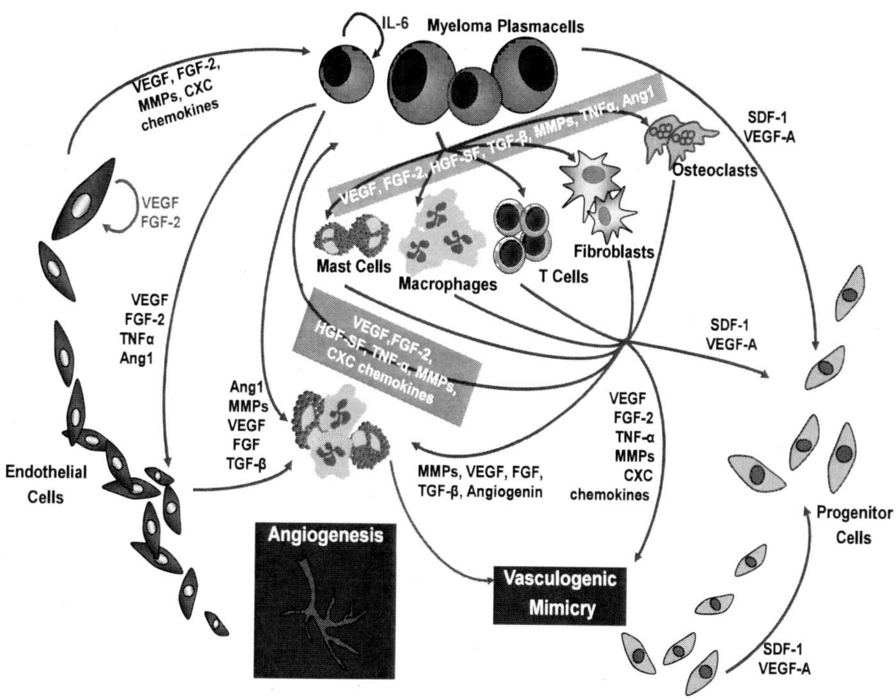

Figure 1.

The new treatment strategies have significantly improved the quality of responses with higher complete Remission (CR) rates in all subsets of patients, thus increasing long-term Progression-Free Survival (PFS) and OS. Achieving CR and sustaining it within a period of three years from the start of the treatment, is usually associated with a high survival rate. It is agreed that "The more profound the remission is, the longer the duration of response"[5]. Moreover, the use of more sensitive parameters such as free light-chain and multi-parameter flow cytometry can better define the depth of response. The Spanish group's prospective analysis of elderly patients receiving novel agents showed that achieving an immunophenotypic response translated into better PFS compared with conventional CR or stringent CR [5].

Old drugs such as the alkylating agent melphalan still play a central role in myeloma treatment and many issues remain unresolved. The treatment strategy should be personalized and 'risk-adapted'. The presence or absence of specific prognostic factors may determine the choice of therapy both at diagnosis and relapse. The treatment options for newly diagnosed patients are based on transplantation eligibility (relies on age and co-morbidities) and risk stratification. In general, high risk-patients are characterized by t(14;16), t(14;20), t(4;14), 17p or 13q deletion while all other patients have a standard-risk [1]. Newest drugs are emerging and are being tested in clinical trials such as immunomodulatory agents (pomalidomide) and new oral proteasome inhibitors (carfilzomib) with encouraging results [3, 6, 7].

New Treatments and Strategies

Development in MM biology has led to changes to the rationale of modern therapy [8]. In fact, the role of microenvironment in myeloma pathogenesis and progression has been well established [9], and the new drugs are designed to target simultaneously myeloma plasma cells and their microenvironment. This different approach has changed the natural history of MM, which still remains an incurable disease even though survival has significantly improved.

MM treatment strategies have largely changed in recent years with numerous new combinations available for initial approaches. A plethora of randomized data enable physicians to choose the best regimen for initial therapy but most available randomized trial data are comparisons of newer regimens with older alkylator- or anthracycline- based regimens. Only few trials have compared modern regimens between each other. Moreover, in these studies surrogate end points, such as response rates and PFS, were used. No randomized data with OS or quality-of-life end points are available. PFS cannot represent a good surrogate for clinical benefit. In numerous instances, PFS has proven to be a poor indicator of clinical benefit: the arm with PFS advantage showed [10, 11] inferior OS [12]. The choice of therapy is driven by surrogate end points such as CR or PFS that were primary end-points of worldwide randomized trials. OS or patient-reported quality-of-life remains the primary end-points that should drive the rational choice of treatment when a patient with MM needs initial therapy.

Moreover, an optimal treatment strategy for the newly diagnosed myeloma patients should be also based on the evaluation of risks and benefits [13]. The actual "cure versus control" debate on whether we should treat myeloma with an aggressive multidrug strategy targeting CR or a sequential disease control approach is primarily based on this aspect [13, 14]. The risk-adapted stratification of patients can be a good indicator for personalized treatments [15].

In standard-risk patients bortezomib-based regimens seem to be reasonable options for initial therapy. Higher CR rates, low toxicity, and the lack of any adverse effect on stem cell mobilization are the principal advantages compared to immunomodulatory-based regimens. The risk of neurotoxicity early in the disease course represents the major unfavorable factor. However, recent studies show that the neurotoxicity of bortezomib can be greatly diminished by administering bortezomib on a once-weekly schedule [16, 17] or by administering the drug subcutaneously [18].

In intermediate or high-risk patients, bortezomib-containing regimens followed by double ASCT and eventually maintenance therapy are able to overcome the poor prognosis with good CR rates and sustained CR [19, 20, 21]. Therefore, a bortezomib-containing regimen would be the preferred choice in this subset of patients.

The combination Bortezomib/Lenalidomide/Dexamethasone (VRD) is a rather expensive regimen and even though response and CR rates are very high it cannot be suggested as standard therapy outside clinical trials due to the lack of data from randomized trials regarding its safety and efficacy. However, it may represent a reasonable treatment option in high-risk myeloma patients since other current options appear inadequate.

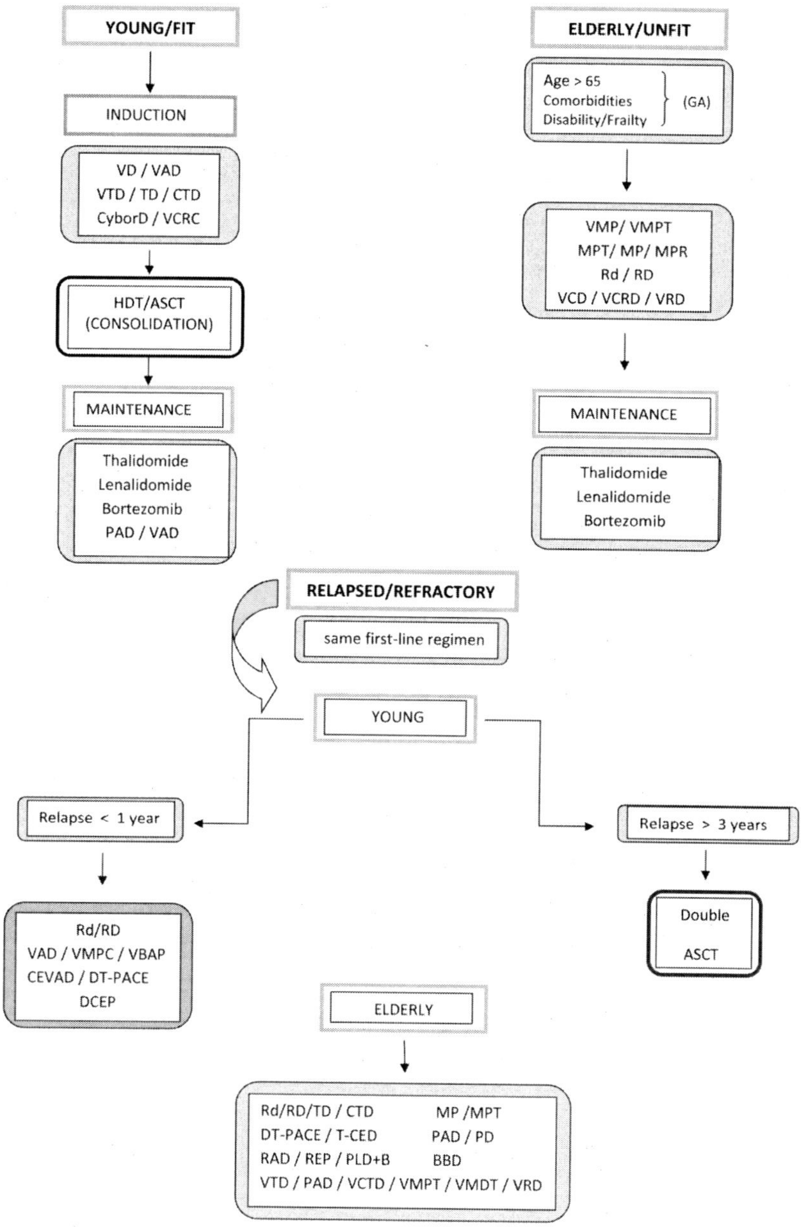

Figure 2. Treatment Algorithm.

At present, no sufficient data are available to recommend any quadruplet regimen as initial therapy outside of clinical trials. The multiagent combination regimen Bortezomib/ Dexamethasone/ Thalidomide/ Cisplatin/ Doxorubicin/ Cyclophosphamide/ Etoposide (VDT-PACE) may be a good choice in very high-risk patients with extensive extramedullary disease or plasma cell leukemia at the time of initial diagnosis [22].

In patients with acute renal failure due to suspected light-chain cast nephropathy, bortezomib-based regimens are of particular value and preferred as initial therapy [23].

In patients who are not candidates for ASCT, melphalan-containing regimens such as Melphalan/Prednisone/Thalisomide (MPT), Bortezomib/ Melphalan/Prednisone (VMP), and Melphalan/Prednisone/Lenalidomide (MPR) are indicated.

Finally, elderly patients are more susceptible to side effects and may be unable to tolerate full drug doses [24]. For these patients, lower dose-intensity regimens improve the safety profile and thus optimize treatment outcomes. The occurrence of serious hematological and non-hematological adverse events during treatment should be carefully taken into account in order to adjust doses and optimize the outcome.

Newly-Diagnosed Multiple Myeloma

Autologous Stem Cell Transplant

Induction therapy followed by ASCT has been regarded as standard therapy for younger patients with good health condition [25]. There is no formal definition of a young patient with MM, although this term is commonly used to identify a person for whom ASCT is planned as part of the treatment program [26]. Patients who are considered potential candidates for ASCT receive 2-4 cycles of a non-melphalan-containing regimen and then proceed to stem cell harvest [27]. Subsequently many patients undergo ASCT. However, depending on the response to initial therapy and the patient's choice, initial therapy can be resumed after stem cell harvest, delaying ASCT until first relapse. The role of early versus delayed ASCT is an argument of debate [28]. Although in a pilot study the OS for patients receiving early or late ASCT after conventional induction chemotherapy was equivalent. Furthermore early auto transplantation was associated with a longer event-free survival (EFS) and better quality of life. In the novel agent era, the issue of early versus late ASCT needs to be reevaluated in the context of large randomized clinical trials [29].

On the contrary, the second ASCT in patients who do not achieve almost a Very Good Partial Response (VGPR) after the first transplant, seems to be the best option[30].

Elderly or unfit patients who are not eligible for ASCT must undertake a treatment for approximately 9-18 months, some of which, such as lenalidomide/low dose dexamethasone (Rd), may be continued until progression if the patient tolerates it [31].

The introduction of novel agents into the induction regimens significantly improves the outcome of patients with newly diagnosed MM [32], probably because of increased rates of immunophenotypic and/or molecular remissions compared with that reported in the recent past.

The role of Bortezomib, the first proteasome inhibitor used in clinical practice in MM, alone and in combination with dexamethasone (VD), was initially explored in patients who were either eligible or ineligible for ASCT [33]. VD shows superior response rates when compared with vincristine/ doxorubicin/prednisone (VAD) with a VGPR rate of 38% vs. 15% after induction therapy in young patients. The higher VGPR rate was confirmed after transplantation (54% vs. 37%), with a PFS improvement (36 vs. 30 months) [10], but the improvement of OS has not been revealed. Sensory neuropathy is the most frequent bortezomib-related toxicity [34]. Studies that compared the 3 drug combination Bortezomib / Thalidomide / Dexamethasone (VTD) with Thalidomide / Dexamethasone (TD) or VD [19,

35] have shown the ability of VTD plus double ASCT followed by bortezomib-based consolidation to overcome the poor prognostic effects of t(4; 14) translocation [35]. After three cycles of induction therapy, VTD was superior to TD with respect to all categories of response, including CR, CR-nCR (31% versus 11%), and at least VGPR (62% vs. 28%). Beyond the best response rates in terms of PFS, it was demonstrated that the use of VTD is particularly useful in patients with acute renal failure as it acts quickly without dose reduction [35]. The addition of thalidomide, lenalidomide, or cyclophosphamide to bortezomib and dexamethasone has been associated with high response rates and longer progression-free survival (PFS). The three drug-combination Bortezomib/Cyclophosphamide/ Dexamethasone (CyBorD or VCD) and the four-drug combination Bortezomib/Cyclophosphamide/ Lenalidomide/Dexamethasone (VCRD) [11] have been studied in the randomized phase 2 trial EVOLUTION [36] in newly diagnosed myeloma patients. VCD was well tolerated with similar activity compared with the combination bortezomib/lenalidomide/dexamethasone (VRD), a combination which produces remarkably high overall and complete response rates [37]. The CR was achieved in 22% and 47% of patients treated with two different schedules of VCD versus 24% of patients treated with VRD. Although highly active, CR rates with VCRD were similar compared with either VCD or VRD. The "immunomodulatory" drugs thalidomide and its derivate lenalidomide have a complex mechanism of action. They target both tumor plasma cells and their microenvironment [38]. Their activity seems to be mediated through cereblon, the putative primary teratogenic target for thalidomide [39]. Thalidomide has a direct tumoricidal activity, an antiangiogenic effect and modulates tumor necrosis factor (TNF)-α signalling through direct and/or indirect effects on the tumour microenvironment [40], reduces Fibroblast Growth Factor (FGF)-2 [41], VEGF and IL-6 secretion in bone marrow stromal cells and by MM cells [42]. It also stimulates the activation and expansion of T cells and augments NK-cell-mediated cytotoxicity through its direct effect on T cells with a consequent increase in IL-2 and Interferon Gamma (IFN-γ) secretion [43], and interferes with NF-κB activity by blocking its ability to bind to DNA or suppresses IκB kinase activity, thus abrogating normal inflammatory cytokine production [44]. Thalidomide also disrupts the host marrow-MM cell interactions by selective modulation of the density of cell surface adhesion molecules [45]. Treatment with thalidomide is associated with sedation, fatigue, constipation, rash, deep-vein thrombosis, and peripheral neuropathy [46]. Lenalidomide is less toxic and more potent than thalidomide [47]. In patients with relapsed or refractory MM, lenalidomide can overcome resistance not only to conventional chemotherapy but also to thalidomide [48; 49]. In newly diagnosed MM, TD produces response rates of 65%-75% [50, 51]. Two randomized trials found TD to be superior to dexamethasone alone [52]. Patients receiving thalidomide-based regimens require deep vein thrombosis prophylaxis with aspirin, low-molecular weight heparin, or Coumadin [53]. In the transplant setting, there are some trials which aim to clarify the role of lenalidomide as induction therapy [54]. Although its use during induction determines good response rates, it seems to impact on the mobilization of stem cells [55, 56, 57].

Allogeneic Stem Cell Transplantation

Allogeneic transplantation (allo-SCT) is an alternative therapy that may improve survival for very high risk and selected patients. The role of allo-SCT remains controversial due to the

Treatment-Related Mortality (TRM) (10–20%) and Graft-Versus-Host Disease (GvHD) rates. Young patients with High-Risk disease, ISS II and III associated with del 1p/1q gain, t(4;14), del(17p) or t(14;16), in whom projected 4-year PFS and OS do not exceed 11% and 33%, respectively may potentially benefit from allo-SCT. Clinical trials with long-term follow up are important to prove that allo-SCT should not be abandoned in MM [58].

Elderly/Unfit Patients

Patients older than 65 years of age are generally not considered eligible for transplantation, although an age cut off for ASCT at 65 years does not reflect standard practice throughout the world. Biologic age can differ from chronologic age, thus it should be taken into account when determining whether a patient is fit for ASCT. A careful geriatric assessment (GA) to define fit versus unfit patients and consequently select and/or dose-reduce therapy is mandatory in this setting [58, 59]. Selected patients with good performance status can be considered for reduced-dose intensity transplantation (melphalan 100 mg/m2, Mel100). For patients aged 65 to 75 years, full-dose conventional therapy is recommended. Patients with significant comorbidities (serious heart, lung, renal, or liver dysfunction) or older than 75 years should receive treatments with appropriate dose reductions. The expected treatment-related side-effects should always be considered when choosing the appropriate treatment. The latter should be immediately discontinued when serious adverse events arise. When serious adverse events are completely resolved, treatment should be restarted with an appropriate dose reduction [59]. Useful treatment strategies and dose-adjustment recommendations have been evaluated in several clinical trials.

In the phase 3 VISTA trial, the combination of Bortezomib/Melphalan/ Prednisone (VMP) compared with Melphalan/Prednisone (MP) was associated with significantly improved OS which persisted with long-term follow-up [60,61]. A subsequent randomized trial showed no significant advantage of Bortezomib/Thalidomide/Prednisone (VTP) over VMP [62]. The principal toxicity of VMP is peripheral neuropathy, which can be reduced using the once a week regimen or the subcutaneous administration of bortezomib [62, 63, 64].

The Italian GIMEMA [63] group compared the combination Bortezomib/ Melphalan/Prednisone/Thalidomide (VMPT) with VMP in a randomized phase 3 trial. The 3-year PFS rate was 56% and 41% respectively. However, patients in the VMPT arm received maintenance therapy with bortezomib and thalidomide, whereas patients in the VMP arm did not receive any additional therapy beyond 9 months. Furthermore, no OS differences were observed: the 3-year OS was 89% and 87% respectively, thus confirming that the use of VMPT as initial therapy has no advantage.

Lenalidomide-based regimens are superior in terms of activity and toxicity when compared to TD. In a Mayo Clinic study of 411 newly diagnosed patients lenalidomide plus dexamethasone showed higher response rates, PFS, and OS [64]. Another phase 3 study has demonstrated TD to be inferior to MP in newly diagnosed elderly patients in terms of OS [65]. MP can be considered a suitable option for initial therapy in patients with acute renal failure, and in combination with bortezomib.

Several randomized trials have shown better response rates with MPT compared to MP [66, 67, 68, 69, 70, 71, 16]. A significant prolongation of PFS and an OS advantage was also observed with the MPT combination [66, 67, 68, 70]. Thromboprophylaxis is mandatory due to the considerable risk (20%) of deep vein thrombosis related to MPT.

Rd is active in newly diagnosed myeloma patients [72] and related to less toxicity and better patient's compliance and OS compared to lenalidomide plus high-dose dexamethasone (RD) [73]. Furthermore high-dose dexamethasone is difficult to incorporate into combination regimens due to its toxicity. The 3-year OS rate with Rd in patients older than 70 who did not receive ASCT is 70% [74], and is comparable to results with MPT and VMP. All patients receiving Rd require antithrombosis prophylaxis [53].

The combination Melphalan/Prednisone/Lenalidomide (MPR) has been recently compared to MP in a randomized trial of 65 years of age or older MM patients [75]. The median PFS was similar between the two groups, 14 versus 13 months respectively. The lack of improvement in PFS with MPR may be related to the dose reductions of both melphalan and lenalidomide often needed when the 2 agents are combined.

The EVOLUTION trial [36, 37] showed similar activity and CR rates between the three combinations VCD, VCRD and VRD in newly diagnosed MM patients. Multiagent combination regimens such as Bortezomib/ Dexamethasone/Thalidomide /Cisplatin /Doxorubicin/Cyclophosphamide/Etoposide (VDT-PACE) have been tested extensively at the Myeloma Institute for Research and Therapy at Arkansas [22], and are particularly useful in patients with aggressive disease.

Cytogenetic abnormalities have been found in approximately 25% of elderly MM patients. High-risk cytogenetic profiles include del(17p), t(4;14), and/or t (14;16) and are associated with a high risk of disease progression and very poor prognosis. Patients with high-risk cytogenetic abnormalities enrolled in the trial in which Len-Dex was compared with Len-dex, were less likely to reach VGPR and showed shorter 2-year OS. In the VISTA trial (VMP versus MP), patients with high cytogenetic risk had the same CR rate and similar TTP and OS times as patients with standard risk, thus suggesting the ability of bortezomib to overcome the poor prognosis of these patients. The GIMEMA group showed a PFS benefit in response to VMPT plus VT maintenance over VMP in patients with high and standard cytogenetic risk patients. The Spanish trial (induction with VMP/VTP and maintenance with VP/VT) showed similar results. However, these bortezomib-based regimens were unable to overcome the negative impact of high-risk cytogenetics, since the PFS and OS were significantly shorter in patients with t(4;14) and/or del(17p). Recently, the IFM group reported similar results: t(4;14) and del(17p) were associated with shorter PFS and OS regardless of the treatment received. These data indicate that the first generation of novel agents do not overcome the negative prognosis of high-risk cytogenetic abnormalities in newly diagnosed elderly patients with MM [2].

Relapsed/Refractory Multiple Myeloma

The time and type of relapse, the efficacy and toxicity of drugs used in prior therapies, age, comorbidities, and patient preferences, bone marrow reserve and renal function must be taken into account in the therapeutic strategy at the time of relapse. Patients with a long first plateau phase after their initial therapy may benefit from the same first-line regimen. Drugs that have shown little or no efficacy and which would only contribute to increase toxicity should be avoided [75].

In young patients with relapse occurred after 3 years from the first autologous stem cell transplantation, a second ASCT is a viable option if the patient has good performance status and whether the patient has responded well to the first transplant procedure. The overall response rates in recent studies, in small sample size, range from 55% to 69%, with a 100-day mortality rate of 10% [76, 77]. Very few relapsed/refractory MM patients (< 1 year) are ultimately cured with allogeneic transplant which shows limited clinical benefit with long-term, disease-free survival of 10% to 20% and high toxicity [21, 78]. In this setting multidrug combinations and high-dose chemotherapy may include high-dose melphalan; high-dose methylprednisolone; high-dose dexamethasone; VAD; Vincristine/Melphalan/Cyclophosphamide/Prednisone (VMPC) alternating with Vincristine/ Carmustine/Doxorubicin/Prednisone (VBAP); Doxorubicin/Vincristine/Dexamethasone/ Etoposide/Cyclophosphamide (CEVAD); Cisplatin/ Doxorubicin/ Cyclophosphamide/ Etoposide (DT-PACE); Dexamethasone/ Cyclophosphamide/ Etoposide/Cisplatin (DCEP) [20; 79-85]. With these therapies overall response rates are between 25% and 65%. Morbidity and mortality are related to the intensity of therapy.

Patients with renal impairment should be considered eligible for bortezomib-containing regimens, since they determine a rapid reduction in light chain load to the kidneys, and maximize the chance of regaining renal function. At each relapse should be considered the possibility to be enrolled in a clinical trial.

In elderly patients, the best choice after the first relapse should be a different regimen from the previous one. If the first remission is long enough, retreatment with the same scheme can be considered. At second or subsequent relapse a clinical trial with experimental agents should be encouraged. If the patient is not eligible for active therapies, palliative treatment with oral cyclophosphamide (50 mg on alternating days) and prednisone (30 mg/day) is recommended [75]. The introduction of thalidomide, bortezomib, and lenalidomide has markedly improved the outcome of patients with relapsed/refractory multiple myeloma.

Thalidomide was the first novel agent to be evaluated in these patients and it has been successfully combined with multiple conventional cytotoxic agents. When compared with thalidomide alone, the addition of dexamethasone resulted in higher response rates of about 50% [86]. Also the addition of cyclophosphamide to thalidomide, with or without dexamethasone, led to higher responses (>PR: 57%– 84%) [87,88]. Furthermore the efficacy of thalidomide in relapsed/refractory MM has been improved by the combination with melphalan (>PR: 59%), MP (>PR: 42%), melphalan/dexamethasone (PR: 70%), Pegylated Liposomal Doxorubicin/Dexamethasone (>PR in 76%), Pegylated Liposomal Doxorubicin/ Vincristine/Dexamethasone (>PR: 75%), DT-PACE (>PR: 32%), or Cyclophosphamide/ Etoposide/ Dexamethasone (TCED; >PR: 68%) [89-93].

Bortezomib regimens have demonstrated marked activity in rrMM, particularly when combined with dexamethasone demonstrating superior response rates (43%v18%; P<.001), TTP (6.2 months v 3.5 months; P<.001), and 1-year OS (80%v66%;P<.003) in the randomized phase III APEX with a survival benefit in patients who had received a median of two prior therapies [94]. Multiple chemotherapeutic agents have been successfully combined with bortezomib in relapsed/refractory MM, such as the combination with pegylated liposomal doxorubicin (>PR: 44%), Low-Dose Dexamethasone/ Pegylated Liposomal

Doxorubicin (PAD) (>PR: 67% to 85%), oral or intravenous melphalan (>PR: 47% to 68%), and Low-Dose Cyclophosphamide/Prednisone/Dexamethasone (>PR: 68% to 82%) [95-98].

An attractive combination partner for bortezomib can be represented by bendamustine. A phase 2 study has demonstrated that the 3 drug combination Bendamustine-Bortezomib-Dexamethasone (BBD) is effective for patients with relapsed/refractory myeloma. The regimen induced responses in two thirds of patients and produced a PFS of 9.7 months and OS of 25.6 months in patients with a median of 2 prior treatment lines, frequently containing bortezomib and/or lenalidomide, and is active in patients with FISH-defined high-risk cytogenetics. Generally the regimen was well tolerated [99].

In 2006, the US Food and Drug Administration approved lenalidomide for use in combination with dexamethasone in patients with relapse/refractory MM. As a single agent at the maximum dose of 25 mg once a day, Lenalidomide determined response rates ranging from 29% to 39% in patients who had received a median of three prior therapies [100].

The two trials MM-009 and MM-010 compared RD vs. dexamethasone alone with improved overall response (60.6% v 21.9%; P>.001), TTP (13.4 months v 4.6 months; P>.001), and OS (38.0 months v 31.6 months; P>.045) for patients treated with RD [101-103]. This combination appears to be effective also in elderly (>75 years) patients, demonstrating overall response rates of 62% and median PFS of 14 months [104]. Currently, all new dexamethasone combination trials use low-dose dexamethasone instead of high dose dexamethasone.

Lenalidomide demonstrates efficacy in relapse/refractory MM patients also when combined with other agents such as doxorubicin/dexamethasone (RAD; >PR: 73%), Low-Dose Cyclophosphamide/Prednisone (REP; minimal response or better [>MR]: 64.3%), Cyclophosphamide/Dexamethasone (>MR: 75%), and Pegylated Liposomal Doxorubicin/ Vincristine/Dexamethasone (>PR: 75%) [105-108].

The combination of two established novel agents with conventional and/or cytotoxic drugs in the relapsed/refractory setting [109-114] has been investigated in several studies. Bortezomib has been successfully combined with thalidomide and other drugs: VTD >PR: 63%, PAD >PR: 74%, VCTD >PR: 88%, VMPT >PR: 67%, and VMDT >PR: 66%. Other studies have evaluated the combination of VRD with good response rate (>MR: 61% to 86%) even in patients resistant to thalidomide, lenalidomide, or bortezomib [7]. Lenalidomide enhances the activity of both bortezomib and dexamethasone, probably through a dual caspase 8 and 9–mediated apoptotic pathway. The combination shows activity in patients previously refractory to bortezomib and IMIDs. Thus, it may resensitize resistant tumor cells. The addition of dexamethasone contributes to rescue patients with progressive disease, showing ≥ 67% PR when using bortezomib, lenalidomide, and dexamethasone in relapse/refractory patients with MM, vs. 39% PR obtained with the doublet bortezomib/lenalidomide [115]. Despite these considerations recent studies have demonstrated that the sequential use of bortezomib and lenalidomide is better than their simultaneous use [75].

Maintenance Therapy

Historically, maintenance therapy was performed with corticosteroids, interferon, and thalidomide. Prolonged PFS, but not OS, significant morbidity and high discontinuation rates were observed. Actually this topic represents one of the most controversial debates in the care of MM patients [116, 117]. Although new therapies have improved the response and survival rates, all MM patients relapse due to residual disease. Latest evidence suggests that consolidation or long-term treatment is able to sustain remission keeping the disease under control [2]. Route and frequency of administration, patient-specific elements such as potential toxicities, end-organ function, quality of life, cytogenetics, and previous treatment should be considered when selecting a maintenance therapy strategy. In elderly patients, the effectiveness of long-term treatment should be balanced against tolerability and patient compliance [118]. The use Thalidomide or lenalidomide as maintenance therapy following ASCT has recently been evaluated in clinical trials with improvements in PFS and OS. A PFS benefit, but no OS advantage, have been also observed with the use of dexamethasone, thalidomide, lenalidomide, or combination bortezomib with thalidomide in patients who did not undergo transplantation [118]. Maintenance therapy with Lenalidomide, a more tolerable IMiD, has been explored in recent randomized, placebo-controlled trials in patients after ASCT compared with placebo, and in older patients initially treated with melphalan-based regimens. Only one of these studies has shown a survival benefit [75, 119, 120]. Available data are not sufficient to recommend routine maintenance with lenalidomide for all patients outside clinical trials. Nevertheless it can be considered in patients whose benefits appear to overcome the risks (e.g., standard-risk patients who are known to be lenalidomide responsive and who are not in VGPR or better after completion of initial therapy).

A recent trial has compared PAD with VAD. Patients treated with the PAD regimen received maintenance with bortezomib (every 2 weeks) after ASCT, and those in the VAD arm received thalidomide as maintenance. The trial shows benefit of using bortezomib not only for induction but also for maintenance after ASCT [121]. In intermediate- and high-risk myeloma patients, a bortezomib-based maintenance approach may be preferable, but needs further investigation. Preliminary results are encouraging and suggest improved PFS and OS with bortezomib maintenance.

Additional studies are needed to better define the timing for initiation and duration of maintenance therapy, determine the role of cytogenetics and the combinations necessary to achieve an optimal increase in OS, to further characterize possible resistance patterns. Until further data are available, the risks and benefits should be evaluated on a patient-specific basis [118].

New Drugs

IMiDs

Pomalidomide is the most potent IMiD, 100 times more than thalidomide and 10 times more than lenalidomide [122]. Pomalidomide exerts its anticancer effects through angiogenesis inhibition, immunomodulation, impeding cytokine production, and interaction with the bone marrow and tumor microenvironment dependent on Cereblon expression [123].

Pomalidomide appears to remain effective in lenalidomide resistant cells in which a reduction of cereblon mRNA expression is observed [39, 123]. Similarly to lenalidomide, pomalidomide causes both cell cycle arrest and apoptosis [124], by P21 WAF activation independently of P53. This highlights the possibility in using these agents to treat P53 mutated malignancies [125].

Furthermore, similarly to lenalidomide and thalidomide, the addition of dexamethasone induces synergy, improving the response rate and the PFS. A phase 2 study [126] showed 62% response rate with a PFS of 13 months. Interestingly most of the patients had been previously exposed to IMIDs.

The activity of this combination has been explored in lenalidomide- and bortezomib-refractory patients enrolled in clinical trials in which approximately one-third of patients achieved at least partial response (PR) and the PFS ranged from 3.3 to 7.7 months.

The phase 3 trial (MM-003) showed a significant advantage for the pomalidomide arm over dexamethasone in terms of ORR (31% vs. 10%), PFS (4 vs. 1.9 months) and OS (not reached vs. 7.8 months). The patients had previously failed both lenalidomide and bortezomib therapies.

Hematological side effects are the main source of toxicity. Low rates of deep venous thrombosis is observed if prophylactic measures are adopted. Nonhematologic toxicities are seen in 5% of patients: fatigue in 62% of cases (8% grade 3–4), thromboembolic events in 3%, peripheral neuropathy in 13% (up to 33% in patients with pre-existing neuropathy that worsens) [127, 128].

In high-risk patients responses were observed in 74% of cases. Also in extramedullary disease in the phase II study conducted at the Mayo Clinic [129] the response rate was 31%, with two patients achieving CR and two patients achieving PR [130]. Two phase II studies conducted at the Mayo Clinic [126] in which two dosing strategies are compared, suggest that 4 mg daily dosing does not yield superior responses than 2 mg daily dosing(43 versus 49%). 26% of patients achieved at least a PR in both cohorts. In contrast, a trend towards a dose-dependent response was observed in the phase I MM-002 study [127]. Toxicities are similar at the 2 and 4 mg dose levels.

Several trials in relapsed/refractory patients are already testing the activity of pomalidomide and dexamethasone in combination with several agents.

Proteasome Inhibitors

Carfilzomib (PR-171) is a more efficacious and less toxic irreversible proteasome inhibitor, inhibiting the chymotrypsin-like site of the proteasome. It shows additional inhibitory effects on the trypsin-like and caspase-like sites with higher doses [131].

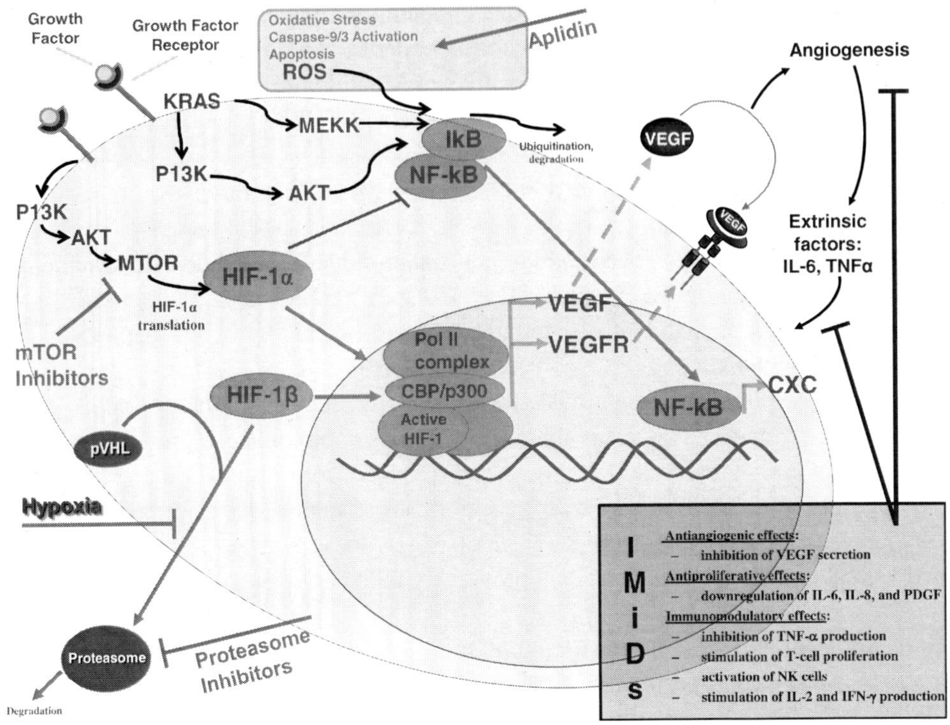

Figure 3.

Carfilzomib has shown single-agent activity in heavily pretreated MM patients in the twice-weekly regimen with dose-reduction (20 mg/m2) in the first cycle to abrogate potential tumor-lysis syndrome [132]. Clinical benefits were observed in one-third of the patients. The outcome was not influenced by adverse cytogenetics, renal impairment, disease stage, or performance score. The response rate was 23.7%, with a median duration of response of 7.8 months, a PFS of 3.7 months, and an OS of 15.6 months. Drug-related adverse events (AEs) of all grades were most frequently fatigue (37%), nausea (34%), and thrombocythemia. Hematologic AE grade 3/4 included anemia (24%), thrombocytopenia (29%) and lymphopenia (20%). Peripheral neuropathy was uncommon (12.4%). Dose adjustment for renal insufficiency was not necessary [133].

In bortezomib-naive patients, carfilzomib showed an impressive single-agent ORR of 52% [134].

The addition of lenalidomide and low-dose dexamethasone to carfilzomib improved the response rate [135, 136] with an overall response of 78-98% and a complete remission rate of 42% after a median of 12 cycles of therapy.

The combination with melphalan and prednisone (CMP) administered on the usual schedule was safe and effective in newly diagnosed elderly patients showed a response rate of 92% [136]. The cyclophosphamide/carfilzomib/thalidomide/dexamethasone (CYCLONE) combination in newly diagnosed MM patients demonstrated a response rate of 100% [137].

Other proteasome inhibitors, such as Delanzomib (CEP18770), Marizomib (NPI-0052) and Ixazomib (MLN9708), are currently being evaluated in phase I and II studies [138]. Marizomib (NPI-0052), an orally active proteasome inhibitor, is a more potent inhibitor of the NF-kB and other cytokines than bortezomib [138]. It interferes with the chymotryptic-like, tryptic-like and caspase-like proteolytic activity of the proteasome. In vitro and in vivo studies show that marizomib overcomes bortezomib resistance and a synergistic effect with the latter has been also observed. Marizomib as a single agent and in combination with bortezomib is being evaluated in clinical trials [139].

Histone Deacetylase Inhibitors

The expression of genes is controlled by DNA/histone interaction. Excessive deactylated level of histones promote the repression of tumor suppressor genes thus favouring cancer development. Overexpression of histone deacetylase (HDAC) by MM cells results in decreased DNA transcription, including transcription of tumor suppressor genes and inhibition of HDAC which reverses these effects [140]. HDAC inhibitors mediate tumor cell death via caspase-dependent and independent apoptosis and autophagy [141], induce cell cycle arrest via p21 up-regulation, block the aggresome complex and induce cell death via the accumulation of ubiquitinated proteins [142].

Currently several HDAC inhibitors have being studied as single agents or in combination with other agents mainly bortezomib and lenalidomide. Vorinostat (SAHA) is an oral HDAC inhibitor that downregulates IGF-1 and IL6 signaling pathways as well as DNA synthesis and repair enzymes [143].

In phase I trials in patients with relapsed/refractory MM disease oral vorinostat was well tolerated. Side effects included fatigue, anorexia, diarrhea and nausea. The combination with bortezomib has shown promising activity [144]. On 23 patients with a median of 7 prior regimens the response rate was 42% including 3 PR among 9 bortezomib-refractory patients.

Panobinostat (LBH589), has been tested in combination with other therapies for relapsed/refractory MM. It is a potent pandeacetylase inhibitor that disrupts aggresome and HSP90 function via inhibition of HDAC6, promoting cytotoxic misfolded/unfolded protein aggregates and MM cell death[142]. In a phase I study the response rate was 68% of patients across all cohorts and, particularly, 62% in bortezomib-refractory patients. Major adverse events included grade 3/4 thrombocytopenia, neutropenia, diarrhea, nausea, pyrexia and fatigue. Various phase I, II and III studies are ongoing to establish the role of panobinostat and its combinations with new agents such as bortezomib, lenalidomide, carfilzomib, in MM treatments.

Romidepsin, Belinostat, ITF2357 and AR 42, other HDAC inhibitors, are still under investigation.

AKT Inhibitors

Perifosine (KRX-0401) is a novel synthetic oral AKT inhibitor [145]. The activation of AKT-pathway induces growth and survival advantage in MM cells through GSK-3β and mTOR phosphorylation. Furthermore it has been associated with advanced stage and poor prognosis in MM patients and resistance to dexamethasone [135].

In a phase I/II study the combination of perifosine and bortezomib, with or without dexamethasone, showed a response rate of 41% (65% in the bortezomib-group vs. 32% in the bortezomib-refractory group) [147] with manageable toxicity. The same combinations in patients with relapsed/refractory MM previously exposed to bortezomib is being evaluated in a phase III randomized trial.

mTOR Inhibitors

The mammalian target of rapamycin (mTOR) is an intracellular serine-threonine kinase that controls cell growth, proliferation, motility, survival and metabolism. mTOR exerts its downstream effects through the formation of protein complexes called mTORC1 and mTORC2 with different functions and target molecules [148]. mTOR acts as a neoplastic switch that is frequently turned on by many mutations found in cancer and hence inhibition of mTOR and its complex offers a promising target.

In a phase II study, temsirolimus showed 38% response rate on 16 patients with relapsed/refractory MM with a TTP of 138 days and a good toxicity profile [149]. The combination of temsirolimus with bortezomib obtains a PR or better in 33% of patients [150]. Everolimus (RAD001) has been studied in MM as a single agent and in combination with lenalidomide, but no encouraging results have been shown. Other mTOR inhibitors such as ridaforolimus are currently being evaluated for their anti-MM activity in preclinical phase I studies.

Emerging data have shown that rapamycin analogs as well as mTOR inhibitors that have activity against mTORC2 do not appear to be effective as monotherapy (only SD or MR obtained in clinical trials with rare PR). They may represent agents that could be evaluated in combination with other anti-myeloma agents in the future.

Heat Shock Protein 90 (HSP 90) Inhibitors

Heat shock protein 90 (HSP90) is a molecular chaperone that facilitates the folding and stability of numerous signaling molecules that control the growth and survival of cancer cells [151]. The client proteins for HSP90 include transcription factors, oncogenic kinases and receptors that are associated functionally with cell cycle control and signaling. HSP90 has been shown to be a key molecular chaperone for signal transduction proteins critical to MM cell growth, survival and drug resistance.

Preclinical studies with tanespimycin (KOS-953) (a small molecule inhibitor of HSP90) have shown a rationale for combining HSP90 inhibitors with bortezomib because of bortezomib-induction of HSP90 along with up-regulation of stress response gene transcripts. HSP90 inhibition increases bortezomib-induced apoptosis in MM cells by blocking the HSP90 stress response. Moreover, tanespimycin may also be protective against bortezomib-associated peripheral neuropathy. The combination tanespimycin/bortezomib in relapsed/refractory MM patients obtained a response rate of 41% in bortezomib-naïve, 20% in bortezomib-pretreated and 14% in bortezomib-refractory patients respectively. Adverse events included diarrhea (60%), fatigue (49%), nausea (49%), thrombocytopenia (40%), and AST elevation (29%). Grade 1-2 peripheral neuropathy was observed in 21% patients with no grade 3-4 peripheral neuropathy, consistent with tanespimycin's neuroprotective effect [152]. Other HSP90 inhibitors are currently in early phase trials in MM.

Monoclonal Antibodies

Monoclonal antibodies (MoAb) represent a new anticancer strategy [153] for patients refractory to new drugs. A large variety of antigen targets can be expressed either on myeloma cells or on components of the bone marrow microenvironment. The majority of them are in preclinical phase/early clinical trials [153, 154].

The use of MoAbs as monotherapy generally do not result in good responses in MM patients. However, preclinical and preliminary clinical data in patients with relapsed/refractory MM suggest that MoAbs act synergistically with dexamethasone, immunomodulators, bortezomib, and show the ability to overcome resistance to these drugs [155]. To date we cannot establish when and in which patients the newest drugs are useful. Their use should be limited to patients enrolled in clinical trials until their conclusion and until the role of these newest drugs in myeloma treatments will be clarified.

Elotuzumab is the best evaluated of these agents in MM. It targets CS1, a glycoprotein that is highly specific to plasma cells. The combination with lenalidomide and dexamethasone has given excellent results with >80% PR in relapsed patients and prolonged PFS. The synergistic action may be attributed to an immune-mediated mechanism: lenalidomide would prepare the natural killer and lymphoid cells to favor the immune recognition, and elotuzumab would modify the plasma cells to be more prone to be targeted by the immune cells. A phase III registration-enabling trial in relapsed myeloma comparing lenalidomide+dexamethasone with lenalidomide+dexamethasone+elotuzumab has just been completed [128].

B-cell activating factor (BAFF) is a member of the tumor necrosis factor superfamily that promotes the survival of malignant B cells, including those in MM. An anti-BAFF monoclonal antibody, tabalumab, a potent and selective fully human IgG4 with neutralizing activity against both membrane-bound and soluble BAFF, has been combined with bortezomib with or without dexamethasone with 46% achieving PR or better [128].

Daratumumab is an anti-CD38 antibody designed to induce the killing of myeloma cells. In the dose-escalation study with daratumumab monotherapy, in a very heavily pretreated population, 42% of them achieved at least PR at doses considered to reach therapeutic levels. These results are highly promising for a drug used in monotherapy in patients with a median of six previous treatments [128].

Aplidin

Plitidepsin (Aplidin) is a cyclic depsipeptide isolated from the Mediterranean tunicate Aplidium albicans that has shown promising in vitro and in vivo antitumor activity in a variety of malignancies. It triggers Fas/CD95-, JNK-, and mitochondrial-mediated apoptotic signaling pathways, showing a strong apoptotic activity on a panel of human MM cell lines, as well as on MM cell cultures from patients, including those resistant to conventional and novel therapies. Phase I and II clinical trials have reported encouraging results with a good toxicity profile [156]. The most important side effects concerned the muscles and bones and were sometimes associated with fatal acute renal failure, transient and reversible transaminases increase was also observed [157]. Phase III trials in MM are still ongoing.

Conclusion

MM treatment strategies and therapies are widely changed over the last decade with the aim to improve patient's survival. The evaluation of treatments must include patient's stratification and personalized therapies. At the same time, it is becoming more important to control the disease in a long-term fashion, maintaining the QoL of the patient.

Our understanding of MM pathogenesis including the intracellular mechanisms as well as the interactions between MM cells and their microenvironment has contributed to the discovery of numerous targets that have become the focus of the development of new drugs. Future studies will focus on the use of these targeted agents in multidrug-combinations: this will maximize their synergism while minimizing toxicities. Several agents and combinations are currently in different clinical studies and are likely to change the natural history of MM in the near future.

Considering the ability of new therapies to modify MM biology, it is reasonable to think of their use as continuous therapy reducing or suppressing the tumor itself.

References

[1] Maes K1, et al. (2013). Epigenetic modulating agents as a new therapeutic approach in multiple myeloma. *Cancers* (Basel). 5(2):430-61.

[2] Mateos MV1 et al. (2013). How should we treat newly diagnosed multiple myeloma patients? *Hematology Am. Soc. Hematol. Educ. Program*: 488-95.

[3] Palumbo A, et al. (2014). New Approaches to Management of Multiple Myeloma. *Curr. Treat. Options Oncol.* (Abstract)

[4] Su J1, et al. (2014). Targeting the biophysical properties of the myeloma initiating cell niches: a pharmaceutical synergism analysis using multi-scale agent-based modeling. *PLoS One*. 9(1):e85059.

[5] Chanan-Khan AA, et al. (2010). Importance of achieving a complete response in multiple myeloma, and the impact of novel agents. *J. Clin. Oncol;* 28: 2612–2624.

[6] Kyle RA1, et al. (2014). An overview of the progress in the treatment of multiple myeloma. *Expert Rev. Hematol.* 7(1):5-7.

[7] Palumbo A & Anderson K. (2011). Multiple myeloma. *N. Engl. J. Med;* 364: 1046–1060.

[8] Borrello I. (2012) Can we change the disease biology of multiple myeloma? *Leuk. Res;* 36: S3–12.

[9] Manier S, et al. (2012). Bone marrow microenvironment in multiple myeloma progression. *J. Biomed. Biotechnol*; 157496.

[10] Harousseau JL, et al. (2010). Bortezomib plus dexamethasone is superior to vincristine plus doxorubicin plus dexamethasone as induction treatment prior to autologous stem-cell transplantation in newly diagnosed multiple myeloma: results of the IFM 2005-01 phase III trial. *J. Clin. Oncol.* : 28: 4621–4629.

[11] Reeder CB, et al. (2009). Cyclophosphamide, bortezomib and dexamethasone induction for newly diagnosed multiple myeloma: high response rates in a phase II clinical trial. *Leukemia*; 23: 1337–1341.

[12] Rajkumar SV, et al. (2010). Lenalidomide plus high-dose dexamethasone versus lenalidomide plus low-dose dexamethasone as initial therapy for newly diagnosed multiple myeloma: an open-label randomised controlled trial. *Lancet Oncol*; 11: 29–37.
[13] Rajkumar SV,et al. (2011). Approach to the treatment of multiple myeloma: a clash of philosophies. *Blood*; 118: 3205–3211.
[14] Rajkumar SV, et al. (2008). Treatment of myeloma: cure vs. control. *Mayo Clin. Proc*; 83: 1142–1145.
[15] Mikhael JR., et al. (2013). Management of Newly Diagnosed Symptomatic Multiple Myeloma: Updated Mayo Stratification of Myeloma and Risk-Adapted Therapy (mSMART) Consensus Guidelines 2013. *Mayo Clin. Proc*. 2013; 88: 360-376).
[16] Beksac M, et al. (2011). Addition of thalidomide to oral melphalan/prednisone in patients with multiple myeloma not eligible for transplantation: results of a randomized trial from the Turkish Myeloma Study Group. *Eur. J. Haematol*; 86: 16–22.
[17] Kapoor P, et al. (2011). Melphalan and prednisone versus melphalan, prednisone and thalidomide for elderly and/or transplant ineligible patients with multiple myeloma: a meta-analysis. *Leukemia*; 25: 689–696.
[18] Moreau P, et al. (2011). Subcutaneous versus intravenous administration of bortezomib in patients with relapsed multiple myeloma: a randomised, phase 3, non-inferiority study. *Lancet Oncol*; 12: 431–440.
[19] Moreau P, et al. (2011). Bortezomib plus dexamethasone versus reduced-dose bortezomib, thalidomide plus dexamethasone as induction treatment before autologous stem cell transplantation in newly diagnosed multiple myeloma. *Blood*; 118: 5752–5758.
[20] Gertz MA, et al. (1995). A phase II study of high-dose methylprednisolone in refractory or relapsed multiple myeloma. *Leukemia*; 9: 2115–2118.
[21] Kröger N, et al. (2004). Relapse to prior autograft and chronic graft-versus-host disease are the strongest prognostic factors for outcome of melphalan/fludarabine-based dose-reduced allogeneic stem cell transplantation in patients with multiple myeloma. *Biol. Blood Marrow Transplant*; 10: 698–708.
[22] Barlogie B, et al. (2007). Incorporating bortezomib into upfront treatment for multiple myeloma: early results of total therapy 3. *Br. J. Haematol.*; 138: 176–185.
[23] San-Miguel J, et al. (2008). Individualizing treatment of patients with myeloma in the era of novel agents. *J. Clin. Oncol*; 26:2761–2766.
[24] Palumbo A, et al. (2011). Personalized therapy in MM according to patient age and vulnerability: a report of the European Myeloma Network (EMN). *Blood*; 118: 4519–4529.
[25] Shuji O & Kazuyuki S. (2014). Autologous Stem Cell Transplantation in Elderly Patients with Multiple Myeloma: Past, Present, and Future. *BioMed Research International*, Article ID 394792(7).
[26] Boccadoro M, et al. (2011). International Myeloma Working Group consensus approach to the treatment of multiple myeloma patients who are candidates for autologous stem cell transplantation. *Blood* 117: 6063-6073.
[27] Gertz MA, et al. (2008). Autologous stem cell transplant in 716 patients with multiple myeloma: low treatment related mortality, feasibility of outpatient transplant, and effect of a multidisciplinary quality initiative. *Mayo Clin. Proc*; 83: 1131–1138.

[28] Moreau P & Rajkumar SV. (2012). Should all eligible patients with multiple myeloma receive autologous stem-cell transplant as part of initial treatment? *Leuk. Res*; 36: 677–681.

[29] Ladetto M, et al. (2010). Major tumor shrinking and persistent molecular remissions after consolidation with bortezomib, thalidomide, and dexamethasone in patients with autografted myeloma. *J. Clin. Oncol.*; 28(12): 2077-2084.

[30] Cavo M, et al. (2007). Prospective, randomized study of single compared with double autologous stem-cell transplantation for multiple myeloma: Bologna 96 clinical study. *J. Clin. Oncol.*; 25: 2434-2441.

[31] Palumbo A & Niesvizky R. (2012). Sustained disease control in transplant-ineligible patients: the role of continuous therapy. *Leuk. Res*; 36 Suppl 1:S19-26.

[32] Kumar SK, et al. (2008). Improved survival in multiple myeloma and the impact of novel therapies. *Blood*; 111: 2516–2520.

[33] Dispenzieri A, et al. (2010). Primary therapy with single agent bortezomib as induction, maintenance and re-induction in patients with high-risk myeloma: results of the ECOG E2A02 trial. *Leukemia*; 24: 1406–1411.

[34] Argyriou AA, et al. (2008). Bortezomib-induced peripheral neuropathy in multiple myeloma: a comprehensive review of the literature. *Blood.*;112(5):1593-1599.

[35] Cavo M, et al. (2010). Bortezomib with thalidomide plus dexamethasone compared with thalidomide plus dexamethasone as induction therapy before, and consolidation therapy after, double autologous stem-cell transplantation in newly diagnosed multiple myeloma: a randomised phase 3 study. *Lancet*; 376: 2075–2085.

[36] Kumar S, et al. (2012). Randomized, multicenter, phase 2 study (EVOLUTION) of combinations of bortezomib, dexamethasone, cyclophosphamide, and lenalidomide in previously untreated multiple myeloma. *Blood*, 119: 4375–4382.

[37] Richardson PG, et al. (2010). Lenalidomide, bortezomib, and dexamethasone combination therapy in patients with newly diagnosed multiple myeloma. *Blood* ; 116: 679–686.

[38] Singhal S., et al. (1999). Antitumor activity of thalidomide in refractory multiple myeloma. *N. Engl. J. Med*; 341: 1565–1571.

[39] Zhu Y, et al. (2011). Cereblon expression is required for the antimyeloma activity of lenalidomide and pomalidomide. *Blood*; 118: 4771–4779.

[40] Sonneveld, P., et al. (2001). Segeren intensified chemotherapy in untreated multiple myeloma: a prospective randomized Phase III [abstract]. *Blood*, 98, 815a.

[41] D'Amato, R. J., et al. (1994). Thalidomide is an inhibitor of angiogemesis. *Proc. Natl. Acad. Sci. U. S. A*, 91-4082-4085.

[42] Ribatti, D. & Vacca, A. (2005). Novel Therapeutic Approches Targeting Vascular Endothelial Growth Factor and its receptors in haematological malignancies. *Curr. Cancer Drug Targets*, 5, 573-578.

[43] Davies, F. E., et al. (2001). Thalidomide and immunomodulatory derivatives augument natural killer cell cytotoxicity in multiple myeloma. *Blood*, 98, 210-216.

[44] Juliusson, G., et al. (2000). Frequent good partial remissions from thalidomide including best response ever in patients with advanced refractory and relapsed myeloma. *Br. J. Haematol.*, 109, 89-96.

[45] Gupta, D., et al. (2001). Adherence of multiple myeloma cells to bone marrow stromal cells upregulates vascular endothelial growth factor secretion: therapeutic application. *Leukemia*, 15, 1950-1961.

[46] Dimopoulos, M., et al. (2007). Lenalidomide plus Dexamethasone for relapsed or refractory multiple myeloma. *N. Engl. J. Med.*, 357, 21.

[47] Marriot, J. B., et al. (2004). The oral combination of thalidomide, cyclophosphamide and dexamethasone (ThaCyDex) is effective in relapsed/refractory multiple myeloma. *Leukemia*, 18, 856-863.

[48] Richardson, P. G., et al. (2002). Immunomodulatory drug CC-5013 overcomes drug resistance and is well tolerated in patients with relapsed multiple myeloma. *Blood*, 100, 3063-7.

[49] Richardson, P. G., et al. (2006). A randomized phase 2 study of lenalidomide therapy for patients with relapsed or relapsed and refractory multiple myeloma. *Blood*, 108, 3458-64.

[50] Weber DM, et al. (2003). Thalidomide alone or with dexamethasone for previously untreated multiple myeloma. *J. Clin. Oncol*; 21: 16–19.

[51] Cavo M, et al. (2004). First-line therapy with thalidomide and dexamethasone in preparation for autologous stem cell transplantation for multiple myeloma. *Haematologica*; 89: 826–831.

[52] Rajkumar SV, et al. (2006). Phase III clinical trial of thalidomide plus dexamethasone compared with dexamethasone alone in newly diagnosed multiple myeloma: a clinical trial coordinated by the Eastern Cooperative Oncology Group. *J. Clin. Oncol*; 24: 431–436.

[53] Palumbo A, et al; (2008). International Myeloma Working Group. Prevention of thalidomide- and lenalidomide-associated thrombosis in myeloma. *Leukemia*; 22: 414–423.

[54] Zou Y, et al. (2013). Lenalidomide versus thalidomide based regimens as first-line therapy for patients with multiple myeloma. *Leuk. Lymphoma;* 54: 2219-2225.

[55] Kumar S, et al. (2007). Impact of lenalidomide therapy on stem cell mobilization and engraftment post peripheral blood stem cell transplantation in patients with newly diagnosed myeloma. *Leukemia*; 21: 2035–2042.

[56] Ria R, et al. (2012). Induction therapy and stem cell mobilization in patients with newly diagnosed multiple myeloma. *Stem Cells Int*; 607260.

[57] Giralt S, et al; (2009). International myeloma working group (IMWG) consensus statement and guidelines regarding the current status of stem cell collection and high-dose therapy for multiple myeloma and the role of plerixafor (AMD 3100) *Leukemia*; 23: 1904–1912

[58] Engelhardt M, et al. (2014). European Myeloma Network recommendations on the evaluation and treatment of newly diagnosed patients with multiple myeloma. *Haematologica*. 99(2): 232–242.

[59] Palumbo A, et al. (2009). How to treat elderly patients with multiple myeloma: combination of therapy or sequencing. *Hematology Am. Soc. Hematol. Educ. Program.*:566-77.

[60] San Miguel JF, et al. (2008). Bortezomib plus melphalan and prednisone for initial treatment of multiple myeloma. *N. Engl. J. Med*; 359: 906–917.

[61] Mateos MV, et al. (2010). Bortezomib plus melphalan and prednisone compared with melphalan and prednisone in previously untreated multiple myeloma: updated follow-up and impact of subsequent therapy in the phase III VISTA trial. *J. Clin. Oncol*; 28: 2259–2266.

[62] Mateos MV, et al. (2010). Bortezomib, melphalan, and prednisone versus bortezomib, thalidomide, and prednisone as induction therapy followed by maintenance treatment with bortezomib and thalidomide versus bortezomib and prednisone in elderly patients with untreated multiple myeloma: a randomised trial. *Lancet Oncol*; 11: 934–941.

[63] Palumbo A, et al. (2010). Bortezomib-melphalan-prednisone-thalidomide followed by maintenance with bortezomib-thalidomide compared with bortezomib-melphalan-prednisone for initial treatment of multiple myeloma: a randomized controlled trial. *J. Clin. Oncol*; 28: 5101–5109.

[64] Mateos MV, et al. (2012). Safety and efficacy of subcutaneous formulation of bortezomib versus the conventional intravenous formulation in multiple myeloma. *Ther. Adv. Hematol*; 3: 117-124.

[65] Gay F, et al. (2010). Lenalidomide plus dexamethasone versus thalidomide plus dexamethasone in newly diagnosed multiple myeloma: a comparative analysis of 411 patients. *Blood*; 115: 1343–1350.

[66] Ludwig H, et al. (2009). Thalidomide-dexamethasone compared with melphalan-prednisolone in elderly patients with multiple myeloma. *Blood*; 113: 3435–3442.

[67] Facon T, et al. (2007). Melphalan and prednisone plus thalidomide versus melphalan and prednisone alone or reduced-intensity autologous stem cell transplantation in elderly patients with multiple myeloma (IFM 99-06): a randomised trial. *Lancet*; 370: 1209–1218.

[68] Hulin C, et al. (2009) Efficacy of melphalan and prednisone plus thalidomide in patients older than 75 years with newly diagnosed multiple myeloma: IFM 01/01 Trial. *J. Clin. Oncol*; 27: 3664–3670.

[69] Palumbo A, et al. (2006). Oral melphalan and prednisone chemotherapy plus thalidomide compared with melphalan and prednisone alone in elderly patients with multiple myeloma: randomised controlled trial. *Lancet*; 367: 825–831

[70] Waage A, et al. (2010). Melphalan and prednisone plus thalidomide or placebo in elderly patients with multiple myeloma. *Blood*; 116: 1405–1412.

[71] Wijermans P, et al. (2010) Phase III study of the value of thalidomide added to melphalan plus prednisone in elderly patients with newly diagnosed multiple myeloma: the HOVON 49 Study. *J. Clin. Oncol*; 28: 3160–3166.

[72] Zonder JA, et al. (2010). Lenalidomide and high-dose dexamethasone compared with dexamethasone as initial therapy for multiple myeloma: a randomized Southwest Oncology Group trial (S0232) *Blood*; 116: 5838–5841.

[73] Rajkumar SV, et al. (2010). Lenalidomide plus high-dose dexamethasone versus lenalidomide plus low-dose dexamethasone as initial therapy for newly diagnosed multiple myeloma: an open-label randomised controlled trial. *Lancet Oncol*; 11: 29–37.

[74] Jacobus S, et al. (2010). Outcome of elderly patients 70 years and older with newly diagnosed myeloma in the ECOG randomized trial of lenalidomide/high-dose dexamethasone (RD) versus lenalidomide/low-dose dexamethasone (Rd) [abstract] *Haematologica*; 95, 0370.

[75] San Miguel JF. (2009). Relapse/Refractory myeloma patient: potential treatment guidelines. *J. Clin. Oncol.*;27(34):5676-7.

[76] Elice F, Raimondi R, Tosetto A, D'Emilio A, Di Bona E, Piccin A, Rodeghiero F. Prolonged overall survival with second on-demand autologous transplant in multiple myeloma. *Am. J. Hematol.* 2006; 81: 426–431 [PMID: 16680735]

[77] Olin RL, et al. (2009). Second auto-SCT is safe and effective salvage therapy for relapsed multiple myeloma. *Bone Marrow Transplant*; 43: 417–422.

[78] Garban F, et al. (2006). Prospective comparison of autologous stem cell transplantation followed by dose-reduced allograft (IFM99 – 03 trial) with tandem autologous stem cell transplantation (IFM99 – 04 trial) in high-risk de novo multiple myeloma. *Blood*; 107: 3474–3480.

[79] Barlogie B, et al. (1987). High-dose chemoradiotherapy and autologous bone marrow transplantation for resistant multiple myeloma. *Blood*; 70: 869–872.

[80] Barlogie B, et al. (1986). High-dose melphalan with autologous bone marrow transplantation for multiple myeloma. *Blood*; 67:1298–1301.

[81] Alexanian R, et al. (1986). High-dose glucocorticoid treatment of resistant myeloma. *Ann. Intern. Med*; 105: 8–11.

[82] Durie BG, et al. (1986). Improved survival duration with combination chemotherapy induction for multiple myeloma: a Southwest Oncology Group study. *J. Clin. Oncol*; 4: 1227–1237.

[83] Giles FJ, et al. (2000). Cyclophosphamide, etoposide, vincristine, adriamycin, and dexamethasone (CEVAD) regimen in refractory multiple myeloma: an International Oncology Study Group (IOSG) phase II protocol. *Am. J. Hematol*; 63: 125–130.

[84] Dadacaridou M, et al. (2007) Dexamethasone, cyclophosphamide, etoposide and cisplatin (DCEP) for relapsed or refractory multiple myeloma patients. *J. Buon*; 12: 41–44.

[85] Lee CK, et al. (2003). DTPACE: an effective, novel combination chemotherapy with thalidomide for previously treated patients with myeloma. *J. Clin. Oncol*; 21: 2732–2739.

[86] Anagnostopoulos A, et al. (2003). Thalidomide and dexamethasone for resistant multiple myeloma. *Br. J. Haematol*; 121: 768–771.

[87] Kropff MH, et al. (2003). Hyperfractionated cyclophosphamide in combination with pulsed dexamethasone and thalidomide (HyperCDT) in primary refractory or relapsed multiple myeloma. *Br. J. Haematol;* 122: 607–616.

[88] Sidra G, et al. (2006). Combination chemotherapy with cyclophosphamide, thalidomide and dexamethasone for patients with refractory, newly diagnosed or relapsed myeloma. *Haematologica*; 91: 862–863.

[89] Offidani M, et al. (2003). Thalidomide plus oral melphalan for advanced multiple myeloma: a phase II study. *Haematologica*; 88: 1432–1433.

[90] Srkalovic G, et al. (2002). Use of melphalan, thalidomide, and dexamethasone in treatment of refractory and relapsed multiple myeloma. *Med. Oncol*; 19: 219–226.

[91] Offidani M, et al. (2006). Low-dose thalidomide with pegylated liposomal doxorubicin and high-dose dexamethasone for relapsed/refractory multiple myeloma: a prospective, multicenter, phase II study. *Haematologica*; 91: 133–136.

[92] Hussein MA, et al. (2006). Phase 2 study of pegylated liposomal doxorubicin, vincristine, decreased-frequency dexamethasone, and thalidomide in newly diagnosed and relapsed-refractory multiple myeloma. *Mayo Clin. Proc*; 81: 889–895.

[93] Moehler TM, et al. (2001). Salvage therapy for multiple myeloma with thalidomide and CED chemotherapy. *Blood*; 98: 3846–3848.

[94] Richardson PG, et al. (2007). Extended follow-up of a phase 3 trial in relapsed multiple myeloma: final time-to-event results of the APEX trial. *Blood*; 110: 3557–3560.

[95] Orlowski RZ, et al. (2007). Randomized phase III study of pegylated liposomal doxorubicin plus bortezomib compared with bortezomib alone in relapsed or refractory multiple myeloma: combination therapy improves time to progression. *J. Clin. Oncol*; 25: 3892–3901.

[96] Jakubowiak AJ, et al. (2009). Phase II trial of combination therapy with bortezomib, pegylated liposomal doxorubicin, and dexamethasone in patients with newly diagnosed myeloma. *J. Clin. Oncol*; 27: 5015–5022.

[97] Berenson JR, et al. (2006). Phase I/II trial assessing bortezomib and melphalan combination therapy for the treatment of patients with relapsed or refractory multiple myeloma. *J. Clin. Oncol*; 24: 937–944.

[98] Reece DE, et al. (2008). Phase I-II trial of bortezomib plus oral cyclophosphamide and prednisone in relapsed and refractory multiple myeloma. *J. Clin. Oncol*; 26: 4777–4783.

[99] Heinz Ludwig, et al. (2014); Bendamustine-bortezomib-dexamethasone is an active and well-tolerated regimen in patients with relapsed or refractory multiple myeloma. *Blood*; 123(7): 985–991.

[100] Richardson P, et al. (2009) Safety and efficacy of single-agent lenalidomide in patients with relapsed and refractory multiple myeloma. *Blood*; 114: 772–778.

[101] Weber DM, et al. (2007). Lenalidomide plus dexamethasone for relapsed multiple myeloma in North America. *N. Engl. J. Med*; 357: 2133–2142.

[102] Dimopoulos M, et al. (2007). Lenalidomide plus dexamethasone for relapsed or refractory multiple myeloma. *N. Engl. J. Med.*; 357: 2123–2132.

[103] Dimopoulos MA, et al. (2009) Long-term follow-up on overall survival from the MM-009 and MM-010 phase III trials of lenalidomide plus dexamethasone in patients with relapsed or refractory multiple myeloma. *Leukemia*; 23: 2147–2152.

[104] Touzeau C, et al. (2012). Efficacy of lenalidomide plus dexamethasone in patients older than 75 years with relapsed multiple myeloma. *Leuk. Lymphoma*; 53: 1318-1320.

[105] Baz R, et al. (2006) Lenalidomide and pegylated liposomal doxorubicin-based chemotherapy for relapsed or refractory multiple myeloma: safety and efficacy. *Ann. Oncol*; 17: 1766–1771.

[106] Knop S, et al. (2009) Lenalidomide, adriamycin, and dexamethasone (RAD) in patients with relapsed and refractory multiple myeloma: a report from the German Myeloma Study Group DSMM (Deutsche Studiengruppe Multiples Myelom). *Blood*; 113: 4137–4143

[107] van de Donk NW, et al. (2010). Lenalidomide (Revlimid) combined with continuous oral cyclophosphamide (endoxan) and prednisone (REP) is effective in lenalidomide/dexamethasone-refractory myeloma. *Br. J. Haematol*; 148: 335–337.

[108] Morgan GJ, et al. (2007). Lenalidomide (Revlimid), in combination with cyclophosphamide and dexamethasone (RCD), is an effective and tolerated regimen for myeloma patients. *Br. J. Haematol*; 137: 268–269.

[109] Ciolli S, et al. (2008) The addition of liposomal doxorubicin to bortezomib, thalidomide and dexamethasone significantly improves clinical outcome of advanced multiple myeloma. *Br. J. Haematol*; 141: 814–819.

[110] Terpos E, et al. (2008). The combination of bortezomib, melphalan, dexamethasone and intermittent thalidomide is an effective regimen for relapsed/refractory myeloma and is associated with improvement of abnormal bone metabolism and angiogenesis. *Leukemia*; 22: 2247–2256.

[111] Palumbo A, et al. (2007). Bortezomib, melphalan, prednisone, and thalidomide for relapsed multiple myeloma. *Blood*; 109: 2767–1772.

[112] Pineda-Roman M, et al. (2008) VTD combination therapy with bortezomib-thalidomide-dexamethasone is highly effective in advanced and refractory multiple myeloma. *Leukemia*; 22: 1419–1427.

[113] Richardson PG, et al. (2009) Multicenter, phase I, dose-escalation trial of lenalidomide plus bortezomib for relapsed and relapsed/refractory multiple myeloma. *J. Clin. Oncol*; 27: 5713–5719.

[114] Palumbo A, et al. (2010) Lenalidomide, melphalan, prednisone and thalidomide (RMPT) for relapsed/refractory multiple myeloma. *Leukemia*; 24: 1037-1042.

[115] Richardson P, et al. (2008) Lenalidomide, bortezomib, and dexamethasone in patients with relapsed or relapsed/ refractory multiple myeloma (MM): Encouraging response rates and tolerability with correlations of outcome and adverse cytogenetics in a phase II study. ASH Annual Meeting Abstracts 111:614a, abstr 1742.

[116] Cunningham D, et al. (1998). A randomized trial of maintenance interferon following high-dose chemotherapy in multiple myeloma: long-term follow-up results. *Br. J. Haematol*; 102: 495-502.

[117] Attal M, et al. (2006). Maintenance therapy with thalidomide improves survival in patients with multiple myeloma. *Blood*; 108: 3289-3294.

[118] Shank BR1, et al. (2014). Multiple myeloma maintenance therapy: A review of the pharmacologic treatment. *J. Oncol. Pharm. Pract*. [Epub ahead of print].

[119] McCarthy PL, et al. (2012). Lenalidomide after stem-cell transplantation for multiple myeloma. *N. Engl. J. Med*; 366: 1770–1781.

[120] Attal M, et al. (2012). Lenalidomide maintenance after stem-cell transplantation for multiple myeloma. *N. Engl. J. Med*; 366: 1782–1791

[121] Scheid C, et al. (2013). Bortezomib before and after autologous stem cell transplantation overcomes the negative prognostic impact of renal impairment in newly diagnosed multiple myeloma: a Subgroup Analysis From the HOVON-65/GMMG-HD4 Trial. *Haematologica*;

[122] Gertz M. (2013). Pomalidomide and myeloma meningitis. *Leuk. Lymphoma*; 54:681-682.

[123] Lopez-Girona A, et al. (2012). Cereblon is a direct protein target for immunomodulatory and antiproliferative activities of lenalidomide and pomalidomide. *Leukemia*; 26: 2326–2335.

[124] Zhu Y., et al. (2013) Molecular mechanism of action of immune-modulatory drugs thalidomide, lenalidomide and pomalidomide in multiple myeloma. *Leuk. Lymphoma*; 54: 683-687.

[125] Escoubet-Lozach L, et al. (2009). Pomalidomide and lenalidomide induce p21 WAF-1 expression in both lymphoma and multiple myeloma through a LSD1-mediated epigenetic mechanism. *Cancer Res*; 69: 7347–7356.

[126] Lacy M, et al. (2011). Pomalidomide plus low-dose dexamethasone in myeloma refractory to both bortezomib and lenalidomide: comparison of 2 dosing strategies in dual-refractory disease. *Blood*; 118: 2970–2975.

[127] Geyer H, et al. (2011). Acute lung toxicity related to pomalidomide. *Chest*; 140: 529–533.

[128] Palumbo A, et al. (2014); International Myeloma Working Group Consensus Statement for the Management, Treatment, and Supportive Care of Patients with Myeloma Not Eligible for Standard Autologous Stem-Cell Transplantation. *JCO*: 32, 587–600.

[129] Short K, et al. (2011) Incidence of extramedullary disease in patients with multiple myeloma in the era of novel therapy, and the activity of pomalidomide on extramedullary myeloma. *Leukemia*; 25: 906–908.

[130] Paul G. Richardson, et al. (2014). Pomalidomide alone or in combination with low-dose dexamethasone in relapsed and refractory multiple myeloma: a randomized phase 2 study *Blood*; 123: 1826-1832.

[131] Demo SD, et al. (2007). Antitumor activity of PR-171, a novel irreversible inhibitor of the proteasome. *Cancer Res*; 67: 6383-6391.

[132] Siegel DS, et al. (2012). A phase 2 study of single-agent carfilzomib (PX-171-003-A1) in patients with relapsed and refractory multiple myeloma. *Blood*; 120: 2817-2825.

[133] Siegel D, et al. (2013) Integrated safety profile of single-agent carfilzomib: experience from 526 patients enrolled in 4 phase 2 clinical studies. *Haematologica*; 98: 1753-1761.

[134] Vij R, et al. (2012) An open-label, single-arm, phase 2 (PX-171-004) study of single-agent carfilzomib in bortezomib-naive patients with relapsed and/or refractory multiple myeloma. *Blood*; 119: 5661-5670.

[135] Niesvizky R, et al. (2013). Phase Ib dose-escalation study (PX-171-006) of carfilzomib, lenalidomide, and low-dose dexamethasone in relapsed or progressive multiple myeloma. *Clin. Cancer Res*; 19: 2248-2256.

[136] Jakubowiak AJ, et al. (2012). A phase 1/2 study of carfilzomib in combination with lenalidomide and low-dose dexamethasone as a frontline treatment for multiple myeloma. *Blood*; 120: 1801-1809.

[137] Mikhael JR, et al. (2012)A phase I/II trial of cyclophosphamide, carfilzomib, thalidomide, and dexamethasone (CYCLONE) in patients with newly diagnosed multiple myeloma. ASCO Annual Meeting Abstracts.

[138] Chauhan D, et al. (2005). A novel orally active proteasome inhibitor induces apoptosis in multiple myeloma cells with mechanisms distinct from Bortezomib. *Cancer Cell*; 8: 407-419.

[139] Chauhan D, et al. (2008). Combination of proteasome inhibitors bortezomib and NPI-0052 trigger in vivosynergistic cytotoxicity in multiple myeloma. *Blood*; 111: 1654-1664.

[140] Ocio EM, et al. (2008). New drugs in multiple myeloma: mechanisms of action and phase I/II clinical findings. *Lancet Oncol*; 9: 1157-1165.

[141] Mitsiades N, et al. (2003). Molecular sequelae of histone deacetylase inhibition in human malignant B cells. *Blood*; 101: 4055-4062.

[142] Dokmanovic M, et al. (2007). Histone deacetylase inhibitors: overview and perspectives. *Mol. Cancer Res*; 5: 981-989.

[143] Mitsiades CS, et al. (2004). Transcriptional signature of histone deacetylase inhibition in multiple myeloma: biological and clinical implications. *Proc. Natl. Acad. Sci. USA*; 101: 540-545

[144] Badros A, et al. (2009). Phase I study of vorinostat in combination with bortezomib for relapsed and refractory multiple myeloma. *Clin. Cancer Res*; 15: 5250-5257.

[145] Kawauchi K, et al. (2009). The PI3K/Akt pathway as a target in the treatment of hematologic malignancies. *Anticancer Agents Med. Chem*; 9: 550-559.

[146] Hideshima T, et al. (2006) Perifosine, an oral bioactive novel alkylphospholipid, inhibits Akt and induces in vitro and in vivocytotoxicity in human multiple myeloma cells. *Blood*; 107: 4053-4062.

[147] Richardson PG, et al. (2011). Perifosine plus bortezomib and dexamethasone in patients with relapsed/refractory multiple myeloma previously treated with bortezomib: results of a multicenter phase I/II trial. *J. Clin. Oncol*; 29: 4243-4249.

[148] Moschetta M, et al. (2014). Therapeutic targeting of the mTOR-signaling pathway in cancer: benefits and limitations. *Br. J. Pharmacol.*

[149] Farag SS, et al. (2009). Phase II trial of temsirolimus in patients with relapsed or refractory multiple myeloma. *Leuk. Res;* 33: 1475-1480.

[150] Ghobrial IM, et al. (2011). Weekly bortezomib in combination with temsirolimus in relapsed or relapsed and refractory multiple myeloma: a multicentre, phase 1/2, open-label, doseescalation study. *Lancet Oncol;* 12: 263-272.

[151] Whitesell L. & Lindquist SL. (2005). HSP90 and the chaperoning of cancer. *Nat. Rev. Cancer*: 5: 761-772.

[152] Richardson PG, et al. (2011). Tanespimycin and bortezomib combination treatment in patients with relapsed or relapsed and refractory multiple myeloma: results of a phase 1/2 study. Br. J. Haematol; 153: 729-740.

[153] Di Bernardo A, et al. (2010). Humoral immunotherapy of multiple myeloma: perspectives and perplexities. *Expert Opin. Biol. Ther*; 10: 863–873.

[154] Bladé J, et al. (2012). Incorporating monoclonal antibodies into the therapy of multiple myeloma. *J. Clin. Oncol*; 30: 1904–1906.

[155] Richardson PG, et al. (2011) Monoclonal antibodies in the treatment of multiple myeloma. *Br. J. Haematol*; 154: 745–754.

[156] Mitsiades et al. (2008). Aplidin, a Marine Organism–Derived Compound with Potent Antimyeloma Activity In vitro and In vivo. *Cancer Res.* 68(13):5216-25).

[157] Mateos M. V, et al. (2010). Phase II Clinical and Pharmacokinetic Study of Plitidepsin 3-Hour Infusion Every Two Weeks Alone or with Dexamethasone in Relapsed and Refractory Multiple Myeloma. *Clin. Cancer Res*;16:3260-3269.

[158] Bruno B, et al. (2005). Novel targeted drugs for the treatment of multiple myeloma: from bench to bedside. Phase III trials in MM are still ongoing. *Leukemia*: 19, 1729–1738.

In: Multiple Myeloma: Risk Factors, Diagnosis and Treatments ISBN: 978-1-63321-514-6
Editor: Steve Holt

Chapter 7

The Role of DNA Methylation in the Genetics and Epigenetics of Multiple Myeloma

Hiroshi Yasui[*1], *Tadao Ishida*[3] *and Kohzoh Imai*[2]
[1]Center for Antibody and Vaccine, Research Hospital,
[2]The Institute of Medical Science, The University of Tokyo, Tokyo, Japan
[3]Department of Gastroenterology, Rheumatology,
and Clinical Immunology, Sapporo Medical University, Sapporo, Japan

Abstract

Multiple myeloma (MM) arises through an accumulation of multiple genetic and epigenetic changes, which play a significant role in tumorigenesis and tumor development. DNA methylation is often found in cancers including MM at the 5-carbon on cytosine residues within CpG islands of genes whose products are associated with the promoter regions of protein-coding genes. This methylation is an epigenetic alteration that leads to heritable changes in gene expression through the recruitment of histone deacetylases and histone methyltransferases. We and other researchers have reported the association of global and regional DNA methylation status with MM. Global DNA hypomethylation is the predominant early change during plasma cell oncogenesis from monoclonal gammopathy of undetermined significance to MM, while regional DNA hypermethylation occurs in tumor relapse and during disease progression. Thus, DNA methylation could be a useful biomarker of MM tumorigenesis and progression. In the current review, we discuss the role of DNA methylation changes; their potential application as epigenetic biomarkers to facilitate risk assessment, diagnosis, prediction of prognosis, and sensitivity to treatment; and epigenetic therapy in MM.

* Correspondence to: Hiroshi Yasui, M.D., Ph.D. Center for Antibody and Vaccine, Research Hospital, The Institute of Medical Science, The University of Tokyo; 4-6-1 Shirokanedai, Minato-ku, Tokyo 108-8639, Japan; TEL: +81-3-3443-8111; FAX: +81-3-6409-2413; E-mail: hiroyasu@ims.u-tokyo.ac.jp

Introduction

Cancers, including multiple myeloma (MM), arise because of an accumulation of multiple genetic changes, which play a significant role in tumorigenesis and tumor development. In addition to genetics, recent studies revealed the role of epigenetics—heritable information that does not affect DNA sequence—in the pathogenesis of cancers, including MM [1-4]. Among epigenetic changes, DNA methylation and histone modification have been well-studied.

DNA methylation occurs at the 5-carbon on cytosine residues in cytosine-guanine pairs known as CpG dinucleotides. DNA methylation is catalyzed by three DNA methyltransferases, including DNMT1, DNMT3A, and DNMT3B, and is a crucial regulator in different biological processes, such as embryonic development, transcription, chromatin structure, X chromosome inactivation, genomic imprinting, genomic instability, and tumorigenesis [5]. Since transcriptionally active regions of the genome are usually CpG rich, methylation of CpG sites is a critical factor affecting gene transcription. DNA hypermethylation of the large clusters of CpG dinucleotides, referred to as CpG islands, at gene promoters and transcription start sites is an epigenetic alteration that can suppress gene expression through the recruitment of methyl-CpG binding domain proteins, histone deacetylases, and histone methyltransferases, thus causing chromatin condensation [6]. Genome-wide hypomethylation and regional hypermethylation are common events in tumors, including hematological malignancies. In MM, DNA hypomethylation was reported as the predominant early change during tumorigenesis that gradually transforms to regional DNA hypermethylation during disease progression [7-9].

In the current review, we discuss the role of alterations in DNA methylation, potential application of epigenetic biomarkers, and target therapeutics in MM.

2. Molecular Mechanism Involved in Tumorigenesis of MM

MM is a neoplastic plasma cell disorder that is characterized by the clonal proliferation of malignant plasma cells in the bone marrow, the presence of monoclonal immunoglobulin in the serum and/or urine in most cases, and associated organ dysfunction, including lytic bone lesions, compromised immunity, anemia, renal failure, and hypercalcemia [10-12]. Recent studies have shown that MM is consistently preceded by a premalignant stage of clonal plasma cell proliferation, termed monoclonal gammopathy of undetermined significance (MGUS) [13,14]. Approximately 1% of MGUS cases evolve to MM per year [15].

MM advances through a multistep transformation process of specific events, including somatic mutations, chromosomal copy-number changes, and non-random chromosomal translocations such as immunoglobulin gene rearrangements involved in cyclin D; furthermore, epigenetic changes drive progression from MGUS, to symptomatic MM, and ultimately to recurrent myeloma, including extramedullary disease and, in some cases, plasma cell leukemia [4,12,16,17] (Figure 1).

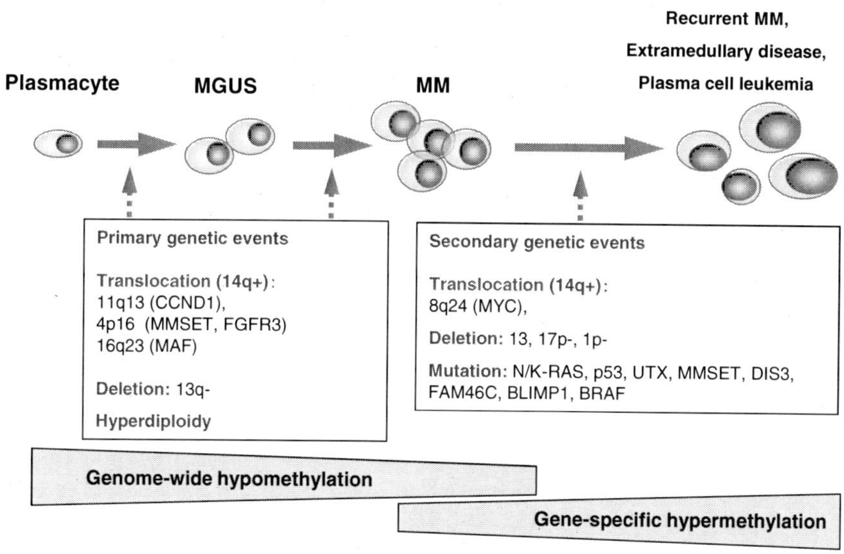

Figure 1. Multiple myeloma (MM) advances through a multistep transformation process due to specific events. These events include somatic mutations, chromosomal copy-number changes, and non-random chromosomal translocations, such as immunoglobulin gene rearrangements involved in cyclin D. Further, epigenetic changes drive progression from monoclonal gammopathy of undetermined significance (MGUS), to symptomatic MM, and ultimately to recurrent myeloma, including extramedullary disease and plasma cell leukemia. Genome-wide hypomethylation occurs during the events indicated by a blue wedge, and gene-specific hypermethylation occurs during the events indicated by a blue wedge.

Recently, several studies using high-throughput sequencing technologies demonstrated heterogeneity of MM genomic evolution and subclonal structure [18-22]. Chapman et al., reported that the analysis of somatic mutations by tumor-genome sequencing in MM cases revealed that, of the numerous genes mutated, identified genes are specifically involved in NFκB activation, protein homeostasis, and histone methylation, which are processes consistent with MM biology [18]. However, the key steps in MM oncogenesis remain unclear [3,4,23,24]. Recent findings also revealed that epigenetics, including DNA methylation and histone modification, is also important in MM pathogenesis. Global methylation analyses in MM have revealed the role of DNA methylation in MM pathogenesis and progress.

2. DNA Hypomethylation in MM

Genome-wide DNA hypomethylation is a common epigenetic alteration in cancer cells. Low levels of DNA methylation in cancer cells is substantially due to the loss of methylation at repetitive sequences such as long interspersed nuclear element-1 (LINE-1; a kind of a retrotransposon), which accounts for 17% of the human genome [19,25]. The following mechanisms have been suggested for DNA hypomethylation in tumorigenesis and tumor development: increased instability of the genome and reactivation of transposable elements (transposons) that can move in DNA [26-28]. Importantly, we and others reported that global methylation levels of DNA repetitive sequences, including LINE-1, progressively decline during the development of MM from MGUS to aggressive myeloma such as plasma cell leukemia [8,9]. We also reported that there is a significant inverse correlation between the degree of genomic loss and LINE-1 methylation levels, and MM cases with LINE-1 hypomethylation had a significantly poor prognosis [9]. Regarding the pathogenesis of MM plasma cells, microarray data examining genome-wide differences in CpG methylation patterns revealed that genome-wide hypomethylation occurs at the transition from MGUS to MM [7].

3. DNA Hypermethylation in MM

DNA hypermethylation at gene promoters and transcription start sites is an epigenetic alteration that suppresses gene expression. Global DNA hypomethylation is the predominant early change during plasma cell oncogenesis from MGUS to MM, while regional DNA hypermethylation occurs in tumor relapse and during disease progression [7]. We and others studied regional DNA hypermethylation in MM and identified certain key genes as targets for epigenetic inactivation (Table 1).

Table 1. Epigenetically silenced genes in multiple myeloma (MM)

Gene	Chromosome	Function	Frequency of DNA hypermethylation of patient MM samples (n > 50)
CDKN2A (p16)	9p21.3	Cell cycle	34% [29]
DAPK1	9q21.33	Apoptosis	52.7% [35]
BNIP3	10q26.3	Apoptosis	5% [36]
RASD1	17p11.2	Cell growth	6–8% [33,40]
SPARC	5q33.1	Cell-extracellular matrix interaction	8–18.2% [36,40]
CD38	4p15	Ectoenzyme	45.9% [40]
GPX3	5q23	Glutathione peroxidase	7.5% [40]
NCAM1 (CD56)	11q23.1	Cell adhesion	5% [40]
PDK4	7q21.3	Regulation of metabolism	15.1% [40]
RBP1	3q23	carrier protein involved in the transport of retinol	16.3% [40]
TGFBI	5q31	Inhibition of cell adhesion	18.2% [40]

These genes include the following: cell-cycle regulators, such as cyclin-dependent kinase inhibitor 2A (*CDKN2A*) [29] and 2B (*CDKN2B*) [30] and checkpoint with fork head and ring finger domains (*CHFR*) [31]; genes involved in cell signaling, such as Ras association

(RalGDS/AF-6) domain family member 1 (*RASSF1*) [32], RAS, dexamethasone-induced 1 (*RASD1*) [33], and transforming growth factor, beta receptor II (*TGFBR2*) [34]; genes involved in apoptosis, such as death-associated protein kinase 1 (*DAPK1*) [35] and BCL2/adenovirus E1B 19kDa interacting protein 3 (*BNIP3*) [36,37]; genes involved in antigen presentation, such as class II, major histocompatibility complex, transactivator (*CIITA*) [38]; genes involved in cell-extracellular matrix interaction, such as secreted protein, acidic, cysteine-rich (*SPARC*) [36]; and genes involved in polycomb repressive complexes, such as enhancer of zeste, drosophila, homolog 2 (*EZH2*) [39].

Recently, Kaiser et al., investigated the association between DNA methylation and MM prognosis using a genome-wide DNA methylation array of 159 patients treated in the Medical Research Council Myeloma IX trial [40]. They identified the following 8 epigenetically regulated genes with changes in DNA methylation status that were significantly associated with prognosis: *CD38*, *RASD1*, *SPARC*, glutathione peroxidase 3 (*GPX3*), neural cell adhesion molecule 1 (*NCAM1*), pyruvate dehydrogenase kinase 4 (*PDK4*), retinol-binding protein 1 (*RBP1*), and transforming growth factor, β induced (*TGFBI*). Importantly, multivariate analysis confirmed that *GPX3*, *RBP1*, *SPARC*, and *TGFBI* are associated with survival, and methylation of the genes is independent of established risk factors for MM. Methylation levels of these 4 genes is low in MGUS, and then increasing methylation is associated with more aggressive MM cellular phenotypes. Walker et al., investigated DNA methylation patterns associated with MM subtypes [7]. They found specific profiles with increased hypermethylation in clinically aggressive subtypes, such as plasma cell leukemia, and in the prognostically unfavorable t(4;14) cytogenetic subtype with overexpressed *MMSET*, which encodes a histone methyltransferase. These findings suggest that methylation changes affect disease biology.

Recent reports correlated hypermethylation of promoter-associated CpG islands with silencing of microRNAs (miRNAs), which are small 18–22 nucleotide RNAs that regulate many intracellular functions [41]. Dysregulation of miRNA genes has been implicated in MM. Moreover, several reports of MM described the role of hypermethylation of tumor-suppressor miRNA genes, including *miR-34b/c* [42], *miR-194-2-192* [43], and *miR-203* [44]. Combined genome-wide analysis of miRNA methylation and miRNA expression profiling is warranted to clarify the role of epigenetic regulation of miRNA in MM.

4. DNA Methylation As an Epigenetic Biomarker in MM

The current prognostic factors in MM include cytogenetic aberrations, such as the nonhyperdiploid, cytogenetically detected chromosomal 13q deletion, t(4;14), t(14;16), 1q gain, and del(17p) detected by fluorescence *in situ* hybridization [10]. Novel therapeutics, such as the proteasome inhibitor bortezomib, can partially overcome adverse outcomes conferred by these abnormalities [45]. However, there has been much less progress in the development of predictive biomarkers for specific treatments [46]. To identify predictive biomarkers for the effect of myeloma therapeutics, appropriate clinical trial designs are necessary. Since some novel MM therapeutics in development have specific molecular targets, the identification of biomarkers that also characterize drug sensitivity is a promising therapeutic strategy [45].

As mentioned above, hypermethylation of *TGFB1*, *SPARC*, *RBP1*, and *GPX3* is associated with significantly shorter overall survival, independent of age, international staging system score, and adverse cytogenetics [40]. Future prospective studies will verify these genes as prognostic MM biomarkers.

We identified *RASD1* as a possible biomarker in MM [33]. *RASD1*, located on chromosome 17p11.2 with frequent loss of heterozygosity in various human tumors, encodes a Ras GTPase with tumor suppressor functions induced by dexamethasone [47,48]. Importantly, MM cells that show *RASD1* methylation are resistant to dexamethasone, and combined treatment with dexamethasone and the hypomethylating agent decitabine (5-aza-2′-deoxycytidine), which inhibits DNA methyltransferase, restores the cytotoxicity of dexamethasone to tumor cells. While the hypermethylation of *RASD1* was observed in approximately 10% of primary MM samples, the methylation levels of *RASD1* were elevated in all of the MM cases that had pair DNAs after repeated antimyeloma therapy, including dexamethasone.

Limited studies have addressed the antitumor effects of the hypomethylating agents decitabine and azacitidine (5-azacytidine) in MM, demonstrating significant *in vitro* antimyeloma activity. The mechanisms involve changes in gene expression and induction of DNA damage [49,50]. Recently, a gene expression-based DNA methylation score was reported, which relates the expression of methylation-regulated genes to predict the efficacy of hypomethylating agents—decitabine and azacitidine—in human MM cell lines and in patient MM cells *in vitro* [51,52]. Phase I/II clinical trials are ongoing to study the side effects and best dose of azacitidine in combination with lenalidomide and dexamethasone in MM; therefore, an investigation regarding association of the methylation score and the response of MM patients could provide promising information [53]. Taken together, these findings suggest the involvement of epigenetic gene silencing in MM progression and drug resistance and the usefulness of demethylation therapy for MM treatment.

Conclusion

In summary, DNA methylation functions in MM tumorigenesis and progression. Several reports have suggested that DNA methylation could be a useful biomarker to predict prognosis and sensitivity to treatment. A further comprehensive analysis using a genome-wide approach with high-throughput sequencing technologies will be necessary to clarify the molecular mechanisms of MM oncogenesis and progression. Epigenetics has become to an essential research area where important challenges should be resolved through further investigations of MM.

Acknowledgments

This study was supported by an Aki Horinouchi Research Grant from the International Myeloma Foundation Japan (H.Y.), a Grant-in-Aid for Exploratory Research (K.I., H.Y.), a

Grant-in-Aid for Scientific Research (C) (T.I., H.Y.), and a Scientific Support Programs for Cancer Research, Grant-in-Aid for Scientific Research on Innovative Areas (K.I., H.Y.) from the Ministry of Education, Culture, Sports, Science, and Technology.

References

[1] Dawson MA; Kouzarides T. Cancer epigenetics: from mechanism to therapy. *Cell* 2012,150,12-27.

[2] Toyota M; Suzuki H; Yamashita T, et al., Cancer epigenomics: implications of DNA methylation in personalized cancer therapy. *Cancer Sci.* 2009,100,787-91.

[3] Yasui H; Ishida T; Maruyama R, et al., Model of translational cancer research in multiple myeloma. *Cancer Sci.* 2012,103,1907-12.

[4] Morgan GJ; Walker BA; Davies FE. The genetic architecture of multiple myeloma. *Nature reviews Cancer* 2012,12,335-48.

[5] Bird A. The essentials of DNA methylation. *Cell* 1992,70,5-8.

[6] Han H; Cortez CC; Yang X; Nichols PW; Jones PA; Liang G. DNA methylation directly silences genes with non-CpG island promoters and establishes a nucleosome occupied promoter. *Human molecular genetics* 2011,20,4299-310.

[7] Walker BA; Wardell CP; Chiecchio L, et al., Aberrant global methylation patterns affect the molecular pathogenesis and prognosis of multiple myeloma. *Blood* 2011,117,553-62.

[8] Bollati V; Fabris S; Pegoraro V, et al., Differential repetitive DNA methylation in multiple myeloma molecular subgroups. *Carcinogenesis* 2009,30,1330-5.

[9] Aoki Y; Nojima M; Suzuki H, et al., Genomic vulnerability to LINE-1 hypomethylation is a potential determinant of the clinicogenetic features of multiple myeloma. *Genome medicine* 2012,4,101.

[10] Palumbo A; Anderson K. Multiple myeloma. *N. Engl. J. Med.* 2011,364,1046-60.

[11] Yasui H; Hideshima T; Richardson PG; Anderson KC. Novel therapeutic strategies targeting growth factor signalling cascades in multiple myeloma. *British journal of haematology* 2006,132,385-97.

[12] Hideshima T; Mitsiades C; Tonon G; Richardson PG; Anderson KC. Understanding multiple myeloma pathogenesis in the bone marrow to identify new therapeutic targets. *Nature reviews Cancer* 2007,7,585-98.

[13] Landgren O; Kyle RA; Pfeiffer RM, et al., Monoclonal gammopathy of undetermined significance (MGUS) consistently precedes multiple myeloma: a prospective study. *Blood* 2009,113,5412-7.

[14] Weiss BM; Abadie J; Verma P; Howard RS; Kuehl WM. A monoclonal gammopathy precedes multiple myeloma in most patients. *Blood* 2009,113,5418-22.

[15] Kyle RA; Durie BG; Rajkumar SV, et al., Monoclonal gammopathy of undetermined significance (MGUS) and smoldering (asymptomatic) multiple myeloma: IMWG consensus perspectives risk factors for progression and guidelines for monitoring and management. *Leukemia* 2010,24,1121-7.

[16] Gonzalez D; van der Burg M; Garcia-Sanz R, et al., Immunoglobulin gene rearrangements and the pathogenesis of multiple myeloma. *Blood* 2007,110,3112-21.

[17] Schmidt-Hieber M; Gutierrez ML; Perez-Andres M, et al., Cytogenetic profiles in multiple myeloma and monoclonal gammopathy of undetermined significance: a study in highly purified aberrant plasma cells. *Haematologica* 2013,98,279-87.

[18] Chapman MA; Lawrence MS; Keats JJ, et al., Initial genome sequencing and analysis of multiple myeloma. *Nature* 2011,471,467-72.

[19] Bolli N; Avet-Loiseau H; Wedge DC, et al., Heterogeneity of genomic evolution and mutational profiles in multiple myeloma. *Nature communications* 2014,5,2997.

[20] Walker BA; Wardell CP; Melchor L, et al., Intraclonal heterogeneity and distinct molecular mechanisms characterize the development of t(4;14) and t(11;14) myeloma. *Blood* 2012,120,1077-86.

[21] Keats JJ; Chesi M; Egan JB, et al., Clonal competition with alternating dominance in multiple myeloma. *Blood* 2012,120,1067-76.

[22] Egan JB; Shi CX; Tembe W, et al., Whole-genome sequencing of multiple myeloma from diagnosis to plasma cell leukemia reveals genomic initiating events, evolution, and clonal tides. *Blood* 2012,120,1060-6.

[23] Stratton MR; Campbell PJ; Futreal PA. The cancer genome. *Nature* 2009,458,719-24.

[24] Hanahan D; Weinberg RA. The hallmarks of cancer. *Cell* 2000,100,57-70.

[25] Huang CR; Schneider AM; Lu Y, et al., Mobile interspersed repeats are major structural variants in the human genome. *Cell* 2010,141,1171-82.

[26] Eden A; Gaudet F; Waghmare A; Jaenisch R. Chromosomal instability and tumors promoted by DNA hypomethylation. *Science* 2003,300,455.

[27] Howard G; Eiges R; Gaudet F; Jaenisch R; Eden A. Activation and transposition of endogenous retroviral elements in hypomethylation induced tumors in mice. *Oncogene* 2008,27,404-8.

[28] Iskow RC; McCabe MT; Mills RE, et al., Natural mutagenesis of human genomes by endogenous retrotransposons. *Cell* 2010,141,1253-61.

[29] Gonzalez-Paz N; Chng WJ; McClure RF, et al., Tumor suppressor p16 methylation in multiple myeloma: biological and clinical implications. *Blood* 2007,109,1228-32.

[30] Ng MH; Chung YF; Lo KW; Wickham NW; Lee JC; Huang DP. Frequent hypermethylation of p16 and p15 genes in multiple myeloma. *Blood* 1997,89,2500-6.

[31] Toyota M; Sasaki Y; Satoh A, et al., Epigenetic inactivation of CHFR in human tumors. *Proceedings of the National Academy of Sciences of the United States of America* 2003,100,7818-23.

[32] Ng MH; Lau KM; Wong WS, et al., Alterations of RAS signalling in Chinese multiple myeloma patients: absent BRAF and rare RAS mutations, but frequent inactivation of RASSF1A by transcriptional silencing or expression of a non-functional variant transcript. *British journal of haematology* 2003,123,637-45.

[33] Nojima M; Maruyama R; Yasui H, et al., Genomic screening for genes silenced by DNA methylation revealed an association between RASD1 inactivation and dexamethasone resistance in multiple myeloma. Clinical cancer research : *an official journal of the American Association for Cancer Research* 2009,15,4356-64.

[34] de Carvalho F; Colleoni GW; Almeida MS; Carvalho AL; Vettore AL. TGFbetaR2 aberrant methylation is a potential prognostic marker and therapeutic target in multiple myeloma. *International journal of cancer Journal international du cancer* 2009,125,1985-91.

[35] Chim CS; Liang R; Fung TK; Choi CL; Kwong YL. Epigenetic dysregulation of the death-associated protein kinase/p14/HDM2/p53/Apaf-1 apoptosis pathway in multiple myeloma. *Journal of clinical pathology* 2007,60,664-9.
[36] Heller G; Schmidt WM; Ziegler B, et al., Genome-wide transcriptional response to 5-aza-2'-deoxycytidine and trichostatin a in multiple myeloma cells. *Cancer research* 2008,68,44-54.
[37] Murai M; Toyota M; Satoh A, et al., Aberrant DNA methylation associated with silencing BNIP3 gene expression in haematopoietic tumours. *British journal of cancer* 2005,92,1165-72.
[38] Morimoto Y; Toyota M; Satoh A, et al., Inactivation of class II transactivator by DNA methylation and histone deacetylation associated with absence of HLA-DR induction by interferon-gamma in haematopoietic tumour cells. *British journal of cancer* 2004,90,844-52.
[39] Croonquist PA; Van Ness B. The polycomb group protein enhancer of zeste homolog 2 (EZH 2) is an oncogene that influences myeloma cell growth and the mutant ras phenotype. *Oncogene* 2005,24,6269-80.
[40] Kaiser MF; Johnson DC; Wu P, et al., Global methylation analysis identifies prognostically important epigenetically inactivated tumor suppressor genes in multiple myeloma. *Blood* 2013,122,219-26.
[41] Wong KY; Huang X; Chim CS. DNA methylation of microRNA genes in multiple myeloma. *Carcinogenesis* 2012,33,1629-38.
[42] Wong KY; Yim RL; So CC; Jin DY; Liang R; Chim CS. Epigenetic inactivation of the MIR34B/C in multiple myeloma. *Blood* 2011,118,5901-4.
[43] Corthals SL; Sun SM; Kuiper R, et al., MicroRNA signatures characterize multiple myeloma patients. *Leukemia* 2011,25,1784-9.
[44] Wong KY; Liang R; So CC; Jin DY; Costello JF; Chim CS. Epigenetic silencing of MIR203 in multiple myeloma. *British journal of haematology* 2011,154,569-78.
[45] Anderson KC. The 39th David A. Karnofsky Lecture: bench-to-bedside translation of targeted therapies in multiple myeloma. *J. Clin. Oncol.* 2012,30,445-52.
[46] Sawyers CL. The cancer biomarker problem. *Nature* 2008,452,548-52.
[47] Kemppainen RJ; Behrend EN. Dexamethasone rapidly induces a novel ras superfamily member-related gene in AtT-20 cells. *The Journal of biological chemistry* 1998,273,3129-31.
[48] Vaidyanathan G; Cismowski MJ; Wang G; Vincent TS; Brown KD; Lanier SM. The Ras-related protein AGS1/RASD1 suppresses cell growth. *Oncogene* 2004,23,5858-63.
[49] Khong T; Sharkey J; Spencer A. The effect of azacitidine on interleukin-6 signaling and nuclear factor-kappaB activation and its in vitro and in vivo activity against multiple myeloma. *Haematologica* 2008,93,860-9.
[50] Kiziltepe T; Hideshima T; Catley L, et al., 5-Azacytidine, a DNA methyltransferase inhibitor, induces ATR-mediated DNA double-strand break responses, apoptosis, and synergistic cytotoxicity with doxorubicin and bortezomib against multiple myeloma cells. *Molecular cancer therapeutics* 2007,6,1718-27.
[51] Moreaux J; Reme T; Leonard W, et al., Development of gene expression-based score to predict sensitivity of multiple myeloma cells to DNA methylation inhibitors. *Molecular cancer therapeutics* 2012,11,2685-92.

[52] Moreaux J; Bruyer A; Veyrune JL; Goldschmidt H; Hose D; Klein B. DNA methylation score is predictive of myeloma cell sensitivity to 5-azacitidine. *British journal of haematology* 2014,164,613-6.

[53] Maes K; Menu E; Van Valckenborgh E; Van Riet I; Vanderkerken K; De Bruyne E. Epigenetic modulating agents as a new therapeutic approach in multiple myeloma. *Cancers* 2013,5,430-61.

In: Multiple Myeloma: Risk Factors, Diagnosis and Treatments ISBN: 978-1-63321-514-6
Editor: Steve Holt

Chapter 8

Bisphosphonate Related Osteonecrosis of the Jaw in Multiple Myeloma

***Kang-Min Ahn**, D.D.S., M.S.D., Ph.D.**
Department of Oral and Maxillofacial Surgery, College of Medicine,
University of Ulsan, Seoul, South Korea

Abstract

Intravenous bisphosphonates are used in multiple myeloma to reduce pathologic bone fracture, bone pain and to correct hypercalcemia. However, bisphosphonates related necrosis of the jaw (BRONJ) has been reported frequently in those who received intravenous bisphosphonates since 2003. Bisphosphonate related osteonecrosis of the jaw is initiated with dental extraction, dental implant surgery, denture wearing, and periodontal surgery or disease, however, it occurs spontaneously. The purpose of this study was to report 15 cases of BRONJ in multiple myeloma. The male to female ratio was 8:7. Six maxilla and nine mandibles were involved. The etiology of the BRONJ was dental extraction (6 cases), dental implant (2 cases), denture wearing (1 case), untreated vertical tooth fracture (1 case), however, five patients did not have any etiology to cause BRONJ. Conservative medical treatment to reduce pain, discomfort and infection is recommended for the initial therapy. However, if there is a sequestrum, which is separated from the basal bone of the jaw, surgical debridement and primary closure is the key to treat the BRONJ. In this study, surgical debridement was performed in 11 patients with success in 9 patients. Six patients died of multiple myeloma during follow-up periods.

* Corresponding author: Kang-Min Ahn DDS, MSD, PhD, Associate professor. Department of oral and maxillofacial surgery, College of Medicine, University of Ulsan, Seoul, South Korea. e-mail: ahnkangmin@hanmail.net. Tel: 82-2-3010-5901. Fax: 82-2-3010-6967.

Introduction

Bisphosphonates (BPs) are potent inhibitors of osteoclasts and are widely used to treat bone diseases such as osteoporosis, metastatic bone lesions of the breast, prostate cancer, and hypercalcemia of malignancy, Paget's disease, osteogenesis imperfecta and multiple myeloma (MM). [1] BPs have revolutionized the treatment of lytic bone lesions and given considerable benefits to prevent lethal pathological fractures.

Multiple myeloma related lytic bone lesion is induced by secondary to increased osteoclastic activity and impaired osteoblastic function. Myeloma cells are known to secrete both stimulators of osteoclasts and inhibitors of osteoblasts. The first one is a receptor activator of nuclear kappa B ligand (RANKL) and the latter one is dickkopf 1 (DKK). [2] BPs have proven ability to reduce skeletal-related events, bone pain and hypercalcemia in MM. [3-9] Established indications of BPs use in MM are pathological fractures, radiographic evidence of osteopenia and lytic bony lesions. [10] The fundamental effect of BPs are the impairment and apoptosis of not only adult osteoclasts but also osteoblast precursors in the bone marrow. It has also been reported that BPs affect osteoblasts, macrophages and endothelial cells and they have anti-angiogenic properties. [11]

There are two types of BPs, which are classified according to having nitrogen components. The first generation of BPs, which do not have nitrogen components, resemble pyrophosphates. There is no report of jaw necrosis related with the first generation of BPs. The mechanism of BPs are not clearly elucidated, however several hypothesis have been suggested. The most commonly accepted mechanism is related with osteoclasts. First, BPs are adhered to the receptors of osteoclasts. In an area of high bone metabolism, part of the bound BPs are endocytosed by activated osteoclasts. Apoptosis of osteoclasts are followed after adhesion to receptors and inhibition of ATP-dependent enzymes. This mechanism is the way that BPs exert their anti-resorptive action. Oral clodronate is the first line of BPs that have been used for the treatment of malignancy-associated bone lesions. However, BPs have an oral resorption of less than 2% and this is further reduced if food is present in the stomach at the time of ingestion. That is why it is recommended to take BPs in the morning before a meal. [12]

The second generation are nitrogen-containing BPs, which are pamidronate (PA) and zoledronic acid (ZA). The potency is 1,000~10,000 times higher than first generation BPs. Following a dose of intravenous BPs injection, about 50% is rapidly bound to the bone surface. [13] In MM, potent BPs such as PA or zoledronic acid (ZA) are the most commonly prescribed. Even though oral BPs of clodronate has been prescribed for prevention of bone fracture, PA and ZA showed superiority in reducing the need for radiotherapy. [14] Such potent intravenous BPs are used to reduce pathologic bone fracture, bone pain and to correct hypercalcemia. [7, 10, 15, 16]

Necrosis of the jaw has been reported frequently in those who received intravenous BPs since 2003. [17] In some case series, oral BPs also resulted in bisphosphonates-related osteonecrosis of the jaw (BRONJ). [18] The true incidence of BRONJ is unknown and there are so many under-reported cases. Until now more than 15,000 cases have been reported. [11] There appears to be an increasing trend in MM patents to develop BRONJ with a very low rate of healing; from 1.9% in 2002~2005 to 3.6% in 2006~2008. [19] BRONJ is defined as exposed bone in the maxillofacial region that persisted for more than 6~8 weeks with current or previous treatment with BPs. There should be no history of radiotherapy to the jaw. [20] The most common etiologic factors for BRONJ are extraction, denture wearing, dental implants, periapical surgery, periodontal surgery and minor oral surgery, however, BRONJ could occur spontaneously. [21] Spontaneous denudation of the jawbone is common in the mandibular area, palatal tori, or the myelohyoid ridge where the overlying mucosa is quite thin.

Although the mechanism of jaw necrosis is elusive, several theories have been proposed regarding the initiation of the jaw necrosis. The prevailing hypothesis focuses on a drug-induced defect in physiologic jawbone remodeling or wound healing by inhibition of osteoclasts. [22] BPs show strong effects on osteoclasts inhibition through adhesion to RANKL, diminishing osteoclast life span, increased osteoclast apoptosis and prevention of osteoclast development from bone marrow precursors. [23-25] The inhibition of osteoclast function inhibits normal bone turnover or remodeling to an extent that local micro-damage from normal mechanical loading or injury such as tooth extraction or dental implant surgery cannot be repaired. The second mechanism of BRONJ of BPs is an inhibitory effect on circulating levels of vascular endothelial growth factor, which is a potent stimulator of angiogenesis. [26] The third mechanism is a direct toxic effect on oral mucosa. [27] The fourth are individual genetic variations in drug metabolism. Since only a minority of BPs users develops BRONJ, there might be individual differences based on genetic variation. [28]

There are several hypothesis of BRONJ in the jawbone only. First, the jaws are a site of constant bone remodeling, receiving continuous mechanical stress during mastication, constant movement of teeth, tooth extraction and dental implant placement, which causes alveolar bone exposure. Constant physical and mechanical stresses in the jawbone stimulate gingival fibroblasts and periodontal ligament cells to express RANKL, which in turn enhances osteoclastogenesis.

Second, the oral cavity is full of micro-organisms. Infection may exert a major role in BRONJ. Microphotographs showed an accumulation of micro-organisms such as Actinomyces and Streptococcus colonies. [29] Third, it is postulated that BPs accumulates in human jaws at higher concentration levels than other skeletons, generally, since bone turnover in the jaws has been demonstrated to be higher. The high turnover rate means high vascularity, which is susceptible to high local concentration of BPs. Fourth, in addition to the effect on osteoclasts, BPs has an anti-angiogenic effect, which may inhibit the regeneration of the mucosal epithelium.

The purpose of this study was to report 15 cases of BRONJ in multiple myeloma patients with its characteristics, bisphosphonate usage, etiology, stages of BRONJ, site of BRONJ, management and its results.

Materials and Methods

The Institutional Review Board of Asan medical center approved this retrospective study. Fifteen consecutive BRONJ patients with MM were referred to the department of oral and maxillofacial surgery from the department of oncology or hemato-oncololgy in Asan medical center, Seoul, Korea. Only the patients who showed jawbone necrosis (e.g., exposed bone, sequestrum) or infection (e.g., gingival swelling, fistula formation) after infusion of BPs were included in this study. BRONJ was clinically diagnosed by the existence of exposed bone, pus discharge, soft tissue swelling, pain and existence of sequestrum. Initial treatment of the BRONJ patients was decided by the stage of BRONJ suggested by the American association of oral and maxillofacial surgeons (Table 1). [30]

Table 1. Stages of bisphosphonate related osteonecrosis of the jaw

Stages	Description
At risk	No apparent necrotic bone in patients who have been treated with either oral or intravenous bisphosphonates.
Stage 0	There is no clinical evidence of necrotic bone, but there are non-specific clinical findings and symptoms such as swelling of the soft tissue, fistula formation.
Stage 1	There is exposed and necrotic bone in asymptomatic patients but there is no evidence of infection
Stage 2	There is exposed and necrotic bone associated with infection as evidenced by pain and erythema in region of exposed bone with or without purulent drainage
Stage 3	There is exposed and necrotic bone with pain, infection and one or more of the following: exposed and necrotic bone extending beyond the region of alveolar bone resulting in 1) pathologic fracture, 2) extraoral fistula, 3) oral antral/oral-nasal communication or 4) osteolysis extending to the inferior border of the mandible or sinus floor.

When BRONJ was suspected, all BPs were stopped after consultation with an oncologist. Treatment protocol of each stage was based on the AAOMS position paper with modifications (Table 2). [30]

Table 2. Treatment protocols of bisphosphonate related osteonecrosis of the jaw in each stage

Stages	Treatment strategies
Stage 0	Oral gargle such as Hexamedin (chlorohexidin 0.12%, Yuhan Pharm, Seoul, Korea) is prescribed to prevent infection. Follow-up of every three months has been scheduled to examine the suspected wound infection or disease progress.
Stage 1	Oral gargle such as Hexamedin (chlorohexidin 0.12%, Yuhan Pharm, Seoul, Korea) is used to prevent infection. Monthly follow-up is scheduled to examine the suspected wound infection or disease progress. Oral hygiene instruction is performed at every visit.
Stage 2	Systemic antibiotics and analgesics are prescribed. If patient has responded well to the systemic antibiotic treatment, monthly follow-up is scheduled. Superficial debridement to relieve soft tissue irritation is recommended to patients who are unresponsive to conservative systemic antibiotic treatment. All the surgical specimens are histopathologically examined and culture of the microorganisms is performed.
Stage 3	Systemic antibiotics, analgesics and oral gargle are prescribed. Surgical debridement of sequestrum is performed. A primary attempt is made to close the wound. If pathologic fracture or persistent extraoral fistula refractory to the surgical debridement or sequestrectomy is detected, complete resection of the lesions and free flap reconstruction is performed after consultation with oncologist. All the surgical specimens are histopathologically examined and culture of the microorganisms is performed.

Results

Demographic data, sites, etiology, treatment, stages, used BPs and frequency of BPs infusion of the patients are listed in Table 3. The male to female ratio was 8:7 and the average age was 66.7±8.8 years old (ranged from 49 to 77 years old). Six maxilla and nine mandibles were involved. Posterior mandible (9 sites), posterior maxilla (5 sites), anterior maxilla (3 sites) and one anterior mandible were involved. The etiology of the BRONJ was dental extraction (6 cases), dental implant (2 cases), denture wearing (1 case), untreated vertical tooth fracture (1 case), however, 5 patients did not have any etiology to cause bone denudation.

All patients had been treated with chemotherapy according to the standard protocol. Standard protocol for MM of Korean national health insurance is followed; patients who are under 65 and do not have major organ complications might receive autologous stem-cell transplantation.

Table 3. Demographic data, sites, etiology, stage, bisphosphonates injection and surgery

NO	Sex	Age	Site	Etiology	Surgery	Surgery	Stage	Drug	NOI
1	M	69	Both Mx	Spontaneous	Yes	Saucerization	2	PA 90mg	11
2	M	58	Ant Mx	implant	Yes	Saucerization	2	PA 90mg + ZA 4mg	14
3	M	69	RtMn	Extraction	Yes	Saucerization	2	PA 90mg + ZA 4mg	12
4	F	75	Lt Mx	Denture	Yes	conservative Tx	2	PA 90mg + ZA 4mg	13
5	F	69	RtMn	Extraction	Yes	Saucerization	2	PA 90mg + ZA 4mg	52
6	F	51	Lt Mn	Extraction	Yes	Saucerization	2	PA 90mg + ZA 4mg	13
7	M	71	Both Mx	Extraction	No	conservative Tx	2	PA 90mg + ZA 4mg	20
8	M	69	both Mn	Spontaneous	Yes	Saucerization	3	PA 90mg + ZA 4mg	21
9	M	60	RtMn	Spontaneous	No	conservative Tx	1	PA 90mg + ZA 4mg	11
10	M	49	Lt Mn	Spontaneous	Yes	Saucerization	2	PA 90mg + ZA 4mg	33
11	M	77	Ant Mx	Spontaneous	No	conservative Tx	2	PA 90mg + ZA 4mg	24
12	F	77	Both Mn	Extraction	Yes	Saucerization	3	PA 90mg + ZA 4mg	27
13	F	65	RtMn	implant	Yes	Saucerization	2	PA 90mg + ZA 4mg	57
14	F	75	Ant Mx	Tooth Fx	Yes	Saucerization	2	PA 90mg + ZA 4mg	19
15	F	67	RtMn	Extraction	Yes	Saucerization	3	PA 90mg + ZA 4mg	16

(M: male, F: female, Rt: right, Lt: left, Mx: maxilla, Mn: mandible, Fx: fracture, Tx: treatment, PA: pamidronate, ZA: zoledronic acid, NOI: number of infusion).

With chemotherapy, all the patients receive steroids (prednisone, Yuhan Pharma, Seoul, Korea) and melphalan (Alkeran 2mg, GSK, Seoul, Korea) for the initial treatment. Bortezomib (Velcade, Janssen Korea, Seoul, Korea) and thalidomide (Thalidomide cap 50mg, Celgene, San Diego, USA) are administrated as a second line of drugs. The third line of drug is lenalidomide (Lenalidomide cap 25mg, Celgene, San Diego, USA). All the patients had received a 4mg zoledronic acid (Zometa, Novartis, Seoul, Korea) or a 90mg pamidronate (Panorin, Hallym Pharma, Seoul, Korea) intravenuously every 4 weeks for prevention of myeloma induced lytic bone lesions and bone resorption.

Fourteen patients received a combination of intravenous ZA 4mg and PA 15mg. One patient received only PA 15mg for 11 times. Mean infusion times were 22.9±14.3 (range from 11 to 57). PA was used only 3~4 times at the beginning of the treatment. Stage 1 was found in only one patient. The other 14 patients showed stage 2 (11 patients) and stage 3 (3 patients). Infection, formation of sequestrum and pain were indications for surgery. Eleven patients showed refractory to the conservative medical treatment and needed surgical debridement. Surgical methods were removing the sequestrum, collagen graft and primary closure. Representative cases are described.

Case 1

A 72-year-old male was referred from department of hemato-oncology to oral and maxillofacial surgery for pain and sinusitis symptoms in both posterior maxillary areas in December 2010. From the medical history, he had traffic accident in 2009 and his neck was injured during the accident. He had been treated conservatively; however, the neck and chest pain was not responsive to the treatment. He was referred to our hospital in February 2010 for further evaluation. Skeletal radiograph showed multiple punch-out lesions in humerus, femur and skull (Figure 1a, 1b, 1c). Bone marrow biopsy had been performed and tissue was confirmed with plasma cell myeloma of plasmablastic type. He had been treated with chemotherapy and received PA (Panorin) every 4 weeks for 11 times from March 2010 to December 2010. He complained about the toothache in the posterior maxillary area in December 2010. Both sides of the posterior maxillary gingiva were inflamed and recessed.

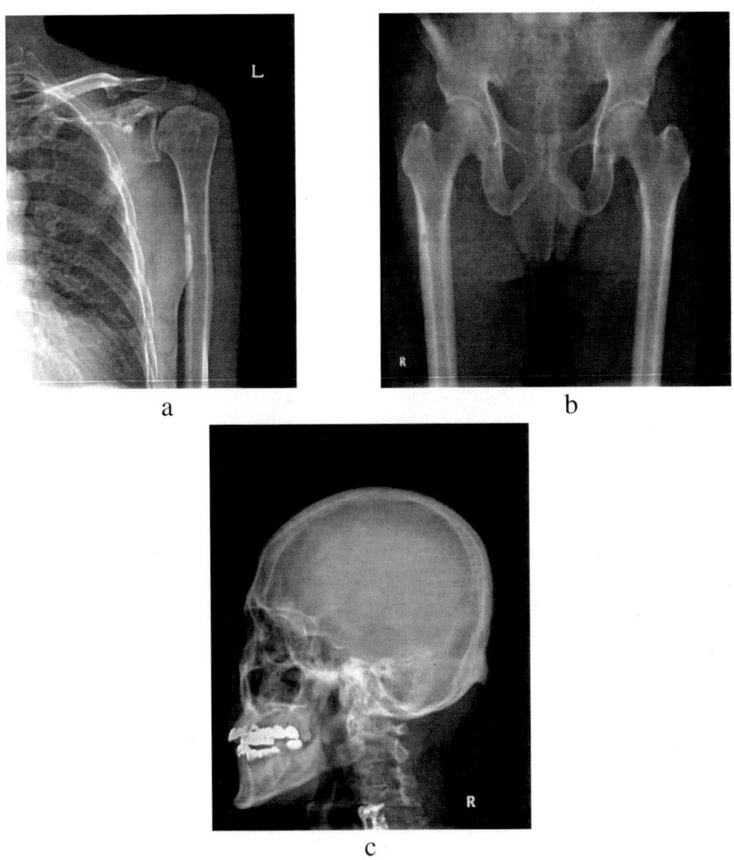

c

Figure 1. Multiple punch-out bony lesions in the humerus(a), femur(b) and skull(c).

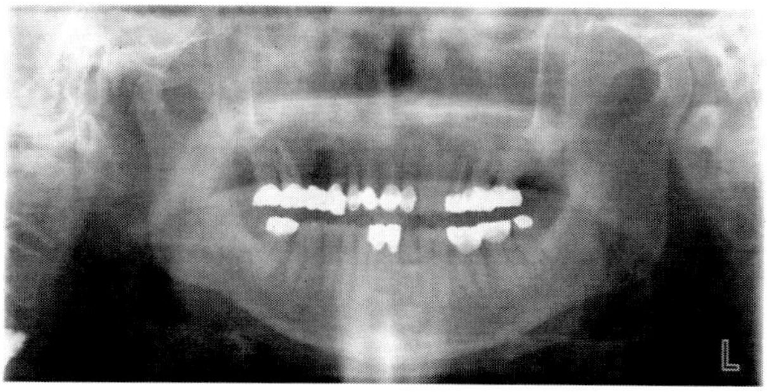

Figure 2. Panoramic radiograph showing radiolucency of both.

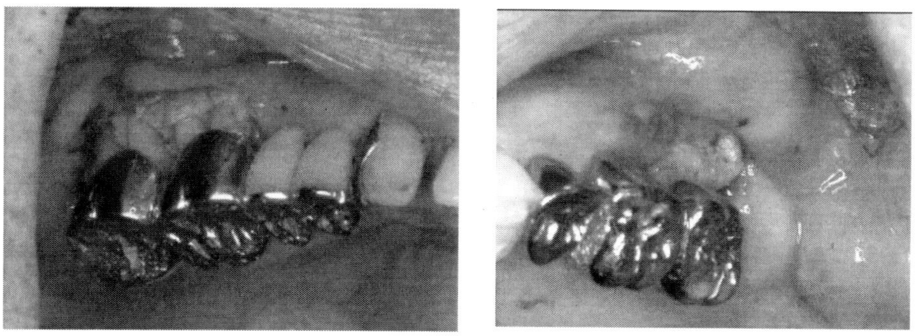

a b

Figure 3. Exposed alveolar bone with gingival inflammation of right (a) and left (b) posterior maxilla.

A panoramic radiograph showed mild bone loss in the right posterior maxilla with apical lesions, and marginal bone loss in the left posterior maxilla with apical lesion of left first molar. (Figure 2) Bone was exposed and bony necrosis was found both in the posterior maxilla. (Figure 3a, b) PA injection was immediately stopped. Stage 2 BRONJ was diagnosed. Antibiotics (Augmentin 375mg, po, bid), analgesics (Airtal 100mg, po, bid) and chlorohexidine mouthwash were prescribed for 2 weeks. Pain was not subsided and gingival recession continued. Extraction of both maxillary molars and sequestrectomy were performed under local anesthesia in January 2011. (Figure 4 a, b) The wound was primarily closed with a layered closure using absorbable sutures (Figure 5a, b).

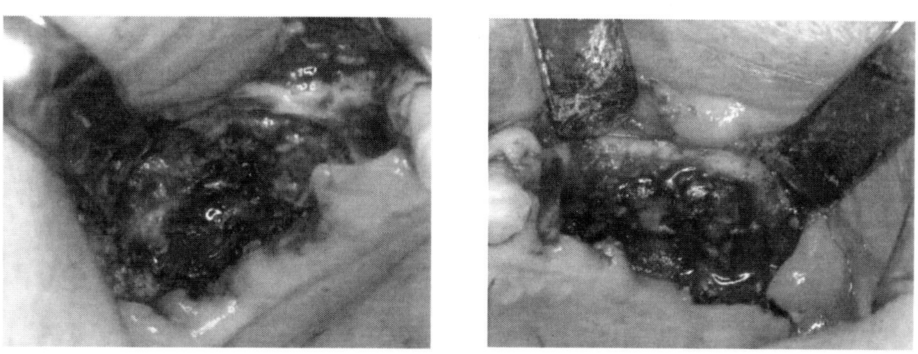

a b

Figure 4. Extraction of #14, 16 and 17 teeth and saucerization of the sequestrum (a) and extraction of #24,25,26 and 27 teeth and saucerization of the sequestrum (b).

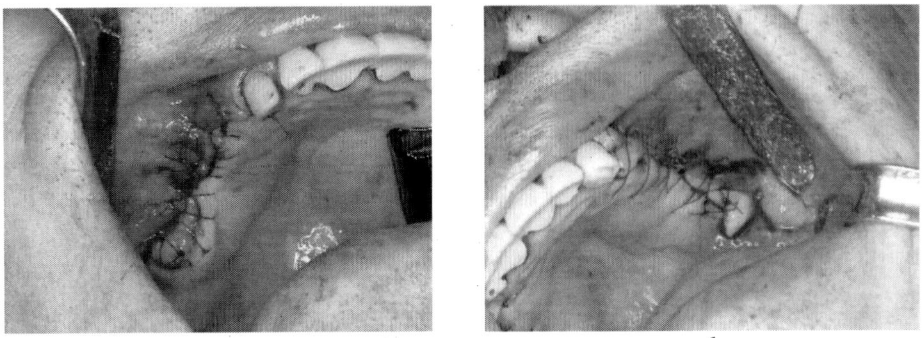

a b

Figure 5. Primary closure of the wound after extraction and saucerization, right (a), left (b).

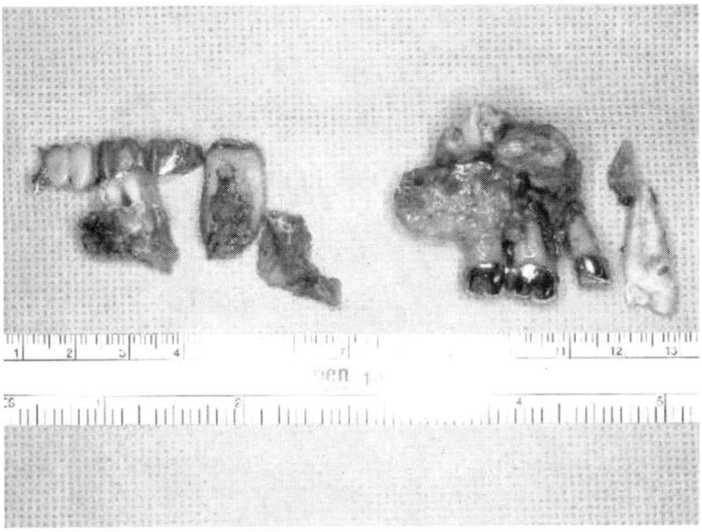

Figure 6. Removed necrotic bone and teeth.

Removed necrotic bone and teeth is shown in Figure 6. The 20-month postoperative follow-up showed complete healing of the both maxillary posterior gingiva and no exposure of the alveolar bone. (Figure 7). Patient wears a partial denture and is satisfied after the operation. Sinusitis symptom has been resolved.

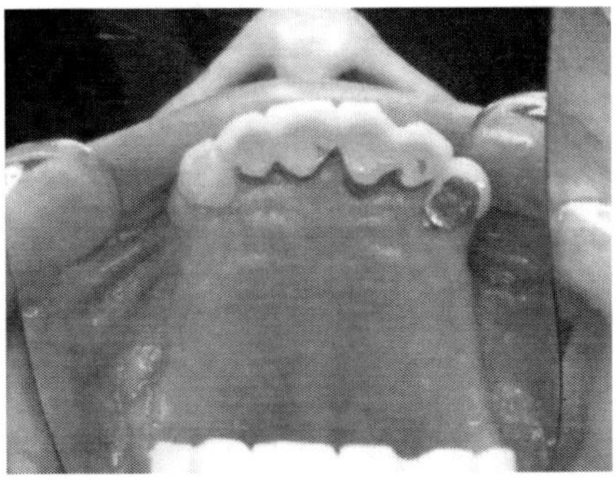

Figure 7. The 20-month postoperative follow-up photograph showing complete healing of the both maxillary posterior gingiva and no exposure of the alveolar bone.

Case 2

A 58-year-old male was referred to our department for pus discharge and pain in the left anterior maxilla area in June 2013. He had been diagnosed as multiple myeloma of plasmablastic type in June 2012. He received PA (1 time) and ZA (13 times) from July 2012 to June 2013. He complained about the toothache and pus discharge in left maxillary lateral incisor.

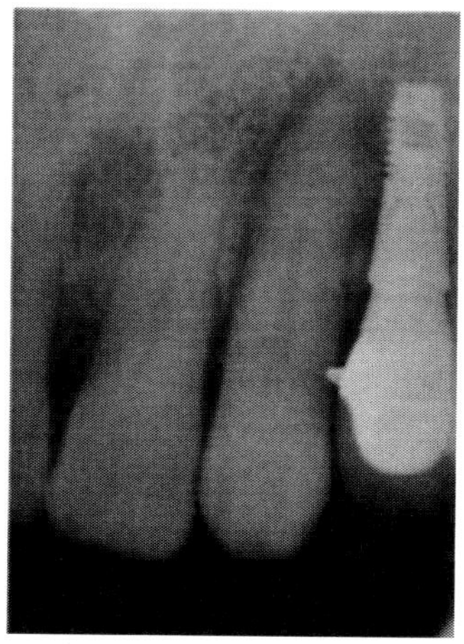

Figure 8. Dental implant is placed in the left maxillary canine area and sequestrum and periapical lesions are found around left maxillary lateral incisor.

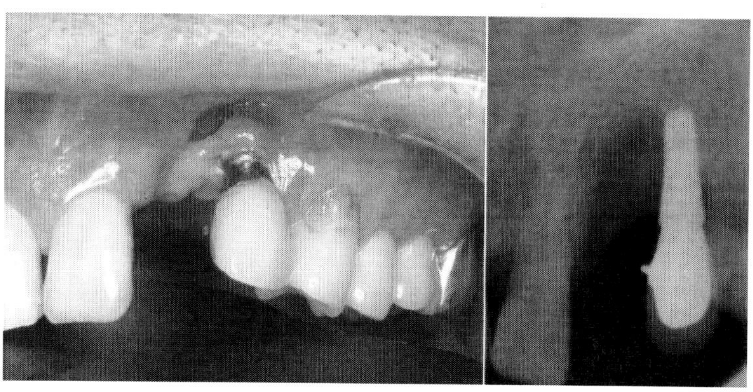

a b

Figure 9. Healed state of extraction site (a) and periapical radiograph showing bony defect in the mesial side of the implant (b).

A dental implant was placed one year ago in the left maxillary canine area. (Figure 8) BPs infusion was ceased after consultation with the oncologist. Consultation with an endodontist concluded that immediate extraction was required to relieve pain and to control infection. Left maxillary lateral incisor was extracted and necrotic bone was removed in October 2013. Patient did not want to remove the implant, so the implant was preserved. Patient was recalled every 3 months for oral hygiene care. The 6-month follow-up after extraction showed healing of the extraction site and resolution of the infection, however, gingival recession and a defect is observed in the medial side of the implant (Figure 9a, b)

Case 3

A 69-year-old male was referred from the department of oncology to our department for treatment of exposed bone and gingival swelling in April 2006. His past medical history included MM (monoclonal gammopathy, IgG lamda type), which had been confirmed by bone marrow biopsy in May 2005, and the use of PA (1 time) and ZA (11 times) from May 2005 to April 2006.

Lateral skull radiograph showed punch out bony lesions and a large destructive mass in the lateral surface of the cervical spine (C1) extended into the left paraspinal muscles from neck computed tomographic scan (CT). Intraoral examination revealed an exposed bone of edentulous ridge in the right mandible and in the retromolar area. (Figure 11) ZA was ceased immediately and conservative treatment with antibiotics (Augmentin 375mg, po, bid), analgesics (Airtal 100mg, po, bid) and 0.12% chlorohexidine mouthwash were performed for 8 weeks.

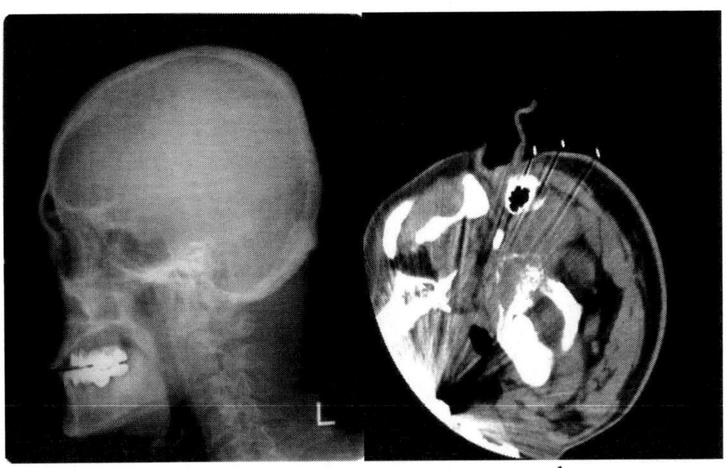

a b

Figure 10. Lateral skull radiograph showing punch out bony lesions (a) and neck CT scan demonstrating osteolytic lesions in the lateral surface of cervical spine (b).

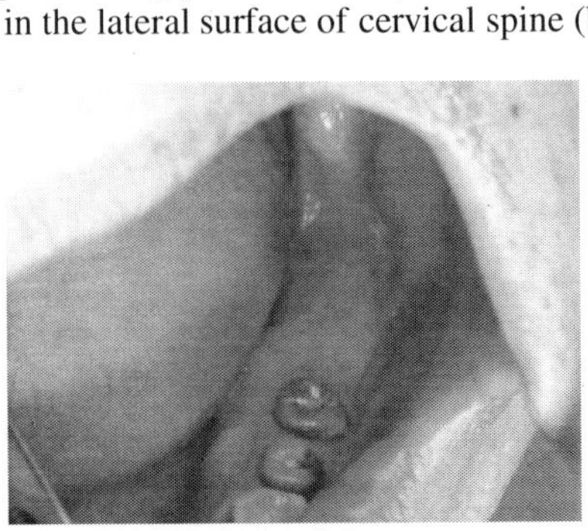

Figure 11. Bone exposure in the right mandible crestal and retromolar area.

Swelling of the vestibule was observed even after conservative treatment and pus was drained through the fistula. (Figure 12) After consultation with the oncologist, debridement, saucerization and primary closure were performed in July 2006.

The six-month follow-up showed complete healing of the exposed bone and fistula. (Figure 13) The patient passed away in August 2008 due to the progression of the MM.

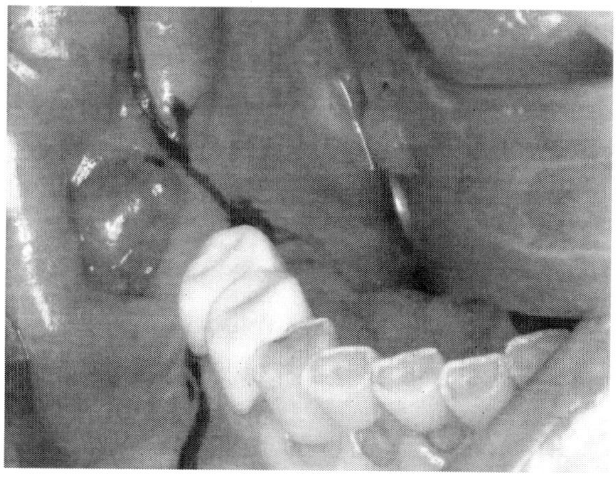

Figure 12. Exposed bone in the lingual side of the posterior right mandible and gingival swelling in the retromolar area.

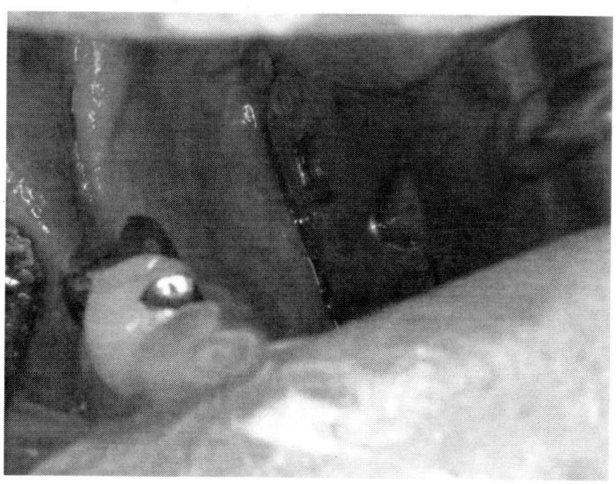

Figure 13. Two-month follow-up of healed gingiva of exposed bone and fistula.

Case 4

A 77-year-old male was referred from the department of oncology for treatment of the gingival pain and recession in December 2013. He had been diagnosed with MM (plasma cell myeloma of plasmacytic type) in October 2011.

Lateral Lumbar spine radiograph showed a compression fracture of L4 and bone destruction of L1 in the initial screening examination. (Figure 14) Whole body PET showed multiple lytic bone lesions with pathologic fractures of right pubic and lumbar bone (L4) and heterogenous hypermetabolic activity in spine (T-L spine). (Figure 15) He had been infused with 4mg ZA for 18 times and 15mg PA for 6 times from October 2011 to October 2013. Intraoral examination showed an exposed necrotic bone of the alveolus in the right anterior maxilla and inflamed gingiva. (Figure 16) Pus was not discharged from the exposed bone, however, patient reported severe pain and discomfort. Aggressive surgical treatment was not indicated due to general condition of the patient, supportive care with 0.12% chlorohexidine oral gargle has been prescribed to prevent infection.

Endodontic treatment had been performed in the right maxillary canine and premolars. (Figure 16) Conservative medical treatment with antibiotics (Augmentin 375mg, po, bid), analgesics (Airtal 100mg, po, bid) and 0.12% chlorohexidine mouthwash were performed for 8 weeks.

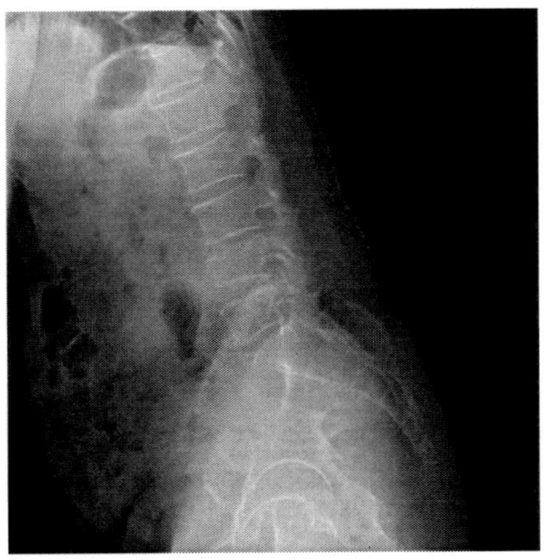

Figure 14. Bone destruction in L1 and compression fracture of L4.

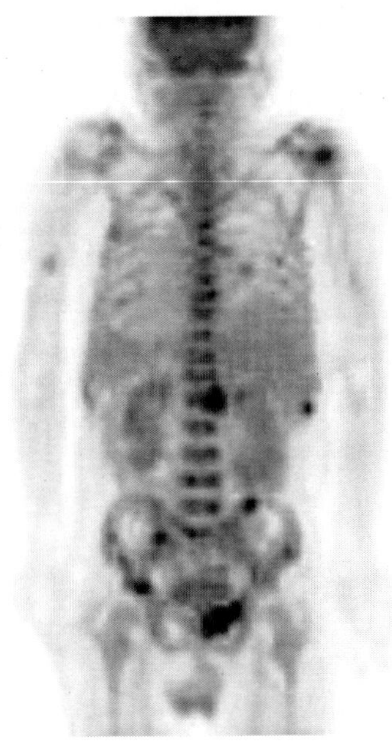

Figure 15. Whole body F-18 FDG-PET showing multiple bony lesions with pubic and lumbar fracture.

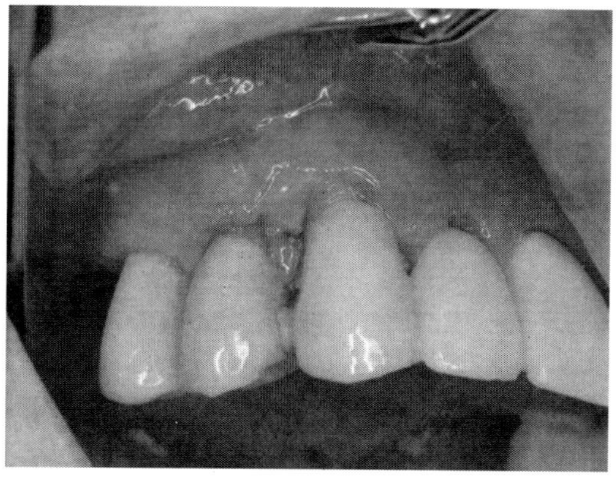

Figure 16. Intraoral photograph showing exposed bone between right maxillary canine and premolar and inflamed gingival.

After medical treatment, pain subsided and inflammation of the gingiva decreased. However, the area of bone denudation had increased and new exposed bone was found on the buccal side of the lateral incisor (Figure 17).

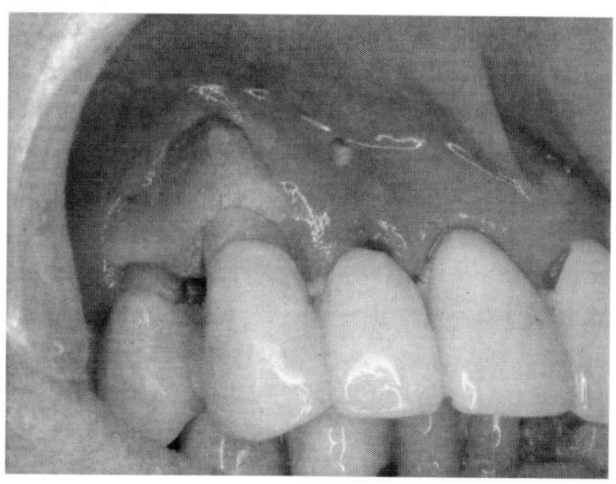

Figure 17. Exposed bone at the buccal side of the canine and first premolar.

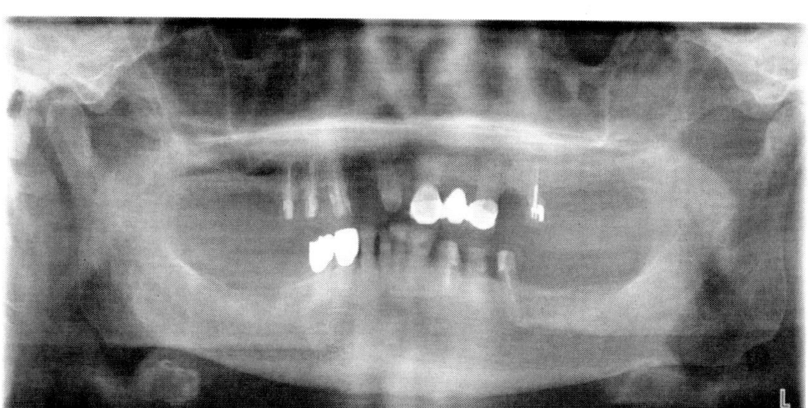

Figure 18. Panoramic radiograph showing multiple bone lesions in the mandible and endodontic treatment of the right maxillary canine and premolars.

Discussion

There is no doubt about the effectiveness of bisphosphonates in multiple myeloma. [4, 5, 31-33] Even though there are complications such as BRONJ, the benefit/risk ratio greatly favors treatment with BPs in MM. BPs reduce bone pain, pathologic fracture and correct hypercalcemia. In our case series of 15 patients, combination of PA 90mg + ZA 4mg or PA 90mg only was infused every 4 weeks. PA was used for the first line of BPs because of lower price. However, ZA has a superior effect to normalize serum calcium in hypercalcemia to PA. Nowadays, ZA has been used as a standard protocol because of the higher potency and less time (15 minutes) than PA (more than 45 minutes), required for infusion. Even though, the risk of the BRONJ increases after 12 months of infusion, five patients developed BRONJ in less than 12 months of infusion. Close follow-up of oral hygiene with regular visits (at least 3 months interval) to a dental clinic is recommended for patients who receive ZA for MM

There are some adverse effects of bisphosphonates, which are fever, osteomalacia, hypocalcemia, bone pain, fatigue, nausea, arthralgia, and renal function impairment. [1] These adverse effects are corrected or prevented by dose adjustment and electrolyte balance. One of the most serious complications associated with bisphosphonates is BRONJ. BRONJ is rare and the incidence ranges from 0.8% to 12%. [20] During past decade, many new findings about bone turnover, bone physiology and pathologic mechanisms have been discovered. Marx recently reported the new findings. [11] First, bone remodeling is the mechanism by which bone adapts to loading stresses and it is the mechanism for bone renewal. Second, osteoclastic bone resorption triggers bone renewal at a rate of about 0.7%/day by its release of growth factors. Third, BPs prevent the renewal of old and injured bone, thus making it brittle and more likely to fracture over time. Fourth, BPs have a half-life in bone of 11 years because of their irreversible binding to bone via their central carbon atom. Fifth, when administered intravenously, BPs load bone and accumulate in bone 142.8 times faster than when administered orally. Sixth, osteoclastic resorption of BPs-loaded bone results in osteoclast death in which the cell bursts, releasing the BPs molecules to reenter the local bone or bone marrow in a re-dosing effect. Seventh, endosteal osteoblasts are dependent on the osteoclastic resorption/growth factor release/new bone formation mechanism of bone renewal, whereas periosteal osteoblasts are not. Eighth, it is likely that endosteal osteoblasts and periosteal osteoblasts have different cell membrane receptors and arise from separate embryologic niches. However, there are many fields that should be proved to clarify the mechanism of jaw necrosis such as half-life of the BPs, maximum dose of tolerance, ideal interval of the BPs injection, selection of BPs according to the stages of the MM.

Suggested potential risk factors are dentoalveolar trauma (e.g., dental extraction), duration of BPs use, potency of BPs(ZA), number of infusions, advanced age and combination of drug such as steroid therapy. The most common risk factor of BRONJ is dentoalveolar trauma such as tooth extraction. In our case series, extraction was the first etiology of BRONJ with 6 patients. However, five patients developed BRONJ without any etiology. Spontaneous denudation of the gingiva had happened in the maxilla and mandible. Direct toxic effect to oral mucosa or anti-angiogenic effect to inhibit epithelial regeneration might be a role in the development of BRONJ.

High potency, frequent dosing schedule and duration of medication are also main risk factors. Potent PA and ZA are most commonly implicated BPs. Retrospective studies reported a 2.4~9.5 times increased relative risk of BRONJ when comparing monthly ZA and PA. [34-37] Also, risk of BRONJ significantly increases after 12~24 months of intravenous injection on a monthly dosing regimen. In our case series, five patients who had BRONJ received BPs infusion in less than 12 months. More studies about the maximum dose of the BPs and individual genetic variations are needed to elucidate the early onset of BRONJ.

Although the incidence of BRONJ in MM is unknown, patients with MM have a higher incidence of BRONJ than breast cancer. [36] The mandible is more common than the maxilla by about 2~5 times [38]. In our case series, the mandible was 1.5 times higher incidence than the maxilla. The posterior area is more common than the anterior and in our case series the ratio was 25:4. Chemotherapy with multiple drugs such as thalidomide, corticosteroids, immunosuppressant and potent BPs might explain the higher incidence of BRONJ in MM patients. A progressively improved prognosis of MM (patient's survival has been increased with advanced chemotherapy agents) and extended exposure to BPs explain the higher incidence of BRONJ in MM. There are established risk factors for BRONJ such as tooth extraction, high potency BPs used intravenously, prolonged use of BPs over 12 months, smoking, diabetes mellitus and ill-fitting dentures.

The International Myeloma Foundation reported that the incidence of BRONJ in multiple myeloma is 6.9%. [36] Hoff et al. have reported that the incidence of BRONJ is 6.9% in multiple myeloma. [39] Cetiner et al. reported that the incidence of BRONJ is 15%, which was higher than other reports. [29] Dimopoulos et al. also reported a 15% BRONJ incidence in MM patients. Most of oncologists prescribe ZA and/or PA for MM patients, which are about 5,000 to 10,000 more potent than oral bisphosphonates. When more potent drugs are used, a higher incidence of BRONJ is expected. [36] BRONJ is common in multiple myeloma patients who have a history of tooth extraction, or implant surgery. However, BRONJ may occur spontaneously in the area of thin mucosa. In our case series, two cases of BRONJ occurred after dental implant surgery. [21]

Bone necrosis related with bisphosphonates is only found in jaw bone. There are some bony complications such as femur neck fracture, osteomalacia and arthralgia; however, necrosis of the bone is only found in the jawbone. The suggested hypotheses for only jaw bone necrosis are 1) high turnover rate of jaw bone, which accumulates more bisphosphonates than other bone, 2) risk of bone exposure during extraction, periodontal surgery, implant surgery and apical surgery, 3) presence of oral microflora, 4) high vascularity of jaw bone. [40]

Prevention

It is impossible to completely prevent BRONJ in MM; however, we should make every possible effort to prevent BRONJ. Regular dental checkups, oral hygiene care, education of proper tooth brushing, and extraction of hopeless teeth are the basic treatment before BPs are prescribed. Bad teeth should be extracted and primary closure is recommended after extraction. Patients with periodontal disease and dental caries should be treated before BPs use and all patients should be informed of the risks of BRONJ. Patients with periodontal disease should be recalled every 6 months while on BPs treatment. There are controversies about the cessation of BPs before extraction. The Mayo clinic guideline on BPs in MM recommends BPs cessation for a month before extraction and until healing is complete. [10] A Canadian consensus guideline recommends a 3~6 months cessation of BPs before tooth extraction. [41] The American association of oral and maxillofacial surgeons' position paper reported that the clinician might consider discontinuation of BPs for a 3-month period before and 3-month period after invasive dental surgery to lower the risk of BRONJ. [42] The Myeloma foundation of Australia recommended a 2~3 month BPs discontinuation before and after dental extraction. [38] They also recommended antibiotic prophylaxis with an anti-streptococcal/anti-anaerobic agent and 0.12% chlorhexidine mouthwash before invasive dental surgery. Re-administration of the BPs should start after evidence of complete mucolization and osseous healing of extraction socket. As the risk of BRONJ increases with duration, dose modification should be considered in patients who received BPs for more than 1 year. [38] Elective dentoalveolar surgery such as implant surgery, apicoectomy, corticotomy and orthodontic surgery are not recommended during intravenous BPs therapy for malignancy. [43]

However, there are many patients who need emergency extraction. In such cases, it is not possible to wait 1~3 months for dental extraction. In such an emergency situation, atraumatic extraction is recommended along with insertion of a collagen plug in the extraction socket after an informed consent form of BRONJ. Closure of the socket by suturing should be tried to minimize bone exposure and prevent BRONJ. [21]

The risk of BRONJ in MM correlates with duration of infusion of intravenous BPs, and a number of guidelines have been established to reduce the cumulative dose of BPs. [10, 16, 38] In general, monthly BPs infusion is recommended for MM with active lytic bone lesions, but after the initial treatment phase of about 12~24 months, dose modification or discontinuation is considered such as substitution into oral BPs, three-monthly intravenous BPs infusion or cessation of the BPs.

Treatment

BRONJ is closely related to the quality of life and difficult to treat. To eradicate BRONJ with a single treatment modality is not usually achieved in most cases. It is important to inform patients that a cure of BRONJ is not a realistic expectation. The goal of BRONJ management should be to improve the quality of life by reducing pain, infection and prevent occurring new areas of BRONJ. This conservative management should be done under consultation with oncologists or endocrine doctors.

There is controversy about stopping BPs when BRONJ has been detected. The so-called "drug holiday" is a temporary discontinuation of BPs to allow bone marrow recovery and the formation of new osteoclasts. Although intravenous BPs have been incorporated within bone for many years, the effect of short-term discontinuation has not yet been proven. However, when BRONJ has been observed, discontinuation of BPs is recommended except with uncontrolled hypercalcemia. [38] In case of treatment-resistant hyerpcalcemia, 3 monthly injections of ZA or oral BPs are recommended. [38, 44] Reinstitution of BPs are recommended after the complete resolution of BRONJ.

Conservative treatment with systemic antibiotic administration is recommended in stage 0~1 BRONJ. Debridement of necrotic bone which is not isolated from basal bone tends to exacerbate rather than improve the BRONJ symptoms, so in most cases therapy should be started conservatively. Patients with stage 2 BRONJ have exposed necrotic bone with infection. These patients benefit from oral antimicrobial gargle in combination with systemic antibiotic therapy. More than 90% of BRONJ patients in stage 1 and stage 2 were stabilized with oral rinses and systemic antibiotic therapy. [45] However, if there are sequestrum, which is separated from basal bone associated with pathologic fracture, extraoral fistula and severe sinusitis (stage 3), it should be removed with surgical debridement. [46] If the sequestrum is not removed, persistent pus drainage and pain is expected. If BRONJ is aggravated, patients have difficulty eating and drinking. Patients may lose their appetite, which is commonly found in patients with chemotherapy. If the patient does not take in enough nutrients, it is hard to continue chemotherapy.

Conclusion

MM patients treated with intravenous BPs are under risk of jaw necrosis. If BRONJ has been detected during follow-up, dentists and oncologists should undertake a multi-disciplinary approach to treat the BRONJ. The oncologist should monitor the prescription of BPs and evaluate the systemic condition of patient who might require a surgical procedure. Dentists should pay more attention to the oral hygiene and existing periodontal disease. Oral and maxillofacial surgeons should be aware of surgical indications of BRONJ.

Invasive dental procedures should be avoided wherever possible in MM patients who receive intravenous BPs for more than 12 months. Prevention is always better than treatment; however, complete prevention is not possible. Discontinuation of BPs is recommended both prior to invasive dental surgery and on development of BRONJ, if the systemic condition permits. Medical and supportive care may be used at the initial stage of BRONJ. However, in the advanced stage when sequestrum is formed, surgical debridement and primary closure after “drug holidays” are the keys for successful healing.

References

[1] Dunstan CR, Felsenberg D, Seibel MJ. Therapy insight: the risks and benefits of bisphosphonates for the treatment of tumor-induced bone disease. *Nat. Clin. Pract. Oncol.* 2007;4(1):42-55.

[2] Glass DA, 2nd, Patel MS, Karsenty G. A new insight into the formation of osteolytic lesions in multiple myeloma. *N. Engl. J. Med.* 2003; 349(26):2479-80.

[3] Berenson J. Pamidronate in the treatment of osteolytic bone lesions in multiple myeloma patients--the American experience. *Br. J. Clin. Pract. Suppl.* 1996;87:5-7; discussion 13-4.

[4] Berenson JR. Bisphosphonates in multiple myeloma. *Cancer* 1997;80(8 Suppl): 1661-7.

[5] Berenson JR, Hillner BE, Kyle RA, et al. American Society of Clinical Oncology clinical practice guidelines: the role of bisphosphonates in multiple myeloma. *J. Clin. Oncol.* 2002; 20(17):3719-36.

[6] Djulbegovic B, Wheatley K, Ross J, et al. Bisphosphonates in multiple myeloma. *Cochrane Database Syst. Rev.* 2001(4): CD003188.

[7] Levy J, Roodman GD. The role of bisphosphonates in multiple myeloma. *Curr. Hematol. Malig. Rep.* 2009;4(2):108-12.

[8] Man Z, Otero AB, Rendo P, Barazzutti L, Sanchez Avalos JC. Use of pamidronate for multiple myeloma osteolytic lesions. *Lancet* 1990; 335(8690):663.

[9] Pozzi S, Raje N. The role of bisphosphonates in multiple myeloma: mechanisms, side effects, and the future. *Oncologist* 2011;16(5):651-62.

[10] Lacy MQ, Dispenzieri A, Gertz MA, et al. Mayo clinic consensus statement for the use of bisphosphonates in multiple myeloma. *Mayo Clin. Proc.* 2006; 81(8):1047-53.

[11] Marx RE. A decade of bisphosphonate bone complications: what it has taught us about bone physiology. *Int. J. Oral Maxillofac. Implants* 2014; 29(2):e247-58.

[12] Licata AA. Discovery, clinical development, and therapeutic uses of bisphosphonates. *Ann. Pharmacother.* 2005;39(4):668-77.

[13] Fleisch H. Bisphosphonates: mechanisms of action. *Endocr. Rev.* 1998; 19(1):80-100.

[14] Ross JR, Saunders Y, Edmonds PM, et al. A systematic review of the role of bisphosphonates in metastatic disease. *Health Technol. Assess* 2004; 8(4):1-176.

[15] Mhaskar R, Redzepovic J, Wheatley K, et al. Bisphosphonates in multiple myeloma. *Cochrane Database Syst. Rev.* 2010(3):CD003188.

[16] Kyle RA, Yee GC, Somerfield MR, et al. American Society of Clinical Oncology 2007 clinical practice guideline update on the role of bisphosphonates in multiple myeloma. *J. Clin. Oncol.* 2007; 25(17): 2464-72.

[17] Marx RE. Pamidronate (Aredia) and zoledronate (Zometa) induced avascular necrosis of the jaws: a growing epidemic. *J. Oral Maxillofac. Surg.* 2003;61(9):1115-7.

[18] Park W, Kim NK, Kim MY, Rhee YM, Kim HJ. Osteonecrosis of the jaw induced by oral administration of bisphosphonates in the Asian population: five cases. *Osteoporos. Int.* 2010; 21(3):527-33.

[19] Pozzi S, Marcheselli R, Falorio S, et al. Bisphosphonates-associated osteonecrosis of the jaw: A long-term follow-up of a series of 35 cases observed by GISL and evaluation of its frequency over time. *Am. J. Hematol.* 2009; 84(12):850-2.

[20] Colella G, Campisi G, Fusco V. American Association of Oral and Maxillofacial Surgeons position paper: Bisphosphonate-Related Osteonecrosis of the Jaws-2009 update: the need to refine the BRONJ definition. *J. Oral Maxillofac. Surg.* 2009; 67(12):2698-9.

[21] Tam Y, Kar K, Nowzari H, Cha HS, Ahn KM. Osteonecrosis of the Jaw after Implant Surgery in Patients Treated with Bisphosphonates - A Presentation of Six Consecutive Cases. *Clin. Implant. Dent. Relat. Res.* 2013.

[22] Ruggiero SL. Bisphosphonate-related osteonecrosis of the jaw: an overview. *Ann. N Y Acad. Sci.* 2011;1218:38-46.

[23] Hughes DE, MacDonald BR, Russell RG, Gowen M. Inhibition of osteoclast-like cell formation by bisphosphonates in long-term cultures of human bone marrow. *J. Clin. Invest.* 1989;83(6):1930-5.

[24] Rogers MJ, Gordon S, Benford HL, et al. Cellular and molecular mechanisms of action of bisphosphonates. *Cancer* 2000;88(12 Suppl): 2961-78.

[25] Hughes DE, Wright KR, Uy HL, et al. Bisphosphonates promote apoptosis in murine osteoclasts in vitro and in vivo. *J. Bone Miner. Res.* 1995; 10(10):1478-87.

[26] Santini D, Vincenzi B, Avvisati G, et al. Pamidronate induces modifications of circulating angiogenetic factors in cancer patients. *Clin. Cancer Res.* 2002; 8(5):1080-4.
[27] Landesberg R, Cozin M, Cremers S, et al. Inhibition of oral mucosal cell wound healing by bisphosphonates. *J. Oral Maxillofac. Surg.* 2008; 66(5): 839-47.
[28] Sarasquete ME, Garcia-Sanz R, Marin L, et al. Bisphosphonate-related osteonecrosis of the jaw is associated with polymorphisms of the cytochrome P450 CYP2C8 in multiple myeloma: a genome-wide single nucleotide polymorphism analysis. *Blood* 2008;112(7):2709-12.
[29] Cetiner S, Sucak GT, Kahraman SA, et al. Osteonecrosis of the jaw in patients with multiple myeloma treated with zoledronic acid. *J. Bone Miner. Metab.* 2009; 27(4):435-43.
[30] Ruggiero SL, Dodson TB, Assael LA, et al. American Association of Oral and Maxillofacial Surgeons position paper on bisphosphonate-related osteonecrosis of the jaw - 2009 update. *Aust. Endod. J.* 2009; 35(3):119-30.
[31] Henk HJ, Teitelbaum A, Perez JR, Kaura S. Persistency with zoledronic acid is associated with clinical benefit in patients with multiple myeloma. *Am. J. Hematol.* 2012; 87(5):490-5.
[32] Kanis JA, McCloskey EV. Bisphosphonates in multiple myeloma. *Cancer* 2000; 88(12 Suppl):3022-32.
[33] McCloskey EV, Guest JF, Kanis JA. The clinical and cost considerations of bisphosphonates in preventing bone complications in patients with metastatic breast cancer or multiple myeloma. *Drugs* 2001; 61(9): 1253-74.
[34] Bamias A, Kastritis E, Bamia C, et al. Osteonecrosis of the jaw in cancer after treatment with bisphosphonates: incidence and risk factors. *J. Clin. Oncol.* 2005; 23(34):8580-7.
[35] Dimopoulos MA, Kastritis E, Anagnostopoulos A, et al. Osteonecrosis of the jaw in patients with multiple myeloma treated with bisphosphonates: evidence of increased risk after treatment with zoledronic acid. *Haematologica* 2006;91(7):968-71.
[36] Durie BG, Katz M, Crowley J. Osteonecrosis of the jaw and bisphosphonates. *N. Engl. J. Med.* 2005;353(1):99-102; discussion 99-02.
[37] Mavrokokki T, Cheng A, Stein B, Goss A. Nature and frequency of bisphosphonate-associated osteonecrosis of the jaws in Australia. *J. Oral Maxillofac. Surg.* 2007; 65(3):415-23.
[38] Dickinson M, Prince HM, Kirsa S, et al. Osteonecrosis of the jaw complicating bisphosphonate treatment for bone disease in multiple myeloma: an overview with recommendations for prevention and treatment. *Intern. Med. J.* 2009;39(5):304-16.
[39] Hoff AO, Toth BB, Altundag K, et al. Frequency and risk factors associated with osteonecrosis of the jaw in cancer patients treated with intravenous bisphosphonates. *J. Bone Miner. Res.* 2008;23(6):826-36.
[40] Pichardo SE, van Merkesteyn JP. Bisphosphonate related osteonecrosis of the jaws: spontaneous or dental origin? *Oral Surg. Oral Med. Oral Pathol. Oral Radiol.* 2013; 116(3):287-92.
[41] Khan AA, Sandor GK, Dore E, et al. Canadian consensus practice guidelines for bisphosphonate associated osteonecrosis of the jaw. *J. Rheumatol.* 2008;35(7):1391-7.
[42] Ruggiero SL, Dodson TB, Assael LA, et al. American Association of Oral and Maxillofacial Surgeons position paper on bisphosphonate-related osteonecrosis of the jaws--2009 update. *J. Oral Maxillofac. Surg.* 2009;67(5 Suppl):2-12.

[43] Khosla S, Burr D, Cauley J, et al. Bisphosphonate-associated osteonecrosis of the jaw: report of a task force of the American Society for Bone and Mineral Research. *J. Bone Miner. Res.* 2007; 22(10):1479-91.

[44] Chen T, Berenson J, Vescio R, et al. Pharmacokinetics and pharmacodynamics of zoledronic acid in cancer patients with bone metastases. *J. Clin. Pharmacol.* 2002; 42(11):1228-36.

[45] Marx RE, Sawatari Y, Fortin M, Broumand V. Bisphosphonate-induced exposed bone (osteonecrosis/osteopetrosis) of the jaws: risk factors, recognition, prevention, and treatment. *J. Oral Maxillofac. Surg.* 2005; 63(11): 1567-75.

[46] Holzinger D, Seemann R, Klug C, et al. Long-term success of surgery in bisphosphonate-related osteonecrosis of the jaws (BRONJs). *Oral Oncol.* 2013; 49(1):66-70.

In: Multiple Myeloma: Risk Factors, Diagnosis and Treatments
Editor: Steve Holt
ISBN: 978-1-63321-514-6

Chapter 9

The Mechanism of Action of Novel Antimyeloma Agents and Newer Therapeutic Strategies

Yossi Cohen*
Institute of Hematology, Asaf Harofhe University Hospital, Zerifin, Israel
Sackler, Faculty of Medicine, Tel Aviv University, Israel

Abstract

Several decades of "stagnation" in the introduction of new antimyeloma agents beyond the traditional corticosteroids and alkylating agents have been occupied from the late nineties by an exciting new era characterized by rapid or even 'explosive' development of a variety of new agents starting from the dramatic comeback of thalidomide, this time as a novel agent against multiple myeloma (MM) followed by the appearance of completely new classes of agents directed against specific molecular targets. The revolution in drug development since then has been manifested by the growing number of clinical trials assessing numerous combinations of older and new first and second generation agents and more recently also by modified routs of drug administrations. Despite this, the progress in elucidation of the basic mechanism of action of many of the novel agents in use has been lagging behind the clinical data acquired and this knowledge gap is becoming an obstacle for the ability to improve the available treatments against resistant disease or to design newer molecules which target the desired pathways more directly. This chapter will summarize the current knowledge on the mechanism of action of some of the mostly used classes of novel agents and those under advanced stage of evaluation. It is noteworthy that in many instances modern research failed to support the general idea standing behind the mechanism offered originally and new theories came instead. Thalidomide is one of the most fascinating examples in all times, for which the obscure binding site and the unknown molecular pathway mediating its diversified physiological effects turned much of the attention towards the clinical manifestations seen and the biological changes observed under experimental conditions,

* Corresponding author: Tel: +972 8 9778223, Fax: +972 8 9779772, Email: yosefc@asaf.health.gov.il.

whether of clinical relevance or just another speculation as also happened with the second generation IMiDs. The proteasome inhibitors in contrast have their binding site recognized already from the first introduction to clinic but even there the means by which the proteasome blockade translates into tumor cell killing remains largely unknown considering the failure to confirm the historical attribution of the cytotoxicity to NFkB inhibition. Another therapeutic modality that has gained a lot of success in the treatment of cancer but in myeloma is still seeking for its place is targeted therapy using monoclonal antibodies directed against specific tumor associated antigens or extracellular factors. The limited benefit of the antibodies studied so far in myeloma is an indication that our targets are not optimally selected and we have to improve our knowledge on myeloma initiating cells and their unique immunophenotype. All these issues will be addressed comprehensively and new insights will be introduced, which will be many times inconsistent with the established literature dogmas.

The IMiDS

More than a half of all pregnant women tend to experience morning sickness. With this statistic in mind, a German company Grunenthal developed a drug for expecting mothers in the late 1950s called thalidomide. Several years after its introduction, more than 10,000 babies were born with severe birth defects. These malformations included stunted or missing limbs, deformed ears and valvular abnormalities. More than 40% of births were still-born or the infants died shortly after birth. This devastation created a huge scare and sparked decades of research in order to figure out what caused these severe birth defects and how to prevent this from occurring again. However, after years of interrogation, in 2006, thalidomide was approved by the FDA for the treatment of multiple myeloma (MM), in addition to its off-label use since the seventies for the treatment of miscellaneous inflammatory conditions.

Structurally, thalidomide contains a phtalimide ring linked to a glutarimide ring via an asymmetric carbon atom. Several factors joined to make the thalidomide binding site and its mode of action so difficult to decipher and one of the most devastating medical mysteries ever: 1. Its peculiar spectrum of biological activities that involve many organs, including the central nervous system (sedation, hypnosis), the peripheral nervous system (neuropathy), the immune system (immunomodulation and reduction of TNFα levels), the cardiovascular system (arrhythmias), the coagulation system (thrombosis), the hematopoietic system (e.g., lenalidomide efficacy in the 5q- dysplasia) and of course the teratogenicity, which as a group are lacking any apparent common denominator. 2. The lack of activation of any known proapoptotic pathway and the few measurable changes observed in treated organisms, excluding the variable decrease in TNFα levels, which remains the best recognized biomarker. 3. The large number of circulating metabolites, exceeding 100 byproducts, which contributed to the complexity in working with this compound. 4. The species specificity that characterized the thalidomide embryopathy, which later turned to be one of the ultimate criteria required to be fulfilled in any explanation for the teratological effects of the drug. The last character limited animal modeling to pregnant rabbits, chickens and monkey until recently, but also implied that the teratogenicity is not necessarily exerted by the parent drug itself but is possibly mediated by one of its active metabolites, generated after processing by microsomal enzymes in a species specific manner. Over the years, the withdrawn from the markets and the difficulties mentioned minimized the global effort invested on the subject, and fade the motivation to solve the thalidomide mystery ever, even though the continues progress in the developmental research and occasional breakthroughs in relevant fields generated new insights, from time to time, leading to new interpretations of the findings combined with "fresh" speculations, suited for the contemporary knowledge, which eventually matured into acceptable models based on discoveries on limb patterning, oxygen-stress related apoptosis, neurotoxic and vasculotoxic effects of thalidomide, which will be discussed in detail below. However, it seems that the most exciting discovery, as far as can be appreciate today, occurred in the year 2010, when a protein called cereblon (CRBN), previously implicated in mental retardation was unexpectedly found to be the thalidomide binding protein. Moreover, knockdown of the zebrafish paralogue of CRBN, i.e., zCRBN induced analogous teratologic malformations to the human embryopathy, including retardation of pectoral fin and otic vesicle (ear) formation, and inhibition of Fgf8 expression in fin buds. This discovery was more recently followed by the demonstration that lenalidomide-bound cereblon acquires the ability to target the proteasomal degradation of two specific B cell transcription factors, Ikaros family zinc finger proteins 1 and 3 (IKZF1 and IKZF3). In addition it was found that in myeloma cell lines, the loss of IKZF1 and IKZF3 is both necessary and sufficient for lenalidomide's therapeutic effect, suggesting that the antitumor and teratogenic activities of thalidomide-like drugs are dissociable. Therefore, it is becoming more and more realistic that we are standing now very close to the end of the mystery. But, are we really there? The documented history of the drug thought us that the thalidomide mystery was "deciphered" too many times over the last decades and it is also too early to propose possible connections between the initial molecular events mentioned, starting with the drug binding and the variety of clinical manifestations observed. For the latter purpose however, it might be constructive to reorganize the numerous pieces of data acquired over the past decades (which are accessible from more than 8,200 PubMed titles on the value "thalidomide") and try to extract relevant information, which will aid integrating old and new findings under a common evidence based frame.

Here I summarized the data, which was looking the most pertinent to our goal, separated into several different categories, which will be discussed below. Although it could sound more natural for the aim of this chapter to start directly from the antiangiogenic subject, which has been already accepted as the leading explanation for the antimyeloma activity of the IMiDEs, I preferred keeping the teratological issue always a step forwards and from there spreading elsewhere, due to the explicit molecular findings discovered during investigation of the thalidomide embryopathy and the ability to connect some of them with the non teratological effects of the IMiDEs. Moreover, the wired collection of non-antitumoral effects of the IMiDs, which include the mysterious propensity of thalidomide to the developing limbs, its efficacy against drug reaction following dapsone administration in erythema nodosum leprosum (ENL), the unique hypnotic properties of this agent characterized by increase in the REM sleep duration and its usefulness against congenital and acquired vascular malformations togetether with the impressive antitumoral properties of the IMiDEs, which eradicate myeloma cells specifically (~15% complete response to lenalidomide + dexamethasone combination in relapsed/refractory patients), and induce hematological and cytogenetic response in the 5q- dysplasia; all of the above effects might be coexistent of course secondary to drug or metabolite activities on completely different molecular pathways, but on the other hand such a selective collection of target sites could also imply for the existence of as yet unrecognized common thread (e.g., cereblon targets), responsible for many of the drug activities mentioned. Our journey will start with lessons from the thalidomide embryopathy, subcategorized into vascular, neurological, oxygen-stress, adhesion molecules and developmental findings, which will be extended if possible and compared to corresponding findings in myeloma in order to find possible molecular targets which are modified in a stereotypical manner by the IMiDEs.

Lessons from the Thalidomide Embryopathy

By far, the most characteristic features of the thalidomide embryopathy were the unique pattern of distribution of embryological defects and the short sensitive period; embryotoxicity with limb defects noted from the 27th to 40th gestational day of exposure; all cases of phocomelia occurred from the 27th to 42nd gestational day. Unfortunately, the last character was also one of the great contributors to the disaster extent by giving the impression that the malformation is sporadic and thereby delaying its linkage with the drug. For the researchers however, the time interval mentioned made easier to delineate the embryonic structures involved and to determine their developmental stage during the incident, so even before the modern molecular biology era a remarkable progress was made, which occassionally yielded fascinating discoveries. Another distinctive feature was the strict species specificity, which will gain special attention latter owing to its great discriminative value. Of more than 30 theories elaborated in attempt to explain the thalidomide mystery in terms of molecular or pathophysiological mechanisms I preferred to concentrate on five and ignore those which were not supported by sufficient evidence. As already mentioned, the five leading hypotheses could be classified, in the most simplistic manner, into vascular, neuronal, oxygen-stress, adhesion molecule and patterning defects on the basis of the suggested etiologies. Each of these hypotheses will be introduced first in its pure teratological context and then if supported by evidence it will be evaluated in the context of myeloma.

a. Angiogenesis and the IMiDs

Based on the negative impact of thalidomide or its derivatives on angiogenesis under certain experimental conditions, the antiangiogenic properties of the IMiDs turned to be one of the most acceptable explanations for both the teratogenic insults as well as for the antimyeloma activities of the IMiDS. The earliest description of vascular injuries induced by application thalidomide was documented in 1966. In this forgotten article, Arthur Jurand from the Institute of Animal Genetics, Edinburgh incubated fowl eggs until Hamburger-Hamilton (HH) stage 17 or 18. The egg's shells were then slightly opened and thalidomide in suspension (0.2 ml of thalidomide 10 or 20 mg/ml) was introduced into the egg-white in close proximity to the embryo or injected into the yolk sac and then sealed with Parafilm (1). Thalidomide introduced into chicken eggs preincubated for 64-68 h causes dilation of the axial limb-bud artery in 24 h after treatment i.e., at stages 21-25. The injured endothelial cells became extremely thinned and formed vesicular projections into the lumen. In some cases there was necrosis in the mesoblast outside the dilated artery. In the most extreme degree of injury the mesoblast was almost completely destroyed. At the ultrastructural level the mitochondria in the endothelial cells of the dilated artery became swollen and vacuolated. These results suggested that the primary cause of thalidomide abnormalities is an injury of the endothelial lining of the axial limb artery. However, it took almost 30 years to rediscover the negative influence of thalidomide on vascular vessels and the seminal work on this topic was done by Robert D'Amato et al. from the Harvard Medical School and reported in 1994. The authors examined the effect of thalidomide on growing vasculature in the chicken chorioallantoic membrane and in the rabbit cornea and they were able to show that orally administered thalidomide can inhibit the angiogenesis induced by basic fibroblast growth factor (b-FGF) in the rabbit cornea [2]. Specifically, chicken chorioallantoic membrane assay was performed by implantation of 0.5% carboxymethylcellulose pellet containing 650 ng of the potent angiogenic protein b-FGF bound to sucralfate on the chick embryo chorioallantoic membrane through a hole cut in the egg shell. After 48 h incubation, neither thalidomide nor EM-12, a related teratogenic analog, exhibited any inhibitory activity on blood vessel growth and this observation was consistent with the known species specificity. Corneal neovascularization was induced by implantation of a similar pellet into corneal micropockets of New Zealand White rabbit, 2 mm from the limbus. Histological examination demonstrated progressive blood vessel growth into the cornea toward the pellet with only rare inflammatory cells evident. This angiogenic response was not altered by severe immune suppression with total body irradiation, and pellets with sucralfate alone did not induce angiogenesis. Oral treatment with a teratogenic dose of thalidomide (200 mg/kg) resulted in an inhibition of the area of vascularized cornea that ranged from 30 to 51% in three experiments with a median inhibition of 36%. The teratogenic analog EM-12 was also inhibitory, with a median inhibition of 42%, while nonteratogenic analogs of thalidomide exhibited no activity. Electron microscopic examination of the corneal neovascularization of thalidomide-treated rabbits revealed specific ultrastructural changes similar to those seen in the deformed limb bud vasculature of thalidomide-treated embryos. During the following years, similar results were reported by other groups, using alternative angiogenic stimulators and/or different thalidomide derivatives and in 1998, a German group showed comparable results using vascular endothelial growth factor (VEGF) (500 or 750 ng) instead of b-FGF in a corneal neovascularization model in rabbits. In that study, animals received two daily feedings of thalidomide (200 mg/kg) and after the 5th day of treatment a significant inhibition of corneal angiogenesis could be recognized, which persisted for more than 16 days [3]. Later they repeated the investigation using thalidomide and two of its derivatives, supidimide and EM12 and applied either b-FGF or VEGF for initiation of the neovascular response [4]. It was demonstrated that all of the three compounds examined inhibit neovascularisation induced by either b-FGF or VEGF containing pellet. EM12, the most teratogenic derivative was also the most potent inhibitor of angiogenesis in this model. In 1997, the Harvard's group reutilized their original corneal neovascularization model but now in mice and they were able to show that in this species, intraperitoneal but not oral administration of thalidomide can inhibit b-FGF or VEGF-induced corneal neovascularization [5]. Notice that this finding negates the species specificity criterion, which will be discussed in detail latter, albeit route of administration was different in this particular instance. The species specificity criterion was also missing in a guinea pig model of foreign body granuloma in which oral administration of thalidomide reduced vascular density [6]. In some more recent studies, an attempt has been made to delineate also the molecular mechanisms underlying the effects of the IMiDs on vascular vessels. A North American group used for this purpose the thalidomide analogue cc-1069, which inhibits endothelial cell proliferation more efficiently than thalidomide. This inhibition was associated with a marked decrease in the activity of the nuclear factor SP1 and a moderate inhibition of NFkB activation in nuclear extracts of endothelial cells [7]. The same compounds however did not impair the viability of the endothelial cells and there was no effect of thalidomide or the thalidomide analogue on the proliferation of a glioma cell line (U251) in vitro. A German group examined the effects of thalidomide on the development of capillary structures in embryoid bodies differentiated from murine embryonic stem cells. At a concentration of 100 μg/ml thalidomide significantly inhibited blood vessel development, when administered during the period of vasculogenesis and angiogenesis, known to occur between day 4 and 8 of embryoid body development [8]. However, 10 μg/ml of the compound did not exert significant effects on the formation of capillary structures. Examination of the intracellular REDOX state indicated that thalidomide exerts its anti-angiogenic properties via the generation of reactive oxygen species (ROS). An Italian group demonstrated in 2003 that thalidomide can inhibit the proliferation of endothelial cells induced by b-FGF and VEGF in-vitro, more so if the cells are grown on vitronectin [9]. At the molecular level, exposure to thalidomide reduced the release of the angiogenic factors MMP-2 and IL-8 by endothelial cells, suggesting a further pathway for the antiangiogenic activity of drug. A Japanese group studied the antiangiogeneic properties of thalidomide in zebrafish [10]. At a concentration of 800 μM for 40 hours, thalidomide caused shortness in length and loss of blood flow in 93% of the zebrafish embryos. The vascular defect was accompanied by additional complications such as severe pericardial edema and heart failure, and subsequently the embryos died by 5 days of development. Except for reduced body length, no deleterious effects were observed on the general morphology of embryonic structures. Vascular defects in the region corresponding to the dorsal artery and vein could be visualized both morphologically and immunohistochemically by the loss of expression of VEGF receptors and these changes appeared only after transient increase in the ceramide content through activation of neutral sphingomyelinase (nSMase). Moreover, the synthetic cell-permeable ceramide, N-acetylsphingosine (C2-ceramide) inhibited the embryonic angiogenesis in a similar fashion as thalidomide. Finally, the blockade of ceramide generation by antisense morpholino oligonucleotides for nSMase prevented the thalidomide-induced ceramide generation and the vascular defect. In contrast, sphingosine-1-phosphate (S1P) inhibited nSMase-dependent ceramide generation and restored the thalidomide-induced embryonic vascular defect with an increase of expression of VEGF receptors. Similar results were observed in human umbilical vein endothelial cells (HUVECs), on which thalidomide induced inhibition of cell growth, generation of ceramide through nSMase, and depletion of VEGF receptors, that could restored to the control levels by pretreatment with S1P. These results implied therefore that the antiangiogenic activity of thalidomide is regulated by the balance between ceramide and S1P signal.

In the year 2009, more than 40-years after Jurand reported his vascular findings in chick embryos, Christina Therapontos et al. from Harvard, returned to this embryonic model and showed that thalidomide derivatives can induce limb defects by preventing angiogenic outgrowth during early chick limb formation [11]. Therapontos et al. applied thalidomide and various thalidomide metabolites over the upper body and amniotic fluid of HH stage 17–19 embryos, at a similar or lower concentration relative to the therapeutic dose of thalidomide used in humans (chick = 160–1,280 μg/kg; human = 700–2,000 μg/kg). This method of drug application preferentially treats the right limb, allowing using the left limb as a control. Anti-inflammatory and thalidomide hydrolysis byproducts (5,6-OH thalidomide; 5′OH-thalidomide; PG Acid (N-phthaloylglutamic acid) had no effect on embryonic or limb development at any concentration tested. However, CPS49, a tetrafluorinated analogue of thalidomide that is chemically and structurally related to thalidomide breakdown products, induced severe limb defects similar to those seen in thalidomide victims. Specifically, CPS49 (100 μg/mL; 160 μg/kg), which has potent antiangiogenic and antitumor effects in vitro, induced defects in 82% (n = 250/306) of forelimbs and 10% (n = 32/306) of hind limbs. No defects were observed in any other regions of the embryo. To determine the effects of CPS49 on the development of the forming limb vasculature, the vascular network was visualized with Indian ink. Within 2 h of treatment, before obvious changes in limb morphology were observed, CPS49 consistently induced a 20% reduction in vessel density relative to controls. Vessel density continued to decrease and was reduced by 34% and 45% by 3 h and 6 h post treatment, respectively, whereas limb area was unaltered or only mildly reduced. By 24 h, vessel density was decreased by 64% and the limb bud itself was severely truncated. Remarkably, other blood vessels and the structure of other tissues in the embryo were unaffected. Embryos that were viable at day 10 were stained to investigate limb cartilage patterns. CPS49 treatment resulted in 4 main truncation phenotypes that resemble the range of limb defects seen in thalidomide-affected children: complete forelimb loss (amelia; 21%), a short humerus-like structure (36%), a shortened humerus with short ulna (21%), or a severely truncated limb with 2 shortened cartilage elements articulating with each other (21%). The expression patterns of genes essential for limb outgrowth like Fgf8 in the apical ectodermal ridge and Fgf10 in the underlying mesenchyme, were decreased significantly, but only after the changes apparent in blood vessels. Expression of Tbx5, required for forelimb initiation, was detectable at all-time points. In contrast, expression of sonic hedgehog, involved in digit patterning, and Msx1, a marker of the progress zone, was normal until 6 h, but reduced or undetectable by 24 h. In summary, this model was consistent with the concept that vascular insult is underlying the thalidomide embryopathy from the aspects of tissue specificity and the sequence of detectable changes, which were evident in blood vessels prior to the pathological and molecular manifestations which appeared later in the primordial tissue. This model however, was limited to thalidomide analogue, which leaves a room for skepticism concerning the implication to humans, as will be discussed in more detail latter.

Not far from the discovery of the antiangiogenic properties of thalidomide [2], the therapeutic implications of this finding were sought in the malignancy setup. In the experimental level, an Israeli group injected B16-F10 melanoma and CT-26 colon carcinoma cells to mice subcutaneously, intravenously and intraperitoneally, combined with daily gavage of 0.3-1.0 mg thalidomide from day two or ten after tumor cell injection [12]. However, in this model, no inhibition of tumor growth or metastasis was noted in thalidomide treated mice as compared to control mice. In addition, both the control and the treated mice developed an intact network of new blood vessels. Nevertheless, a few years later the antitumoral activities of thalidomide were also examined in the clinical setup. In one study, oral thalidomide 800 mg/d given to 39 adults with previously irradiated, recurrent high-grade gliomas resulted in two objective radiographic partial responses (6%), two minor responses (6%), and 12 patients with stable disease (33%). Eight patients were alive more than 1 year after starting thalidomide, although almost all with tumor progression [13]. In another phase II trial, which included 18 patients with recurrent glioma, who had failed radiotherapy and chemotherapy regimens, only 6% of the patients achieved any clinical response and the median survival from the start of thalidomide treatment was 2.5 months only [14]. In contrast, the IMiDEs demonstrated extreme therapeutic efficacy in MM, and this discovery marked the beginning of a new era for patients and provided researchers an opportunity to address the antiangiogenic properties of the drug in situ, which led to interesting conclusions that will be discussed below.

Angiogenesis and the IMiDS in MM

The assumption that the activity of thalidomide on its target sites is mediated via its antiangiogenic properties became assessable in the malignancy setup owing to the availability of authentic specimens from thalidomide treated patients. Two methods have been adopted for this purpose in MM, the first was measurement of the cytokine levels and the second utilized BM biopsies to answer this question directly. Baseline cytokine levels were associated in some of the studies with the tumor load and with the outcome. For example, in a Spanish study that included 38 patients with relapsed/refractory MM, baseline serum levels of VEGF were significantly higher and levels of hepatocyte growth factor (HGF) were significantly lower in thalidomide responders, whereas serum levels of b-FGF and IL-6 did not correlate with the response to treatment [15]. In an Australian phase II trial that included 75 patients with relapsed/refractory myeloma, elevated VEGF levels were also predictive for a superior response to thalidomide and in responders VEGF levels decreased significantly from a median of 65.8 pg/mL (range: 9.2–562.4) to 43.3 pg/mL (range: 0–208.1) at best response [16]. Because serum cytokine levels is derived from secretion by both the normal and the tumor cells, the influence of the IMiDEs on cytokine release from the tumor cells proper can be estimated only by direct assessment of this question in a pure population of tumor cells. To this end, a French group analyzed the modulation of the expression pattern by lenalidomide (a second generation IMiDE),using real-time quantitative PCR, in a collection of 23 MM cell lines (17). Surprisingly, although lenalidomide inhibited the proliferation of two-thirds of the myeloma cell-lines examined, as measured by ^{3}H-thymidine incorporation, it paradoxically increased the expressions of TNFα, insulin-like growth factor-1 (IGF-1) and IL-8 (an angiogenic factor) in both lenalidomide sensitive and lenalidomide resistant MM cells. The last observation doubted therefore the assumption that the IMiDEs work in myeloma through inhibition of angiogenesis. However, relying upon cytokine levels might be misleading because stimulation of angiogenesis might be mediated via direct cell-cell contact between tumor and endothelial cells or alternatively could be exerted by unmeasured cytokines. For this discrimination we will need also the micro vessel density (MVD) data.

In contrast to the cytokine levels, the MVD provides a direct estimation of the vascular density in the tissue and it can be also repeated during the course of treatment. To this end, Yaccoby et al. utilized their severe combined immunodeficiency-human (SCID-hu) host system and examined the effect of thalidomide on MVD in a mice model of myeloma [18]. In this model, tumor cells interact with the human microenvironment to produce typical myeloma manifestations in the hosts, including stimulation of neoangiogenesis. To "humanize" the metabolism of thalidomide, SCID-hu mice received implants of fetal human liver fragments under the renal capsule in addition to subcutaneous implants of a fetal human bone. It was found that daily thalidomide given by peritoneal injection significantly inhibited myeloma growth in 7 of 8 experiments, each with myeloma cells from a different patient, in hosts implanted with human liver. In contrast, thalidomide exerted an antimyeloma effect in only 1 of 10 mice without liver implants thus confirming that human-like metabolism is required for the antimyeloma effects of thalidomide, a reminiscence of the species specificity in thalidomide teratogenicity. In addition, human bone MVD in the untreated controls was higher than in thalidomide-responsive hosts but not different from nonresponsive ones. Also the expression of VEGF by MM cells and by other cells in the human bone was not affected by thalidomide treatment in any experiment. In conclusion, although the response to thalidomide was correlated with MVD reduction, there was definitely no indication that the decrease in MVD was the cause of the tumor reduction rather than being secondary to reduced tumor burden. In agreement with the findings described, serial MVD measurements in BM samples from MM patients before and after starting thalidomide treatment led virtually to the same conclusion. For example, a Japanese group evaluated BM biopsies from 51 patients with untreated myeloma or monoclonal gammopathy of undetermined significance (MGUS) and found as expected that BM MVD is higher in MM and is correlated with the tumor load. After starting thalidomide the monoclonal component decreased by at least 30% in seven of 11 evaluable patients whereas MVD decreased in only three of the responders (19). A Spanish study from 2008, examined the same issue in a group of 44 patients (14 newly diagnosed, 30 refractory/relapsed), who were treated with novel agents (thalidomide, lenalidomide, bortezomib) combined with dexamethasone. In 19 of the patients, a pretreatment BM biopsy was available and MVD was examined using anti-CD34 antibody. In addition, serum levels of various angiogenic factors (VEGF, b-FGF, and HGF) and cytokines (IL-6 and TNFα) were also measured. Despite the correlation found between MVD and the tumor load, MVD was not significantly correlated with either disease stage or response to therapy. Also baseline serum levels of the cytokines measured were not correlated with the response to treatment and no significant correlation was found between BM MVD and the serum levels of angiogenic cytokines. In fact, b-FGF serum levels even increased after starting therapy. The final conclusion therefore, was that no correlation exists between MVD and the serum levels of angiogenic cytokines, neither between each of them and the response to therapy [20]. Similar conclusions could be drawn from the Australian phase II trial mentioned, which included overall 75 patients with relapsed/refractory myeloma [16]. For example, before treatment some of the patients had high MVD levels without having a large marrow infiltrate and vice versa. After treatment, the MVD fell significantly in responders from a median baseline count of 21 (range: 7–71) to 10 (range: 4–20) at best response; and increased in patients who progressed during the study from 10 at baseline or best response (range: 1–130) to 20 at first progression (range: 1–113). However, the MVD did not decrease in all thalidomide responders and six of the 19 responders who had serial MVD measurements showed no change or even some increase in their MVD despite the clinical response. In addition, in the majority of responders in whom MVD did decrease, this was not follow a strict linear pattern but after an initial decrease the MVD often reached a plateau or even increased despite an ongoing response to therapy.

In conclusion, the lack of reduction of MVD levels in the myelomatous BM prior to the cytoreduction induced by the IMiDEs undermines the prevailing concept that the antimyeloma activity of the IMiDs is mediated via inhibition of angiogenesis. Also the cytokine levels measured were inconsistent with primary suppression of angiogenic stimulation as the explanation for the antimyeloma activity of the IMiDEs. Therefore, outside the context of research, MVD or cytokine measurements are lacking any beneficial value. An exception to the last statement is concerned for the subset of patient with the Polyneuropathy, Organomegaly, Endocrinopathy, M-protein and Skin changes (POEMS) syndrome, a rare variant of plasma cell dyscrasia; for which patient's group, serum VEGF levels are strongly correlated with the response to thalidomide [21, 22].

The failure to link the antitumoral effects of the IMiDEs to inhibition of angiogenesis should not let us forget that the vascular meshwork is not just a transporter but it also participates in many physiological and pathological processes in the marrow such as homing, migration, proliferation and tumor invasion and recent data even placed BM vessels in the center of a provisional "vascular niche" entity, at least for the hematopoietic stem cell [23]. Therefore, it is still possible that the IMiDEs are doing part of their antitumural work via modification of the vascular wall endothelium. Although this possibility has not been examined as yet, it is noteworthy that the IMiDEs modify gene expression [24] and enhance endothelial cells maturation status. The significance of this differentiation in its broader sense will be elaborated at the end of this section but some of the clinical applications of the cell maturating property of thealidomide will be presented here. For example, in hereditary hemorrhagic telangiectasia (HHT) thalidomide reduced the severity and frequency of nosebleeds (epistaxis) in the majority of treated subjects [25]. The blood hemoglobin levels increased due to reduced hemorrhage and enhanced vessel wall stabilization. In mice heterozygous for a null mutation in the Eng gene (encoding endoglin), used as an experimental model of HHT, thalidomide treatment stimulated mural cell coverage and through this rescued vessel wall defects. Thalidomide also increased platelet-derived growth factor-B (PDGF-B) expression in endothelial cells and stimulated mural cell activation. The effects of thalidomide were partially reversed by pharmacological or genetic interference with PDGF signaling from endothelial cells to pericytes. Biopsies of nasal epithelium from individuals with HHT showed that similar mechanisms can explain the protective effects of thalidomide on humans. Thalidomide showed protective effects also in non-hereditary vascular malformations, as demonstrated in an open-label, randomized controlled trial [26]. On the molecular levels, stabilization of vessel wall was associated in one study with downregulation of Hif-1α, Ang2, Notch1 and Dll4, which are all tending to become overexpressed under hypoxic conditions [27]. Finally, thalidomide was protective for cultured endothelial cells, which were injured by preincubation with doxorubicin. In this model, doxorubicin induced a dose- and incubation time-dependent and caspase-3-mediated apoptosis of endothelial cells [28]. Thalidomide alone caused no changes in intact endothelial cells in terms of morphology, cell viability or activation of caspase-3. In contrast, when thalidomide was added to doxorubicin-injured endothelial cells, there was protection from cell death, increase in viability of endothelial cells, induction of differentiation and formation of neotubules.

In summary, although the antimyeloma effects of the IMiDs could not be explained in terms of quantitative vascular changes, the impact of the IMiDs on endothelial cell maturation may imply that MVD is not the real player here but qualitative changes on vascular endothelium may represent one of the mechanisms behind the antimyeloma activity of this class of agents. This possibility may be supported by the marked induction of vascular modulating genes like IL8, PTGS2 (encoding for COX-2) and AREG (encoding for amphiregulin) in primary MM cells after their removal from the BM niche in contrast to low and stable expression of the strong vasculogenic genes like VEGF and b-FGF, which are known to induce angiogenesis quantitatively [29]. The induction pattern mentioned actually reflects the response of the tumor cells to the interruption of their interactions with integral niche structures and signals, which are missing in vitro. The lack of induction of strong angiogenic factors such as VEGF and b-FGF in vitro, also suggests that in niche the angiogenesis is not a limiting factor but on the other hand the tumor cells have to stimulate their vessels to function according to their needs in terms of niche signaling in analogy to the vascular niche model.

b. Oxidative Stress and the IMiDs

The growing interest on oxidative stress during the last decades did not skip the thalidomide mystery and the seminal work on this topic was published in 1999 by Parman et al. In that study, Parman et al. showed in rabbits that thalidomide stimulates embryonic DNA oxidation and teratogenicity, both of which were abolished by pre-treatment with the free radical trapping agent α-phenyl-N-t-butylnitrone (PBN). In contrast, in mice, a species resistant to thalidomide teratogenicity, thalidomide did not enhance DNA oxidation, even at a dose 300% higher than that used in rabbits [30]. Therefore, the authors concluded that these results constitute direct evidence that the teratogenicity of thalidomide may involve free radical-mediated oxidative damage to embryonic cellular macromolecules. In 2002, Hansen et al. located the oxidative damage to the limb bud itself [31]. They treated thalidomide-resistant Sprague-Dawley rat embryos (gestation day 13) with thalidomide in utero (300 mg/kg/day) and found no changes in intracellular glutathione (GSH) distribution in the limb bud tissue whereas thalidomide-sensitive New Zealand White rabbit embryos (gestation day 12) showed selective intracellular glutathione (GSH) depletion in the limb bud progress zone after treatment with thalidomide (300 mg/kg/day). This finding was accompanied by preferential decrease in NFkB expression in rabbit limb bud cells but not in rat limb bud cells. In addition, PBN rescued NFkB expression in thalidomide-treated cultures of limb bud cells compared with cultures that received thalidomide only. In situ hybridization showed a preferential decrease in expression of the limb patterning molecules Twist, Fgf8, and Fgf10 after thalidomide treatment (400 mg/kg per day) in rabbit embryos while the expression in rat embryos was not affected. Intravenous co-administration of thalidomide and PBN restored normal patterns and localization of these molecules in rabbits. These findings were considered as indicating that NFkB binding is diminished due to selective thalidomide-induced REDOX changes in the rabbit, resulting in a significant attenuation of the expression of genes necessary for limb outgrowth. Later, in 2004, the same group reported that the failure of the progress zone mesenchyme to express Fgf10 and Twist resulted from the failure of NFkB to bind to its DNA promoter [32]. In contrast, Knobloch et al. suggested in 2007 that the oxidative damage is mediated by bone morphogenetic proteins (Bmps). They injected thalidomide (50 µg) into the extraembryonic blood vessels of HH 19 chick embryos (750 µg/kg egg weight) and of total 309 treated embryos, the forty-seven (15%) which survived until day 7 showed uni or bilateral limb truncations including amelia
[33]. Of note, both proximal and distal structures were affected in all cases and uni or bilateral microphthalmia was seen in 21% of the embryos but as expected, phthalimide did not cause limb or eye defects. On the molecular level, they decided to check the expression of Dkk1 and found a remarkably higher expression of this gene in the limb buds from thalidomide treated HH 23/24 chick embryos compared to controls as well as in human but not in mouse embryonic fibroblasts. Since Dkk1 is controlled by Bmp signaling during early limb development, they continued to check the upstream regulation and showed that indeed there was induction of Bmp4, Bmp5 and Bmp7 following injection of thalidomide into the extraembryonic blood vessels of HH 19 chick embryos. In addition, in primary embryonic

cells isolated from the mesenchyme of chicken limb buds as well as in primary embryonic chicken fibroblasts thalidomide (38.7 μM = 10 μg/ml) increased the apoptotic rate x6 compared to controls but it did not increase apoptosis in primary mouse embryonic fibroblasts. As in whole limb buds, thalidomide induced the expression of both Bmp4 and Dkk1 in progress zone limb bud cells and in human embryonic fibroblasts but not in mouse embryonic fibroblasts whereas recombinant Noggin and anti-Dkk1 antibody completely neutralized thalidomide-induced cell death as also did Gsk3β inhibitors. In-vivo, Dkk1 and Gsk3β inhibitors reduced the truncation and microphthalmia proportions induced by thalidomide. Altogether, the results of this study suggested that limb bud cell apoptosis induced by thalidomide is initiated by ROS and mediated by blocking of Wnt/β-catenin signaling. Later, in 2008, the same group revealed that PTEN/Akt pathway participates in the apoptotic signaling cascade induced by thalidomide and that PTEN stabilization contributes to the limb anomalies via Akt suppression and caspase activation [34]. Finally, the discovery of Tbx5 and Sall4 gene abnormalities in congenital limb defects (Holt-Oram and Okihiro syndrome, respectively), prompted Knobloch et al. to investigate these genes also in the context of thalidomide limb defects and indeed RT-PCRs done on RNA extracted from wing buds of HH 23/24 chick embryos as well as from human embryonic fibroblasts revealed reduced transcription of Tbx5 and Sall4 in response to thalidomide [35]. When considering the vascular and oxidative insults together, it makes sense that both phenomena are related or in other words that the vascular insult was secondary to the oxidative stress, as demonstrated in embryoid bodies [8]. It is also noteworthy that the oxidative-stress hypothesis has not been extended to myeloma so far.

c. Adhesion Molecule and the IMiDs

The earliest referral to thalidomide in the context of adhesion was documented in 1984 and the finding was that the thalidomide metabolite EM12 inhibits the attachment of tumor cells to concanavalin-A coated surface [36]. Since1994, more data have been acquired, especially from German studies. Initially, it was found in human volunteers that thalidomide modulates the expression of many adhesion molecules such as CD18 (the common beta-chain of the beta 2-integrins), CD54 (ICAM-1), CD49b (VLA alpha 2) and CD49d (VLA alpha 4) [37]. In 1996, the same group demonstrated that EM12, triggers dramatic downregulation of several surface adhesion molecules (e.g., CD11a/CD18, CD49d/CD29, CD61, etc.) on early limb bud cells and on cells from some other primordia during early organogenesis of a primate (marmoset, Callithrix jacchus) [38], whereas oral administration of two daily doses of EM12 (2 x 50 mg/kg body weight) to Wistar rats from day 7 to 10 of pregnancy did not downregulatethe same adhesion molecules in limb bud cells from that species [39]. The species specificity demonstrated was considered by the authors as representing causal relationships between the downregulation of adhesion molecules and the teratogenic action of thalidomide. Based on the observation that thalidomide can bind at the N-terminal domain of N-cadherin by mimicking a tryptophan residue another German group suggested in the year 2000, that thalidomide might disturb cellular recognition and migration during morphogenesis by interaction with the N-terminal domain of N-cadherin, which is critical for the homodimerization of the adhesion molecule [40]. When considering the relationships found between the thalidomide embryopathy and adhesion molecule modulation it is readily seen that species specificity was the main association in favor of the suggested mechanism and even that was in conflict with the tissue specificity criterion required to be fulfilled in any explanation for the thalidomide embryopathy, as will be elaborated in detail latter.

Nevertheless, when speaking of myeloma, adhesion molecule modulation becomes much more meaningful and therefore this issue will be summarized briefly. The major proteins involved in the interactions between MM cells and the extracellular matrix include CD44, very late antigen 4 (VLA-4), VLA-5, leukocyte function-associated antigen 1 (LFA-1, CD11a), neural cell adhesion molecule (NCAM, CD56), intercellular adhesion molecule 1 (ICAM-1, CD54), vascular cell adhesion molecule 1 (VCAM-1, CD106), syndecan-1 (CD138), and monocyte chemoattractant protein (41). The initial homing of MM cells to the BM milieu is mediated by binding of the stromal-derived growth factor (SDF-1α) in the BM to its C-X-C chemokine receptor (CXCR-4) located on MM cells. The interaction between MM cells and BM stromal cells leads to increased production of IL-6, a myeloma cell growth and survival factor, as well as additional growth factors. In addition, SDF-1α also modulates the expression of VLA-4, LFA-1, VCAM-1, and ICAM-1 that mediate the adhesion between MM cells and BM stromal cells. Furthermore, adhesion of MM cells to BM stromal cells enhances NFκB activity that further upregulates IL-6 and VEGF. Also TNFα, which is secreted by MM cells, enhances the expression and secretion of IL-6 from BM stromal cells [42]. TNFα also activates NFκB and induces the expression of LFA1, ICAM-1, VCAM-1, VLA-4, and MUC-1 on MM cell lines as well as VCAM-1 and ICAM-1 on BM stromal cells. The IMiDs diminish IL-2, interferon-γ, and IL-6 regulator suppressor of cytokine signaling (SOCS) expression in immune (CD4T, CD8T, natural-killer T, natural-killer) cells from both BM and peripheral blood (PB) of MM patients [43]. In pre-clinical models, inhibition of adhesion molecules by statins restored drug sensitivity to cultured MM cells by reducing cell adhesion mediated drug resistance (CAM-DR), however the effects of the IMiDEs on CAM-DR has not been examined as yet.

d. The Nervous System and the IMiDs

The mechanisms discussed so far were purely hypothetical based and relied upon experimental models to support the feasibility of the suggested insults in terms of species and organ specificity. The last two hypotheses are much more complex and apart from species and tissue specificity they are trying to face with the unique distribution of deformities based on diagnostic findings like x-rays from thalidomide victims. The first of the two hypotheses linked the teratogenesis with the neuropathy which is frequent in thalidomide users.

The earliest attribution of the thalidomide embryopathy to a neurological insult was documented in 1966. Gavin Gordon from Cumberland, UK was impressed from the fact that the thalidomide neuropathy is predominated by sensory symptoms while weakness is usually mild and involves proximal rather than distal muscles [44]. Gordon explained: "The wide variety of deformities in neonates following the use of thalidomide as a sedative by the mother can only be the result of a toxic factor acting on the initial nerve impulses to muscles in the organogenetic phase of development. This explanation is developed to cover all the deformities seen in 'thalidomide babies' and is correlated with the pathogenic picture in adults following prolonged dosage". In 1968, Fullerton et al. described the clinical and laboratory findings in 22 patients who suffered from thalidomide neuropathy, during follow up periods between four to six years after stopping the drug. Symptoms and signs were unchanged in approximately 50% of cases; have improved in a quarter, and the remainder have recovered. Sensory nerve action potentials were recorded and found to be closely related to the clinical state. Sural nerve biopsies from six patients, performed two to six years after stopping thalidomide, showed selective loss of large diameter fibers. There was no segmental demyelination. In two of the nerves a marked increase in number of small fibers was taken to indicate regeneration. In 1973, Janet McCredie and William McBride revived Gordon's hypothesis (probably unaware of it) and created the basis for the axonal substraction theory [46]. Their assumption was based on detailed radiological review of five cases, supported by a summary of 50 similar children in Britain, which revealed that the bones and joints of thalidomide victims are absent, hypoplastic, tapered, or fused, and the surface area of skin is reduced. These signs were considered analogous to the trophic changes in adult sensory peripheral neuropathy. The authors put forward the hypothesis that the teratogenic action of thalidomide is exerted on the neural crest and its derivatives, and that the reduction deformities of the limbs represent embryonic peripheral neuropathy. During the next years, McBride developed an experimental model which supported the neurological etiology of dysmelia [47]. Thalidomide was administered to pregnant rabbits in dosages of 150-250 mg/kg/day on days 8-12 of gestation. These females produced 40 offspring, 21 of which were deformed. Four control females produced 34 offspring, none of which was deformed. Degenerative changes were found in the neurons and axons of dorsal root ganglia in day-13 experimental embryos, i.e., at least 16 hours before the earliest signs of thalidomide dysmelia have been reported in rabbits. Since the dorsal root ganglia form in rabbits on days 11 and 12, the changes evident on day 13 indicated that degeneration of neurons and axons may be a pathogenetic factor in thalidomide-induced peripheral deformities. McBride and Stokes also proposed that the size of nerve injury is the factor which determines the extent of deformity: damage to peripheral sensory nerves results in preaxial abnormalities while a greater damage results in amelia [48]. Further support to the toxic neuropathy explanation for the embryopathy came from the study by McCredie et al. which was published in 1984 [49]. Pregnant rabbits were given oral thalidomide (150 mg/kg/day) on days 7-11 of gestation and seven fetuses with partial or total absence of the tibia, five treated fetuses without deformities, and four untreated controls were examined. The sciatic nerves were dissected and transverse sections were taken from an identical site. In all treated animals there was a significant reduction in total fascicular area and in the number of large diameter fibers. However, in deformed fetuses a significant depletion of total fiber numbers was evident as compared with the controls. It was concluded therefore that dysmelic deformities of the limbs are secondary to toxic embryonic neuropathy occurring when damage to the nerves reduces the transverse fascicular area below a critical threshold. The toxic neuropathy demonstrated experimentally, encouraged McCredie and Willert to go a step forwards and try to explain also the deformity distribution pattern and in 1999 they reported their findings, based on comparisons between the limb defects as appeared in x-rays from thalidomide victims and the sclerotome map [50]. The sclerotomes are areas of segmental sensory innervation of the limb skeleton defined by the radiation of referred pain. According to the sclerotome subtraction theory, injury to the sixth cervical nerve in the embryo will affect the sixth cervical sclerotome, resulting in defects in parts of the thumb, radius, humerus and scapula. Likewise, damage at the level of the fourth lumbar nerve will reduce or subtract the fourth lumbar sclerotome, sparing the foot but reducing the tibia, femur and pelvis. As expected, there was a high overlap (73.5%) between the skeletal deformities seen and the sclerotome map and these results were considered as confirming the principles of skeletal reduction according to the sclerotomes with involvement of the sensory nervous system in the process of limb morphogenesis and teratogenesis. Further support to the sclerotome subtraction theory came from the investigation of limb development by Stephen et al. The author placed tantalum foil barriers either lateral to the mesonephric duct or parallel to the long axis of the chick embryo in the wing field of stage-12 to -15 chick embryos [51]. These barriers blocked the somatopleure's communication with more medial tissues at specific somite levels. The results of these experiments indicated that the limb is not induced from one specific point, and portions of the humerus appear to be induced segmentally along the entire limb field. It was proposed then, that the humerus is originated from several separate components which fuse to form the definitive bone. The "segmentation" of limb development in this study could fit the sclerotome subtraction theory, however several findings contradicted this theory. First, a German publication from 1982, showed that removal of axolotl nerve 4 (the largest brachial nerve, estimated to contribute 50-60% of the forelimb axons) by repeated resection resulted in pronounced reduction deformities with impaired regeneration of skeletal limb elements [52]. However, removal of nerve 3 or 5 gave less pronounced phenotype and although the dependency of skeletal element formation upon nerves was verified it did not follow a strict segmental subtraction, probably due to overlapped innervation of nerves 3, 4, and 5 to all four axolotl digits. More strikingly, Streker and Stephens placed a foil barrier into early chick embryos lateral to the neural tube in order to block brachial plexus-level neural crest cells from reaching the limb [53]. However, despite the interrupted innervation to the limb, the limb skeleton developed normally. Thus, the proposals that the segmental pattern of the limb is determined by level-specific nerves and that diminished levels of innervation will result in skeletal malformations were both refuted.

It is now well agreed that mesenchymal rather than ectodermal insult stood behind the thalidomide limb deformity, as first suggested by William McBride. It is also clear that the contribution of the neurological findings described to the understanding of the mechanism of action of the IMiDEs is small because both the physiological findings and the histological data acquired from affected nervous specimens of thalidomide users were not specific and molecular investigation was not done.

The situation is slightly different in respect to the CNS, since thalidomide has unique influence on the REM (rapid eye movement) sleep pattern, which its control is largely established. It is also important to recognize the general influence of thalidomide on the CNS, as described in 1960: "Thalidomide is a new sedative hypnotic drug which produces no toxic effects when administered orally to animals in massive doses. The drug has a quieting effect on the CNS, reducing the voluntary activity of laboratory animals and promoting sleep. Unlike the barbiturate drugs it does not cause an initial excitation in mice, incoordination or narcosis. It potentiates the actions of other CNS depressants, in particular the barbiturates. Its sedative effects are counteracted by CNS stimulants. Thalidomide proved to be virtually non-toxic. Mice tolerated the maximum oral dose (5 g/kg) that could be administered, without ill effects. Sleeping mice could be easily aroused, and then they resumed normal but slow movements and showed little interest in their surroundings. In contrast, both phenobarbitone and glutethimide caused initial excitation, marked ataxia, and incoordination of movement followed by narcosis and death. CNS stimulants rapidly counteracted the depressant action of thalidomide in mice. They quickly resumed normal motility and with increasing doses of methylamphetamine they became hyperactive and convulsed. The motility of mice made hyperactive with methylamphetamine (5 mg/kg, subcutaneously) was not depressed by an oral dose of thalidomide (500 mg). The interaction of methylphenidate (Ritalin) with thalidomide was very similar to that of methylamphetamine [54].

Almost forty years later, it was shown that thalidomide aggravates canine cataplexy, a pathological manifestation of REM sleep atonia seen in narcolepsy [55]. Specifically, after intravenous injections of thalidomide (0.25-8.0 mg/kg) to six narcoleptic and four control Dobermans from the Stanford Canine Narcolepsy Colony, long episodes (30 minutes) of complete muscle atonia appeared in all narcoleptic animals but not in control animals. Polysomnographic recordings in two narcoleptic animals demonstrated a de synchronized electroencephalogram (EEG) pattern with silent electromyogram (EMG), a typical polygraphic pattern of cataplexy. In contrast, intravenous diazepam, a commonly used hypnotic with GABAergic activity, had no effect on cataplexy in narcoleptic animals. In vitro receptor binding and enzymatic assays revealed that thalidomide does not bind to or enzymatically modulate the neurotransmitter systems reported to be involved in the regulation of cataplexy [56].

In order to find possible molecular targets of thalidomide in the CNS, based on its physiological activity, which will later serve us to define the connection between the various activities of the drug the control of REM-sleep will be briefly describe. The REM sleep consists of a dreaming state in which there is activation of the cortical and hippocampal EEG, rapid eye movements, and loss of muscle tone. In humans, thalidomide significantly increased the time spent in REM and stage 3-4 sleep as compared with placebo. On the other hand, thalidomide significantly decreased the time spent in stage 1, while the time spent in stage 2 was unchanged. The effect of thalidomide on REM and stage 3-4 sleep is unique as compared with other hypnotics [57]. A key molecule in the physiology of REM sleep is orexin (hypocretin). A series of studies have suggested that loss of hypothalamic neurons which produce orexin causes narcolepsy in humans while in other mammalian species orexin plays an extremely important role in the regulation of sleep/wakefulness states, especially in the maintenance of wakefulness [58]. The orexin neuropeptides produced by lateral hypothalamic neurons play a critical role in the maintenance of wakefulness by activating two distinct receptors, the orexin-1 (OX1R) and the orexin-2 (OX2R) receptor that are widely distributed throughout the brain. The orexin system is believed to stabilize the wake-sleep flip-flop switch in wake-active structures consisting of histaminergic, monoaminergic, and cholinergic neurons, and also to regulate the onset of REM sleep and associated muscular atonia in the brainstem. In accordance with the prominent function of orexins in sustaining wakefulness, pharmacological blockade of both OX1R and OX2R (OX1/2R) has been shown to promote sleep in various species, and the dual OX1/2R antagonists almorexant, SB-649868 and suvorexant have been clinically validated for the treatment of insomnia. Further investigations conducted in rodent models on the specific role of OX1R and OX2R in sleep modulation indicate that selective blockade of OX2R seems to be sufficient to initiate and prolong sleep [59].

The brainstem flip-flop switch is consisting of mutually inhibitory REM-off and REM-on areas in the mesopontine tegmentum. Each side contains GABA (gamma-aminobutyric acid)-ergic neurons that heavily innervate the other. The REM-on area also contains two populations of glutamatergic neurons. One set projects to the basal forebrain and regulates EEG components of REM sleep, whereas the other projects to the medulla and spinal cord and regulates atonia during REM sleep. The mutually inhibitory interactions of the REM-on and REM-off areas may form a flip-flop switch that sharpens state transitions and makes them vulnerable to sudden, unwanted transitions-for example, in narcolepsy [60]. The principle nuclei mediating REM sleep and their interactions with other brainstem and forebrain nuclei were recently identified by elegant work in rat. The sublaterodorsal nucleus, which is equivalent to the subcoeruleus or perilocus coeruleus in the cat, is the major structure responsible for REM sleep [61]. More recent work has led to the concept of a putative on/off switch for control of REM sleep [60]. In this model, the ventrolateral part of the periaqueductal grey matter and the lateral pontine tegmentum represent the REM-off region; i.e., these nuclei turn off REM sleep. Lesions of these nuclei increase the amount of REM sleep. This region is regulated by multiple afferents, it is *inhibited* by GABAergic and galaninergic projections from the forebrain ventrolateral preoptic nucleus plus the cholinergic projections from the pedunculopontine nucleus/laterodorsal tegmental nucleus. The periaqueductal grey matter and lateral pontine tegmentum REM-off neurons are *activated* by projections from the noradrenergic locus coeruleus, serotonergic raphe nucleus and importantly, by hypocretinergic pathways from the lateral hypothalamus. Narcolepsy is characterized by inappropriate intrusions of REM sleep and severe reductions of brain hypocretin; this could be explained by loss of hypocretin projection, thereby tipping the balance in favor of REM-on firing [62]. In relation to thalidomide, it can be speculated on the basis of the flip-flop model that this compound modulates either the REM-off or REM-on signaling cascade. However, further evaluation of this issues will be presented in the next section.

e. Limb Patterning and the IMiDs

The last hypothesis to be discussed here seems to have very little in common with the known activities of the IMiDs in myeloma. Nevertheless, as will be demonstrated, limb development is controlled by a dynamic signaling sequence and therefore identification of the exact stage where limb development was interrupted will exhibit the signaling system which was active at that stage, which might be the specific target of thalidomide. It is now also the time to refer more comprehensively to the criteria adopted for the elimination of irrelevant information which masked the meaningful findings as outlined by Reinhard Neubert from Freie Universität, Berlin [63]: "Since there seems to be no end to speculations on the possible mode of the teratogenic action of thalidomide, it may be helpful to recall the criteria that should be fulfilled when seriously attempting to explain the teratogenicity of this type of compound. These criteria are essential to provide an explanation of the pronounced species and phase specificity, as well as the malformation pattern associated with the teratogenic action of thalidomide, and they imply that the investigations should be performed:

- In a thalidomide-sensitive species (primates or possibly rabbits)
- At the thalidomide-susceptible stage of embryonic development (a short but well defined period)
- In cells of thalidomide-susceptible primordia (e.g., of the limbs or the heart)
- Under conditions inducing a close to 100% teratogenic effect
- At doses not inducing embryo mortality or a pronounced growth retardation
- To demonstrate that the effect is confined to thalidomide and its teratogenic derivatives and not inducible with non-teratogenic derivatives with a very similar chemical structure (e.g., thalidomide isomers or enantiomers).

In considering each of the four theories described earlier to the spirit of Neubert's perspective, they all failed the dosage criterion owing to the use of non-adjusted doses of thalidomide in respect to the doses used by pregnant women. In such mega dose range, thalidomide generated toxic oxygen injuries within susceptible organs, including the microcirculation due to the oxidizing properties of thalidomide derivatives [64]. Also the species specificity demonstrated in those experiments was likely a reflection of differences among species in neutralizing the ROS generated by oxidizing thalidomide derivatives rather than being specific at the primordial level as have been demonstrated in monkey. For example, in green pregnant monkey, an oral administration of thalidomide in a single or 3-day treatment periods between days 28 and 33 resulted in defects of the limbs which resembled those observed in humans, macaques and baboons [65] and no internal abnormalities were noted in any of the thalidomide-treated fetuses [66, 67]. In baboon, a relatively large series of experiments involving single and multiple dose treatments from 4 to 24 mg/kg/day, defined the sensitive period between days 25 and 29 of gestation. Macaque species have also demonstrated a similar sensitive period to thalidomide. A cranio-caudal gradient of development was also evident, so treatment on day 25 most commonly affected the upper limbs, treatment on day 27 affected the lower limbs, and treatment on day 29 only affected the tail. Limb reduction defects, including amelia and phocomelia, were the most common observation in macaques as well as in baboons. Finally, it has to be emphasized that no clear dose–response was observed in those fetuses [68] and that the thalidomide analog CG 3033 (supimide) did not provoke any teratogenity in this species in a remarkable contrast to the observations in non-primate animals [69].

If we return to the thalidomide doses applied experimentally, recall that 0.25 mg/kg thalidomide was sufficient to aggravate canine cataplexy [55], while in humans, a single 100 mg dose (1-2 mg/kg) during the sensitive period was sufficient to produce malformations (and even 20 mg was documented) [70]. A 100 mg dose of thalidomide given to human volunteers resulted in a plasma concentration of 1 mg/L = 1 μg/ml, while 200-mg thalidomide led to a Cmax of 2.40 μg/ml; tmax, 2.40 h; AUC0-∞, 21.62 μg/h/ml and $t_{1/2}$ of 6.18 h [71]; as well as Cmax 2.00 μg/ml, tmax 3.2 h, AUC0-∞ 19.8 μg/h/ml and $t_{1/2}$ of 6.17 h according to data from another study [72]. In contrast, the thalidomide doses used experimentally were 400 mg/kg in the seminal work by Parman et al. [30], 200 mg/kg in the D'Amato [2] and Kruse [3] et al. studies; 100 μg/ml but not 10 μg/ml inhibited embryoid endothelial cells in the Sauer et al. study [8], while the thalidomide concentration used by the Japanese group in zebrafish was 800 μM = 206.7 μg/ml [10].

Just consider the 35% incidence of phocomelia but also 24% decrease in fetal body weight, 450% increase in the incidence of fetal resorptions and 780% increase in postpartum fetal lethality in the study by Parman et al. [30] as well as the severe systemic complications in zebrafish, which included severe pericardial edema with heart failure and subsequent embryonic death by 5 days of development [10] in comparison to the lack of any apparent abnormality in chick embryos when thalidomide was applied in the range of the human doses (chick = 160–1,280 μg/kg; human = 700–2,000 μg/kg) [11] and the lack of systemic morbidities in mothers of thalidomide babies and in MM patients. Thus, in considering the mega dose range of thalidomide used in the experimental models described earlier, it becomes possible to explain most of the findings, whether speaking of the vascular injuries, neuronal insults or the so called 'species specificity' as derived from the same toxic oxygen-stress generated by thalidomide metabolites in a dose dependent manner. So we are left now with the last chance for getting a feasible explanation to the thalidomide embryopathy and with it to the mechanism of action of the IMiDEs in general. But before proceeding, a short introduction to limb development is needed.

Limb development is proceeding from proximal (humerus) to distal (digits). The limb bud elongates by means of proliferation of the mesenchymal cells underneath the apical ectodermal ridge (AER), a thickening in the limb ectoderm that forms at the distal tip of the growing limb bud. This region of cell division is called the progress zone, and it extends about 200 μm in from the AER. The Fgf released from the AER keeps the progress zone mesenchymal cells dividing. The cellular matrix begins its differentiation by the condensation of cells that will form the cartilage templates of individual bones. As the limb grows outward, the proximal mesenchymal cells that are farthest from the AER and destined to become skeletal elements undergo condensation and initiate chondrogenesis. Thus, the condensations that give rise to proximal limb elements form first while the cells at the tip of the limb bud remain undifferentiated. As the bud continues to enlarge, more distal skeletal elements differentiate sequentially until the complete set of condensations is laid down. In summary, the condensations are proceeding from proximal (early) to distal (late) by the control of Fgfs released from the AER, which promotes proliferation and inhibits condensation and differentiation in mesenchymal cells nearest the apical ectodermal ridge. Experimentally, when AER is removed from an early limb bud, only the most proximal parts of the stylopod (humerus) are made. However, if an Fgf-containing bead is placed in the hole left by the removal of the AER, a normal limb will form [73]. From the findings described above, it becomes clear that the limb deformities seen in thalidomide babies could not result from interruption of AER signaling because these deformities frequently spared distal elements like hand and digits unless the entire limb was missing (Amelia).

In 1998, Cliford Tabin from the Harvard University proposed a new hypothesis based on the progress zone model of limb development [74]. Tabin's hypothesis consisted of two components ("double hit"), the first was familiar and consistent with the general thought that the primary event was an apoptotic insult to the limb bud mesenchyme (e.g., by impaired angiogenesis). The second "hit" tried to explain the sparing of distal-most elements (i.e., fingers) by introducing a secondary developmental defect. The idea was that the primary apoptotic "hit" required time until mesenchymal recovery and thus delayed limb elongation which in turn prolonged the time spent of proximal identity elements within a distalizing signal field (comprised of Fgf) originated from the AER (located in the tip of the limb bud) and consequently re-specified proximal identity cells to distal elements. The need for a secondary developmental "hit" was explained by Tabin: "Perhaps the most striking aspect of this syndrome is phocomelia (a severe shortening of the limbs). The long bones are shorter than normal and more proximal elements are lost, such that in extreme cases the hand or fingers are attached directly to the shoulder, a condition described as resembling the flipper of a sea. Here I show how these defects can be understood in the context of current models for limb patterning. Although the pharmacological basis for thalidomide's effect remains controversial, the net result of thalidomide exposure is a decrease in growth of the limb-bud mesenchyme. From the perspective of pattern formation, the challenge is to understand why the decrease in growth should lead to a specific loss of proximal limb elements. This effect could be viewed as paradoxical, as other perturbations that prevent limb bud growth, such as removal of the specialized AER at the tip of the limb bud, lead to the opposite patterning defect: deletions of distal structures. These truncations induced by AER removal are explained by the 'progress zone' model of proximodistal patterning, and consideration in this context can also explain the distinct proximodistal defect seen with thalidomide. According to the progress-zone model, proximodistal structures are specified sequentially under the influence of a continuous signal, now believed to be a Fgf, produced by the AER. Initially, the entire limb mesenchyme has a proximal identity; left on its own, it would develop into proximal structures. However, the mesenchyme at the tip of the limb bud under the AER — the progress zone — is exposed to Fgf and becomes respecified to a slightly more distal fate. As limb development proceeds, the progress zone cells divide and, as a result of this growth, not all of these cells remain within range of the Fgf signal. Those too far from the AER maintain their already specified proximal fate, whereas those still in close proximity to the AER are once again respecified to a still more distal ate. This model explains the distal truncations seen following surgical removal of the AER: without the source of the distalizing factor Fgf, no further distal patterning occurs and only the proximal elements specified before the AER was removed are formed. The phocomelia observed following thalidomide treatment can also be understood from this developmental perspective. Thalidomide treatment blocks mesenchymal proliferation in the limb bud. I propose that this means that the progress zone does not increase in its number of cells, despite continued exposure to Fgfs from the AER. As a result, no progress-zone cells end up outside the range of the Fgfs, which would be required for them to remember proximally assigned fates. Instead, the entire progress zone is progressively distalized, ultimately programming the entire limb bud to form only the distal-most elements. Consistent with this view, an effect like that of thalidomide can be produced by irradiating the limb mesenchyme, limiting proliferation in the progress zone without affecting the distalizing activity of the AER. Based on these data, a similar mechanism was proposed as a general explanation for phocomelia. Loss of intermediate limb elements, the most common type of limb malformation seen in offspring of women who used thalidomide, is therefore a predicted consequence of altering growth in the progress zone while leaving intact the production of Ffgs by the AER. Many of the pharmacological mechanisms proposed to explain thalidomide's decreasing growth in the early limb bud, such as inhibition of the growth of blood vessels, could also contribute later to decreased growth of the skeletal elements, leading to shortening of the long bones. Although this is not strictly a patterning defect, it is commonly observed in thalidomide cases. Finally, after the period of exposure to thalidomide, the progress zone would recover, leading to the range of patterning defects occasionally seen, including Amelia (absence of limbs), phocomelia, and radial aplasia (lack of development of the radius). The limb patterning defects of thalidomide are therefore the understandable and expected result of decoupling distalization from outgrowth during limb patterning".

Despite being elegant, unique in attempt to explain the deformity distribution pattern, and introducing developmental considerations rather than sticking to toxic insult exclusively, Tabin's hypothesis did not peak too much interest and was even criticized by Reinhard Neubert et al.: "With regard to Tabin's hypothesis, we must consider the fact that the critical period for thalidomide-induced typical limb malformations (amelia and phocomelia) is very early. According to investigations in primates, developmental stages 11 to 14 are affected, reaching (for example in the marmoset *Callithrix jacchus*) a maximum at stages 11 to 12. Upper limb buds start to develop as early as stage 11. The AER, which is critical according to Tabin's hypothesis, does not occur until stage 14, too late to bring about amelia or phocomelia" [75].

In 2009, Tabin's hypothesis from 1999 was tested experimentally. Galloway and Tabin et al. induced apoptosis in limb bud mesenchyme using x-irradiation (first "hit"). However, despite the remarkable apoptosis in limb bud mesenchyme, the phenotype of the embryos was not as they expected: "Here, using a combination of molecular analysis and lineage tracing in chick, we show that x-irradiation-induced phocomelia is fundamentally not a patterning defect, but rather results from a time-dependent loss of skeletal progenitors. Because skeletal condensation proceeds from the shoulder to fingers (in a proximal to distal direction), the proximal elements are differentially affected in limb buds exposed to radiation at early stages. This conclusion changes the framework for considering the effect of thalidomide and other forms of phocomelia, suggesting the possibility that the aetiology lies not in a defect in the patterning process, but rather in progenitor cell survival and differentiation. Moreover, molecular evidence that proximodistal patterning is unaffected after x-irradiation does not support the predictions of the progress zone model" [76]. In other words, Tabin's et al. returned to the single "hit" apoptotic insult...

Now, after rejection of each of the five theories mentioned from one reason or another, we stay again with no a reasonable explanation to this saga. However, the last statement is not precise because limb patterning defect was excluded only in the context of a single speculative hypothesis whereas from almost any other consideration (e.g., the thalidomide doses used, its short half-life, the lack of general morbidities in mothers, MM patients and monkey), limb patterning defect remains the only possible explanation. However, the strongest argument in favor of limb patterning defect is derived from the spatiotemporal sequence of limb element loss (or sparing), which will be elaborated after description of the sequence by the words of Henkel and Willert from 1969: "In the upper limb mild manifestations of the deformity are restricted to the radial ray of the hand. Then follows, with increasing severity, involvement of the radius and only after the radius is either completely absent or its remnants have fused with the ulna is the humerus affected" [77], as well as the description by Smithells and Newman in 1992: "The bones of the upper limb are affected in a remarkably regular order, starting with the thumb, followed by the radius, the humerus, the ulna, and finally the fingers on the ulnar side of the hand (middle., ring, and little fingers) [78].

As readily noticed, the deformity sequence described was definitely non-linear, for the ulna was reduced only after the humerus and the ulnar digits were reduced even later, thereby making the whole sequence difficult to interpret from a developmental perspective. However, much of the confusion was probably caused by the intuitive tendency to relate to limb truncation as a proximodistal insult similar to the truncations produced in AER extirpation experiments, which gave rise to a linear sequence of bone element loss from distal-most to proximal. In contrast, in congenital limb defects for example, truncation deformities result many times from mutations in anteroposterior patterning genes, like Tbx5 in Holt-Oram syndrome, Sall4 in the Okihiro syndrome [79] as well as mutations in Shh, Wnt7a, Wnt5a and Wnt 3a, which are all associated with truncations and reduction deformities. Therefore, it is still possible that thalidomide interrupts the anteroposterior patterning sequence, provided that this sequence overlaps the limb defect sequence described in thalidomide babies.

Some evidence for sequential maturation of limb elements along the anteroposterior axis, came from the study by Koyama et al., which was published in 1966 [80]. Koyama et al. were concerned from the fact that the activities of the ZPA (zone of polarizing activity; essential for anteroposterior patterning) and AER dwindle early in embryogenesis and soon after ceases, when in fact the proximal skeletal elements are still rudimentary in structure and the more distal ones are yet to become recognizable. One possibility was that the chondrocytes formed following mesenchymal condensation start themselves expressing properties similar to those of ZPA and/or AER and in so doing, may bring skeletal development to completion. To answer this question they isolated radius and ulna with attached presumptive periosteum from the stage 29 embryos, subdividing each element into one diaphysis and two epiphyses, and grafted the resulting tissue fragments to the anterior margin of host stage 19-20 wing buds. As negative control, they used fragments of most-anterior non-chondrogenic mesenchyme and overlying ectoderm from the same wings. The results confirmed their basic assumption and also revealed that the fragments of ulna had a much stronger polarizing activity than those from radius at this stage; ulna's diaphysis in fact displayed the strongest activity among all the fragments tested and induced supernumerary digits including digit 4 in about 25% of operated wings. Ulna's epiphyses and radius' diaphysis were weaker and induced digits 2, 3, or both but not digit 4. Tissue fragments of most-anterior non-chondrogenic mesenchyme had no appreciable activity, attesting to the fact that polarizing activity was topographically restricted to the cartilaginous structures. To further assess the specificity of the polarizing activity, they grafted fragments of stage 29 ulna's or radius' diaphysis to the center of host stage 20-21 wing buds rather than to the anterior margin. In that case, no induction of supernumerary digits was observed (0/7). Surprisingly, when they examined stage 31 embryos, the polarizing activity of ulna's diaphysis had decreased significantly compared to that observed at stage 29 while the activity of radius's diaphysis was now higher; indeed, radius' diaphysis induced digit 4 in about 25% of operated wings. The epiphyses of both radius and ulna had comparable moderate activity at this stage 31; however, with further development the activity decreased substantially while it was still significant in developmentally younger distal elements, such as metacarpals and first phalange at stage 34. Clearly, the presence of polarizing activity in developing cartilaginous elements occurs sequentially and transiently along the proximodistal and posterior-anterior axes. In summary, the acquisition of polarizing activity by the cartilaginous structures followed clear proximal-to-distal and posterior-to-anterior routes. Thus, [1] stage 25 cartilaginous humerus had polarizing activity while stage 25 prospective radius did not, [2] posteriorly-located stage 29 ulna had stronger activity than anteriorly-located stage 29 radius, and [3] ulna's diaphysis had stronger activity at stage 29 than 31 while radius's diaphysis was stronger at stage 31 than 29. Prior to inducing extra digit formation, the cartilaginous grafts induced Hoxd-12 and Hoxd-13 gene expression in adjacent competent mesenchymal tissue. Strikingly, the cartilaginous grafts activity also induced expression of Shh and polarizing activity in adjacent mesenchyme, which ZPA grafts cannot do; thus, the cartilaginous structures displayed activities "upstream" of those of the ZPA. The results thus supported the hypothesis that chondrocytes can themselves direct skeletal morphogenesis. In so doing and as a result of their inductive activities, the cells may also have an important role in the completion of limb patterning and morphogenesis.

The relevant conclusion from that study to our subject is that the differentiation of discrete bone elements during the post condensation stage (and probably also before that), is by no means progressing along the proximodistal axis, like the sequence of chondrocyte condensation but each element has its specific timing, likely depending on distance from the AER (which generates the Fgf gradient) and from the ZPA (responsible for the Shh gradient). In fact, the two morphogenic gradients mentioned (or the three if we include the Wnt signaling along the dorsovental axis) might collaborate in the right limb location to create a permissive morphogenic constellation of signals for differentiation. If the maturation sequence described by Koyama et al. is indeed dependent on morphogenic gradients, than the earlier maturation of the ulna and ulnar digits (and therefore their sparing from thalidomide insults), could result from their closer proximity to the ZPA. Anyway, the differentiation sequence reported by Koyama's et al. partially overlapped the limb deformity sequence described in thalidomide victims wherein the radius was always reduced earlier than the ulna and the thumb before the ulnar digits. It was not a perfect match however, because the autopod (digits) differentiated lastly in the Koyama's et al. study in contrast to its most frequent sparing in thalidomide victims. Nevertheless, this instance provided firm evidence that the differentiation sequence of discrete bone elements after the chondrocyte condensation stage turns to be non-linear and therefore can overlap the cumulative sequence of the thalidomide limb defects. In order to find possible patterning factors which their interruption can mimic the phenotypic spectrum observed in thalidomide victims the relevant anteroposterior molecules will be described.

a. Hedgehog signaling: Shh is an example of a morphogen as defined by Lewis Wolpert's French flag model—a molecule that diffuses to form a concentration gradient and has different effects on the cells of the developing embryo depending on its concentration. Shh remains important in the adult. Of the hedgehog homologues, Shh has been found to have the most critical roles in development, acting as a morphogen involved in patterning many systems, including the limb and midline structures in the brain, spinal cord, the thalamus by the zona limitans intrathalamica and the teeth. Mutations in the human Shh, cause holoprosencephaly type 3 as a result of the loss of the ventral midline. Gli3 (the gene implicated in human Greig cephalopolysyndactyly syndrome) is proposed to negatively regulate Shh by restricting its expression and influence to the posterior mesoderm. Genetic analyses in mice showing that Shh and Gli3 are dispensable for formation of limb skeletal elements: Shh(-/-) Gli3(-/-) limbs are distally complete and polydactylous, but completely lack wild-type digit identities. Recently it was shown that the effects of Shh signaling on skeletal patterning and ridge maintenance are necessarily mediated through Gli3. It was propose that the function of Shh and Gli3 in limb skeletal patterning is limited to refining autopodial morphology, imposing pentadactyl constraint on the limb's polydactyl potential, and organizing digit identity specification, by regulating the relative balance of Gli3 transcriptional activator and repressor activities [81]. Ptch1 encodes a 12-pass transmembrane glycoprotein that functions as a negative regulator of the Shh signaling pathway. Binding of Shh ligand to the Ptch1 receptor liberates Smoothened activity, which ultimately leads to the release and nuclear translocation of activator and repressor forms of the Gli family of zinc finger transcription factors (Gli1, Gli2, and Gli3). Inactivation of Ptch1 via loss of function mutation leads to constitutive pathway activation due to unrestrained Smoothened activity. A diverse range of downstream targets have been identified in mammals, including members of other developmental pathways, such as Wnt, Bmp, and Notch, in addition to genes involved in cell cycle progression, apoptosis, and migration. Mice null for Ptch1 die during the early stages of embryonic development (at E9.5) due to severe developmental anomalies in embryonic patterning. Mutations in *PTCH1* cause Gorlin syndrome often with a midline cleft lip and mutations have also been found in holoprosencephaly patients [82, 83]. The family of Gli proteins (Gli 1-3) comprises the intracellular mediators of the hedgehog pathway, which regulates a myriad of developmental processes, one of which is limb development. Whereas

Gli 1 and Gli 2 seem to be dispensable during limb development, Gli 3 is especially crucial since all Gli 3-associated human congenital diseases comprise limb malformations. Furthermore, Gli3(-/-) mouse embryos exhibit pronounced polydactyly in conjunction with a loss of digit identities. Mutations in Gli3 cause several congenital diseases including Greig cephalopolysyndactyly syndrome and Pallister–Hall syndrome. Most of the clinical characteristics of Gli3 associated syndromes are distinct, but all share digit abnormalities. Only Gli3 seems to exert such an irreplaceable function in limb development since Gli1 and Gli2 deficient mouse embryos develop well patterned extremities. The effects of a loss of Gli3 function can be seen in *extra-toes* (*XtJ*) mice, which carry a *Gli3* null allele and represent a mouse model for GCPS. Heterozygous $Gli3^{+/-}$ mice display mild preaxial polydactyly (= supernumerary digits at the anterior side) while the limbs of homozygous $Gli3^{-/-}$ embryos exhibit severe polydactyly associated with a complete loss of digit identities. Consequently, Gli3 is believed to act in the regulation of both the number and the identity of digits [84].

b. Tbx5: The transcription factor Tbx5 is expressed in the developing heart, eyes and anterior appendages. Mutations in human Tbx5 cause Holt–Oram syndrome, a condition characterized by heart and upper limb malformations. Tbx5-knockout mouse embryos have severely impaired forelimb and heart morphogenesis from the earliest stages of their development. However, zebrafish embryos with compromised tbx5 function show a complete absence of pectoral fins, while heart development is disturbed at significantly later developmental stages. Tbx5b gene in zebrafish is co-expressed with its paralogue, tbx5a. Downregulation of tbx5a and/or tbx5b in zebrafish revealed that tbx5 genes have essential roles in the establishment of cardiac laterality, dorsoventral retina axis organization and pectoral fin development [85].

c. Bmps: are multifunctional growth factors that belong to the transforming growth factor beta (TGFβ) multigene family**.** In the vertebrate limb bud, the expression of several members of the Bmp gene family has been documented, namely Bmp2, Bmp4 and Bmp7. Current evidence indicates that Bmp2, Bmp4 and Bmp7 are the main source of Bmp signaling in the developing limb including AER formation, AER regression, cartilage and bone differentiation and interdigital webbing regression because of the early lethality of null mutants for Bmp2 and Bmp4, as well as their receptors, Bmpr1 and Bmpr2. In addition, these Bmps share functional similarities and may display functional redundancy. As a result, the role of one particular Bmp gene may be hidden by the activity of others. For example, although the mutation of Bmp7 by itself has little influence on limb development, it does enhance the Bmpr1b mutant phenotype [86].

d. Wnt7a pathways: Wnt7a is located in the dorsal ectoderm and it has two main pathways: one is via b-catenin (known as the canonical pathway) and the other is not dependent on b-catenin (known as the non-canonical pathway). In the canonical pathway binding of Wnt7a to its receptor (the receptor has two parts: a protein called Frizzled and a co-receptor called LRP5/6), stabilizes intracellular β-catenin by combining to a complex responsible for β-catenin degradation [79]. This complex has many components including APC (adenomatous polyposis coli) and GSK-3b (glycogen synthase kinase). The stabilized β-catenin in the cytoplasm combines with E-cadherin (cell surface protein responsible for cell-to-cell interactions) and the complex plays an important role in chondrogenesis of the developing limb. Stabilized β-catenin enters the nucleus to interact with transcription factors (especially T-cell factor or TCF) and upregulates Shh expression. Shh is initially expressed in the absence of Wnt7a. Later, however, Shh can only be maintained in the presence of Wnt7a. The secreted Shh does not just control anteroposterior patterning (including the development of the ulnar ray). It is also the key inductive signal for Fgf4 in the AER, which acts via a biofeedback mechanism to regulate Shh expression (Fgf4 contributes to the outgrowth of the limb along the proximodistal axis), and it also induces local expression of Hox-D13, which is also required for limb patterning. Isolated suppression of Shh results in ulnar ray deficiency which is always associated with short upper limbs secondary to reduced Fgf4 activity. Animals lacking the Shh gene function have truncated hind limbs and ulnar ray deficiency in the forelimbs. The Wnt7a non-canonical pathway in the upper limb development induces the expression of Lmx-1 in the dorsal mesoderm, which is responsible for the development of dorsal hand structures (hair, nails, extensor tendons, etc.). Isolated mutation of the Lmx-1 results in nail-patella syndrome (absent nails and patella). In the Al-Qattan palmar duplication syndrome there is a mutation of Wnt7a and hence there is lack of development of dorsal hand structures (the dorsum of the hand resembles a palm with absent nails) (Lmx-1 suppression), ulnar ray deficiency (Shh suppression), short upper limbs/truncated lower limbs (severe Fgf4 and Shh suppression). There are two main down-regulating proteins of Wnt7a activity. Dickkopf-1 (Dkk1) is a Wnt antagonist (i.e., an inhibitor of the Wnt canonical pathway) and animals with null allele of Dkk1 get overexpansion of the apical ectodermal ridge (AER) with polysyndactyly. The second protein is Engrailed-1 (En-1) produced in the ventral ectoderm and acts to suppress the activity of Wnt7a. Loss of En-1 allows Wnt7a to be expressed throughout the ectoderm (i.e., along both the ventral and dorsal ectoderm). As a result, no ventral structures will develop and affected mice get duplication of dorsal feet elements with all nails exhibiting the characteristic 'circumferential' nail appearance of the distal ends of the digits because of the presence of a plantar nail and dorsal nail joining at tip of the digit. Furthermore, affected mice have defective cerebellums indicating that En-1 has a role in cerebellar development. In humans, bi-dorsal duplication is usually partially expressed in the little (and sometimes also the ring) fingers and more than 30 cases have been described under different terms such as 'clam nail deformity'.

e. Wnt3/3A pathways: Wnt3 and Wnt3a are closely related. Wnt3 is expressed in the AER of the chick and is necessary for AER formation while Wnt3a is expressed in the limb ectoderm of the mouse and is required for normal limb development. In humans, homozygous Wnt3 mutation causes tetra-amelia. This is expected since the human Wnt3 is responsible for normal development of the AER which is, in turn, responsible for the outgrowth of the limb. The pathway of Wnt3/3a is similar to the canonical pathway of Wnt7a (i.e., via β-catenin). It is interesting to note that LEF-1 is the preferred factor for the Wnt3/3a pathway, while TCF is the preferred factor for the Wnt7a pathway. The normal interaction of β-catenin and LEF-1 will result in normal development of the AER, the production of Fgf8 (an important growth factor for the outgrowth of the limb) and the production of Bmp-2 from the AER. Proper chondrogenesis is known to be balanced by the antagonistic actions of Bmp2 (stimulating effect) and the Wnt7a pathway (inhibitory effect). Mis-expression of Wnt3a causes ectopic expression of AER genes for Fgf8 and Bmp2. Working in conjunction with Wnt3a in the AER is R-spondin-2. R-spondin-2 is a protein which acts synergistically with extracellular components of the Wnt pathway and also functions as a class of ligands independent of Wnt-proteins, leading to downstream activation of β-catenin-dependent genes. Finally, Fgf10 (a mesenchymal inducer for limb formation) is known to induce Wnt3a in the AER, and mice in which both copies of the Fgf10 gene have been disrupted by gene targeting fail to develop limbs. Furthermore, Fgf10 appears to have a positive regulatory loop with Fgf8.

f. Wnt5/5a pathway: We have previously noted that Wnt7a is specifically expressed in dorsal ectoderm and Wnt3/3a in the AER. Wnt5/5a are expressed in two sites: the AER and the limb mesoderm where Wnt5a follows a proximodistal gradient in the mesoderm of the developing limb. It is important to realize that Wnt5/5a act in the early stages of regeneration of the limb bud to control the de-differentiation of stump cells giving rise to regeneration-competent cells. Therefore, it is not surprising to know that Wnt5a is essential for normal chondrogenesis. It is also important to realize that the Wnt5/5a pathway acts mostly via modulation of intracellular calcium and not via stabilization of β-catenin. In fact, the Wnt5a pathway is sometimes called 'the antagonizer' pathway of the Wnt7a canonical pathway [87]. Wnt5a pathway stimulation induces siah 2 which leads to increased b-catenin degradation in the cell. In contrast, Wnt7a canonical pathway stimulation results in decreased β -catenin degradation. As mentioned earlier, Wnt5a is strongly expressed in the distal limb bud and its expression becomes weaker as one goes proximally. Therefore, it is not surprising that experimental limbs with Wnt5a -/- have missing distal digits. In these limbs, the AER has a normal appearance but the distal limb bud has accumulation of β -catenin and lack of expression of Sox9 (an early marker for mesenchymal condensation and chondrocyte differentiation).

When considering all the patterning molecules mentioned, it can be readily noticed that only Wnt3a and Fgf10 signaling interruption could give rise to tetra-amelia, which is part of the spectrum of thalidomide embryopathy. Albeit one can speculate then that interruption of Wnt3a signaling at a certain time point during limb development could result in composite reduction deformities, which involve both the anteroposterior and the proximodistal axes (due to the role of Fgf10), similar to the deformities seen in thalidomide victims, it is improbable that the phenotypic spectrum of such insult will include phocomelia. Therefore, at this stage we have to consider an alternative developmental sequence which is corresponding to the limb deformity sequence described in thalidomide victims. The last spatiotemporal sequence left is the sequence of chondrogenesis.

Chondrocyte maturation sequence: In the limbs, where extensive growth is required for proximodistal extension of the long bones, endochondral development begins with the aggregation of undifferentiated mesenchymal cells to form condensations, which by their position, shape, and size already prefigure the future skeletal elements [88]. In the core of these condensations, cells differentiate into chondrocytes, which secrete cartilage matrix. At the periphery, cells form a perichondrial sheath that surrounds the cartilage model. Proliferation of chondrocytes and perichondrial cells, as well as deposition of new matrix, are responsible for initial growth of these skeletal elements. At a certain stage, which is specific for each element, cells in the center undergo further maturation into hypertrophic chondrocytes, a process characterized by their exit from the cell cycle, enlargement and secretion of a distinct extracellular matrix that becomes progressively calcified. As a result, immature proliferating chondrocytes become restricted to each end of the skeletal element. These changes are accompanied by direct differentiation of perichondrial cells into osteoblasts, followed in turn by the deposition of a calcified bone matrix, the "bone collar," around the cartilaginous core of the future long bone. Changes in the composition and properties of the cartilage matrix in the hypertrophic zone, allow invasion by capillaries, accompanied by apoptosis of terminally differentiated chondrocytes, degradation of the calcified cartilage matrix, and its replacement by the trabecular bone matrix secreted by invading osteoblasts. The ordered progression of the differentiation program and the columnar arrangement of the chondrocytes result in a stratified organization where zones of proliferation, maturation, hypertrophy, calcification, and bone formation can be recognized, proceeding from the articular ends to the shaft of the bone. Continued proliferation of the less mature chondrocytes at the extremities, their differentiation into hypertrophic chondrocytes, and their replacement by trabecular bone near the center results in longitudinal growth of the bone. Continued deposition of cortical bone by the periosteum leads to radial growth. Finally, bone remodeling results from the combined activities of the osteoclasts, bone resorbing cells of hematopoietic origin, and the osteoblasts. Coordinating each of these processes is critical in determining the size, shape, and mechanical properties of the bones.

Before discussing the place of chondrogenesis in the thalidomide story, it has to be emphasized that none of the patterning molecules mentioned could explain how a single dose of thalidomide causes truncation of an entire limb or reduction of several bone elements, considering the short $t_{1/2}$ of the drug and the recovery of limb bud mesenchymal cells following considerable insults like irradiation [76]. To illustrate that, recall the two week sensitive period in humans, in which the 12-hours exposure to effective thalidomide levels represent 3.5% only of the sensitive period and therefore 3.5% of the limb development during that period. In fact, the striking effect of any dose of thalidomide on limb development, leaves only one logical explanation to that 50-year mystery, which is that thalidomide strikes only once, but this strike irreversibly changes cell fate of susceptible primordia. In other words, thalidomide is predicted to behave like a differentiating agent, much like retinoids which are also teratogenic in a dose independent manner. In considering the phenotype and the timing of the catastrophic event, speaking of already defined identities (i.e., humerus, ulna, radius etc.), which must however be prone to immature differentiation or commitment, only condensed chondrocytes could fulfill these criteria. From the chondrogenetic sequence described, it appears that premature differentiation of proliferating chondrocytes to hypertrophic chondrocytes, when already committed segments are being protected (or spared), can explain the truncation deformities induced by thalidomide. Indeed, the differentiation sequence of condensed mesenchymal elements described by Koyama et el. is largely overlapping the limb deformity sequence described in thalidomide babies. Additional support to this scenario might be gained from assessment of radiological images of thalidomide victims. Indeed, careful assessment of radiological images of thalidomide victims from the series of McCredie et al. [51], can give the impression of a “frozen” or fixed maturation state, manifested by a spectrum of maturation figures in the same image, from well-formed elements which were developed normally to formed elements with abnormal features, such as fusions or incomplete shaping as well as to completely absent segments. For example, the image in Figure 8a [51], shows truncation of the proximal part of humerus with an intact distal part and normal shapes of the ulna and fibula, which are however fused at the tips. Figure 7a shows proximal radioulnar fusion alone. Figure 10a, shows humeroulnar fusion between the proximal humerus and the distal ulna, with a relatively normal shape of the fused elements. The interpretation on the basis of premature commitment, is that the missing segments were composed initially of hypertrophic chondrocyte rudiments (which have limited elongation potential), whereas the mineralized tissue between the zeugopod bones (ulna and radius) could result from premature differentiation of intermediate zone chondrocytes to hypertrophic chondrocytes, which were later replaced by osteoblast. The fused humeroulnar bone could result from hypertrophic differentiation of the missing segment in between the two element tips (before humeroulnar separation to two discrete elements by joint formation), leaving the growing tips fused because the prematurely committed segment in between did not elongate and was replaced by osteoblasts which were mineralized later.

Such scenario is also consistent with the pathological findings described in the postmortem (PM) examination of a thalidomide child who was born alive and survived for 13 months [89]. In that case, which was described by Odette Hagen in 1966, it was considered extremely likely that the cause of the deformities was the ingestion of thalidomide by the pregnant mother. Clinically, in addition to severe limb shortening, there was bilateral microtia (abnormally small ears), a midline facial hemangioma, and a systolic heart murmur which disappeared as the child grew older. Radiologically, the baby was considered to have one long bone and three digits in each fore limb, and one long bone with a deformed foot in each inferior limb. It was considered that her death at the age of 13 months was caused by sudden heart failure due to congenital heart disease. In the upper limbs the main defect was an absence of the upper end of the humerus on both sides. Embedded in the deltoid muscle on the right was a small piece of cartilage about 1 cm. long, which on microscopy was identified as hyaline cartilage. The only true long bone in the upper limb was the ulna, to the upper end of which was attached a mass of hyaline cartilage which seemed to represent the lower end of the humerus. The radius, thumb and index finger were absent. The glenoid fossa was absent. The muscles which usually attach to the upper end of the humerus were fused together, and this fused fibrous body was attached to the cartilaginous mass at the upper end of the ulna. The muscles which usually attach to the radius and thumb were absent. The flexor muscles associated with the ulna and medial three digits were normal, except that there was no separation of the flexor digitorum superficialis and flexor digitorum profundus. The extensor muscles were poorly developed and in the hand the tendons fused with the deep fascia. On the left the soft tissues of the two lateral digits were fused. The nerve supply of the upper limbs followed the usual basic pattern, but with certain variations. The arterial supply of the upper limbs appeared very good. The lower limbs showed basically the same defects as did the upper limbs, viz, the upper end of the proximal long bone was absent and muscles which usually attach to it were fused. The acetabulum was absent. The distal end of the femur was present, but the only muscle directly attached to it was the short head of the biceps. In the leg the fibula with its muscles and their nerves was absent on the right, but on the left was represented by a thick strip of fibrous tissue to which the peroneal muscles were attached. This strip fused with the lower end of the tibia. On both sides the soleus arose with the gastrocnemius from the rudimentary femur. On the left the extensor hallucis longus arose from the fascial strip representing the fibula and sent tendons to all five toes. The phalanges of the second and third digits were partially fused, as were the skin and subcutaneous tissue of these digits. The extensor digitorum on this side sent a tendon to the hallux which blended with the periosteum of the first phalanx. There were no other muscles or tendons associated with this digit. The internal auditory meatus was normal, but the auditory nerve ended blindly in the bone. The facial nerve continued on to emerge from the skull at the suture between the mastoid process of the temporal and the parietal bone. There was no styloid process.

In summary, both the radiological images and the PM examination revealed fused bone segments and residual rudiments, which the PM examination identified as hyaline cartilage. This finding is consistent with the suggested catastrophic differentiation insult. In order to find which signaling pathways are controlling chondrocyte maturation and therefore can be the targets of the IMiDEs in the context of differentiation induction we have to recognize the chondrocyte maturation control.

Chondrocytes Maturation Control: At the molecular levels, it is now believed that mesenchymal condensations occur through 'identity' determination signals rather than simple 'core' formation: the humerus under the influence of retinoic acid/Meis-1 genes, and the bones of forearm/hand under the influence of Shh signaling. The zeugopod and autopod may be divided into three zones [88]. The area around the Shh contain descendants of Shh-expressing cells and is responsible for the development of the ulna, digit 5, digit 4 and part of digit 3. The next zone is under the influence of long-range Shh signaling and is responsible for the development of digit 2 and part of digit 3. The third zone is not under the influence of any Shh signaling. In this zone, the radius and digit 1 develop under the influence of other signals including Tbx5 and Sall4. Therefore, experimental mice with deletions leading to lack of Shh expression will have absence of the ulna and digits 2 to 5. The final digital patterning is a very complex process. It includes apoptotic mechanisms within the interdigital tissue and is under the influence of many factors including bone Bmps, Fgf and Hox-7. The transcription factor Msx2 is highly expressed in the interdigital zones and is thought to be a regulator in the Bmp4-mediated programmed cell death pathway. Hox gene interactions also play a role in this 'identity' process with Hox-D9, Hox-A11, and Hox-A13/D13 contributing to the development of the humerus, forearm bones, and bones of the hand respectively.

Hox genes: The 39 human HOX genes are located in four clusters (A-D) on different chromosomes at 7p15, 17q21 (corrected) 12q13, and 2q31 respectively and are assumed to have arisen by duplication and divergence from a primordial homeobox gene. Disorders of limb formation, such as hand-foot-genital syndrome, have been traced to mutations in HoxA13 and HoxD13. Hox genes are expressed in nested patterns along the proximal-distal axis of the limb bud, and mutations of these genes lead to alterations in the sizes and shapes of precartilage condensations in mice and humans, which are normally expressed in a region of the limb that will give rise to the radius and ulna. The result is severe reduction of these elements [90].

Indian hedgehog: Ihh is initially expressed in chondrocytes of the early cartilaginous skeletal elements [88]. On maturation, expression becomes progressively restricted to postmitotic prehypertrophic chondrocytes adjacent
to the PTH/PTHrP-R-expressing proliferative zones. It was demonstrated that ectopic expression of Ihh in developing chick long bones induces up-regulation of PTHrP expression in the articular perichondrium, leading to delayed differentiation of the chondrocytes, and delayed and abnormal ossification, a phenotype opposite to that seen in mice homozygous for null mutations in either PTHrP or its receptor. Furthermore, addition of Hedgehog protein to limb cultures delayed chondrocyte differentiation but only if PTHrP signaling was intact. These results suggest that Ihh and PTHrP regulate chondrocyte differentiation through the establishment of a negative feedback mechanism, in which production of Ihh by prehypertrophic chondrocytes induces PTHrP expression, thereby preventing additional chondrocytes from moving down the differentiation pathway. When prehypertrophic chondrocytes fully differentiate they no longer express Ihh. Consequently, the negative

feedback mechanism is attenuated and new chondrocytes are allowed to initiate the differentiation process. Ihh signaling is also required for chondrocyte proliferation and osteoblast differentiation, independent of PTHrP signaling. Most of the *Ihh*$^{-/-}$ mice die at birth due to respiratory failure resulting from defects in the development of the rib cage.

Dkk1: is a member of the dickkopf family and it functions as an inhibitor of the canonical Wnt signaling. Elevated levels of Dkk1 in the BM, plasma and PB is associated with the presence of osteolytic bone lesions in patients with MM [91]. Recently the role of Dkk1 in limb development was evaluated in a transgenic mouse model overexpressing Dkk1 in the appendicular skeleton [92]. In this model, Dkk1 was expressed under the control of the mesodermal specific enhancer element of Prx1 which its expression is mainly limited to the limbs, interlimb flank, latissimus dorsi muscle, craniofacial mesenchyme, and soft-tissues of the eye during embryogenesis. Prx1-Dkk1 mice exhibit severe shortening to near absence of forelimb and/or hind limbs when compared to their wild type counterparts. Importantly, all of the skeletal deficiencies observed were of the longitudinal type as in all cases absence of distal elements was always associated with reduction of proximal elements. I addition, two-thirds of mice showed some degree of forelimb abnormality, while one-third exhibited hind limb abnormalities and all mice with hind limb abnormalities had some degree of forelimb anomaly. No abnormalities of the cranial skeleton or viscera were noted. The wide spectrum of phenotypes observed from almost normal appearing mice to mice with severely affected and nearly absent limbs was correlated with the degree of Wnt/β-catenin inhibition. Interestingly, Dkk1 expression was readily observed in the osteoblasts lining the bones of Prx1-Dkk1 mice but not in wild-type controls. In BM-derived mesenchymal stem cells from 8-week old Prx1-Dkk1 mice (severe phenotype) there was an almost 80% decrease in total β-catenin in comparison to wild type. Using a β-catenin/TCF-responsive reporter (pGL3-OT/OF), in BM-mesenchymal cells from wild-type cells, β-catenin nuclear activity increases proportionally to the amount of exogenous β-catenin. In contrast the ability of BM-mesenchymal cells from Prx1-Dkk1 to similarly upregulate β-catenin nuclear activity is significantly reduced in direct correlation to the phenotype (i.e., the more severe phenotype the less β-catenin nuclear activity). In addition mesenchymal stem cells from Prx1-Dkk1 mice had limited proliferative ability, but normal differentiation potential.

A Unifying Explanation for all the Thalidomide Effects

Of the various signaling pathways discussed, only Ihh interruption could fully explain the thalidomide embryopathy, whereas mis-expression of Dkk1 resulted in truncation deformity sequence along the proximodistal axis [92]. Ihh keeps condensed chondrocytes undifferentiated and capable of proliferating and premature interruption of Ihh signaling will induce terminal differentiation of the affected segments to hypertrophic chondrocytes, leaving ungrowing chondrocyte rudiments instead of growing bone segments. Ihh mutations are associated with brachydactyly [93] and brachydactyly was also observed in thalidomide treated monkey [94]. However, differentiation of mesenchymal cells to osteoblasts depends on canonical Wnt signaling so a feedback loop must exist between Wnt and hedgehog pathways to ensure one way commitment. Therefore, primary or secondary modification of Wnt signaling by thalidomide might be also the common thread, which connects between the embryopathy, REM-sleep, and the antimyeloma activity of the IMiDEs. For example, in myeloma the overexpression of Dkk1 is associated with myeloma bone disease [91]. In considering the fact that thalidomide is not directly cytotoxic to primary MM cells, together with the findings that endothelial and stromal cells and especially osteoclasts are critical supporters of primary MM cells and can rescue MM cells from apoptosis in vitro [95], my speculation is that thalidomide induces (terminal) differentiation or commitment of endothelial and mesenchymal cells as well as of monocytes, which reduce their ability to support MM cells. Endothelial cell differentiation was already noticed after thalidomide treatment of congenital and acquired vascular malformations. Finally, differentiation of the MM cells themselves is also an option, considering the observation that co-culture of BM-derived mesenchymal stromal cells revert MM cells to less differentiated phenotype by the combined activities of adhesive interactions and interleukin-6 [96]. Thus, it is possible that the antimyeloma activity of the IMiDEs is partly mediated via maturation of BM mesenchymal cells, leading in turn to maturation of the MM cell phenotype from immature to more mature and so less proliferative. The connection between REM-sleep and Wnt signaling, was demonstrated by Millstein et al. using a computationally efficient statistical approach that was applied to relate sleep patterns to gene expression patterns in mouse hypothalamus. The results yielded a set of 11 transcripts associated with 24 h REM sleep. Two of the corresponding genes, Sfrp1 and Sfrp4, are involved in Wnt signaling and several others, Irf7, Ifit1, Iigp2, and Ifih1, have links to interferon signaling. Interestingly, in our GEP analysis of MM cells, Ifit1 and related genes were induced considerably after exposure of the cells to lenalidomide in vitro (unpublished data).

The Thalidomide Binding Site

In 2010, Takumi Ito et al. reported that CRBN, a protein encoded by a candidate gene for mild mental retardation, is a primary target of thalidomide teratogenicity [97]. To purify the bound protein they used ferriteglycidyl beads and after extensive washing their eluate contained two specifically bound polypeptides. After proteolytic digestion and tandem mass spectrometry CRBN and damaged DNA binding protein 1 (DDB1) were identified, respectively and confirmed by immunoblotting. Moreover, in 293T cells CRBN was found to function as a subunit of E3 ubiquitin ligase complex and undergoes autoubiquitination in a Cul4A- and DDB1-dependent manner.

These results suggested that thalidomide inhibits E3 function of the CRBN-containing complex by directly binding to CRBN. To examine the effects of thalidomide on zebrafish development, they transferred dechorionated embryos to media containing different concentrations of thalidomide at 2 hours post fertilization (hpf) and allowed them to develop for 3 days. It was found that in thalidomide-treated embryos, formation of the proximal endoskeletal disc of the pectoral fin was severely inhibited at 75 hpf, and otic vesicle size was significantly reduced at 30 hpf. In addition, the zebrafish CRBN orthologous gene, zCRBN, whose product has ~70% identity to human CRBN was found to interact with DDB1 and was affinity-purified from zebrafish embryos as a major interactor with thalidomide. Embryos injected with an antisense morpholino oligonucleotide for zCRBN exhibited specific defects in fin and otic vesicle development, similar to those of thalidomide-treated embryos. For example, the size of otic vesicles was reduced by half in the knockdown embryos. At the molecular level, Fgf8a expression in the AER was severely reduced or absent in thalidomide-treated 48-hpf embryos, whereas shh expression in the ZPA was affected negligibly. They speculated the existence of an inhibitor to Fgf8 production which is a possible downstream target of thalidomide and the CRBN-containing E3 complex.

In myeloma cells, acquired deletion of CRBN was found to be the primary genetic event determining isogenic MM1.S cell lines to be sensitive or resistant to lenalidomide and pomalidomide. Gene expression changes induced by lenalidomide were dramatically suppressed in the presence of CRBN depletion, further demonstrating that CRBN is required for lenalidomide activity. Downstream targets of CRBN include interferon regulatory factor 4 (IRF4) previously reported to also be a target of lenalidomide. Patients exposed to, and putatively resistant to, lenalidomide had lower CRBN levels in paired samples before and after therapy. In summary, CRBN was found to be an essential requirement for IMiD activity and a possible biomarker for the clinical assessment of antimyeloma efficacy [98]. In addition, in GEP data from the HOVON-65/GMMG-HD4 trial high cereblon expression was associated with better survival in patients with newly diagnosed MM treated with thalidomide maintenance. In this patient set, increase of CRBN gene expression was significantly associated with longer progression-free survival. In contrast, no association between CRBN expression and survival was observed in the arm with bortezomib maintenance [99]. Likewise, in MM patients with which were treated with lenalidomide and dexamethasone, there was significant association between baseline CRBN expression and the response to therapy [100]. More recently, two articles reported independently that lenalidomide promotes the CRBN-dependent destruction of Ikaros proteins [101]. Therefore, it will be interesting to check in the future possible regulation of Ihh by the CRBN complex. However, as argued by Ito et al., cereblon may not be the exclusive thalidomide binding protein.

Two alternative binding proteins for the IMiDEs, if indeed Ihh serves as a primary target of these agents, may include Cyp26a1 and Cytochrome P450 oxidoreductase (POR). Both of these proteins were implicated in teratogenesis and are also known to bind small chemical compounds. In mice, Cyp26a1 knockout exhibits spina bifida and tail truncation as a consequence of patterning defects, and also homeotic transformation of anterior vertebrae has been described. Cyp26b1 knockout mouse embryos display craniofacial defects and reduced limbs. Homozygous mutants die immediately after birth owing to respiratory distress before vertebral defects become obvious, and hence no other bone defects have been reported. In zebrafish, the effects of Cyp26 enzymes have been studied in the context of hindbrain and neural crest patterning. The zebrafish *stocksteif* mutant, exhibits severe over-ossification of the entire vertebral column. *stocksteif* encodes cyp26b1, a cytochrome P450 member that metabolizes retinoic acid. The mutant is completely phenocopied by treating 4 dpf wild-type embryos with either retinoic acid or the pharmacological Cyp26 blocker R115866, thus identifying a role for retinoic acid and *cyp26b1* in osteogenesis of the vertebral column. In conclusion, Cyp26 might be another possible binding site for thalidomide in analogy to the binding of the differentiating factor retinoic acid to the same cytochrome P450 members [102].

In considering the dependence of Ihh in cholesterol biosynthesis, another possibility is that thalidomide perturbs the interaction between Ihh and associated sterol. Cholesterol has been shown to be necessary for the activity of members of the hedgehog family. After being synthesized intracellularly, the N-terminal half of hedgehog proteins becomes conjugated with cholesterol by an autocatalytic reaction that simultaneously cleaves off the inactive C-terminal polypeptide. The mature active hedgehog protein, which is about half the size of full-length hedgehog, can then be anchored to the cell membrane and eventually released from the secreting cell. The inhibition of cholesterol biosynthesis is associated with congenital malformations. Triparanol, an inhibitor of desmosterol Delta24 reductase, produces a high rate of limb malformations in rat fetuses exposed at gestational day 10 to a single oral dose (150-200 mg/kg) given to the pregnant dam. The inhibitor induces the accumulation of desmosterol and zymosterol in embryo tissues. Comparison of the animal model with human syndromes, including limb osseous and skeleton perturbations, suggests a combination of desmosterol and Delta8 unsaturated sterols as being involved in the deleterious influence on limb bone formation [103]. The relations between both the cytochrome system and cholesterol biosynthesis with teratogenicity is exemplified by POR. POR is the electron donor for microsomal cytochrome P450 enzymes and other non-P450 enzymes. Targeted deletion of POR expression in mice leads to a variety of embryonic defects, including bone abnormalities. In addition, POR mutations in humans are associated with impaired steroidogenesis and skeletal malformations. Rat chondrocytes transfected with POR-specific short interfering RNAs exhibited decreased cell proliferation and differentiation and induced apoptosis. In addition, the reduced expression of POR in chondrocytes caused decreased intracellular cholesterol content. The addition of cholesterol in the culture medium prevented the POR small interfering RNA (siRNA)-mediated effects on chondrocyte proliferation, differentiation, and apoptosis. Interestingly, POR siRNA-transfected chondrocytes exhibited reduced Ihh expression, with such effect being neutralized by cholesterol. Lastly, recombinant human/mouse Ihh prevented the POR siRNA-mediated effects on chondrocyte proliferation, differentiation, and apoptosis. These findings suggested that the bone malformations associated with defective POR activity are due to reduced cholesterol synthesis and, in turn, reduced Ihh expression in chondrocytes [104].

Finally, a variety of compounds regulate downstream hedgehog signaling and by this way may also the IMiDEs act. Normally, hedgehog signaling is initiated by the binding of hedgehog ligands (Shh, Ihh, and Dhh) to the 12TM Patched1 (Ptch1) receptor, resulting in accumulation and activation of the G protein-coupled receptor-like protein Smoothened (Smo) within the primary cilium. How Smo regulates Gli transcription factor function remains unclear, but this process involves the scaffolding protein Suppressor of Fused (Sufu), which can directly inhibit the Gli proteins and facilitate their proteolytic processing into N-terminal repressors. Smo is perhaps the most “druggable” target within the hedgehog pathway, and Smo inhibitors have demonstrated efficacy in murine tumor models and human clinical trials [105].

Conclusion Remarks

- Thalidomide is not acting via inhibition of angiogenesis, at least in myeloma. This was clearly shown using BM microvascular density (MVD) measurements in thalidomide treated patients.
- Thalidomide is a known differentiating agent for blood vessel endothelium. This property has been utilized clinically to treat congenital and acquired vascular malformations.
- The teratogenicity of thalidomide can be explained by premature differentiation of limb bud chondrocytes during the sensitive period.
- Interruption of Indian hedgehog/Dkk1 signaling pathways can be the direct cause of thalidomide teratogenicity, which may be mediated by thalidomide binding to cytochrome members or disruption of sterol-Ihh relationships.
- Terminal differentiation of BM monocytes and/or mesenchymal cells, which support MM cells can be responsible for the antimyeloma activities of the IMiDEs

Proteasome Inhibitors

The proteasome is the main nonlysosomal endoprotease enzyme complex present in the cytoplasm and nucleus of all eukaryotic cells. It plays a critical role in the degradation of most short-lived intracellular proteins that control cellular events such as cell cycle, transcription, DNA repair, cell death, signal transduction, metabolism, morphogenesis, differentiation, antigen presentation and neuronal function. The proteasome is also responsible for protein quality control by eliminating damaged and abnormal proteins. Its structure is hollow and cylindrical and this 26S enzymatic complex is assembled from at least 66 proteins with the help of a number of chaperone proteins. It is composed of the catalytic 20S core and two 19S or 11S regulatory units at either ends. The catalytic 20S core is organized into a stack of four seven-subunit rings, with the top and bottom rings formed by seven polypeptides, termed the α-subunits, and the two inner rings of seven β-subunits. Poly-ubiquitination drives the interaction between the 19S (11S) and 20S particles. It requires the activity of three enzymes: ubiquitin-activating enzyme (E1), ubiquitin-conjugating enzyme (E2), and ubiquitin-protein ligase (E3). The mechanisms behind polyubiquitination are still being hotly debated. According to one mechanism, each ubiquitin is added sequentially to the growing chain (termed "elongation"). Other authors support the idea of a poly-ubiquitin chain that is preformed and then added to the target protein. Ubiquitin receptor proteins have an N-terminal ubiquitin-like (UBL) domain, and the 19S regulatory particle has an affinity for and recognizes these UBL domains. After the poly-ubiquitinated protein is recognized by 19S, the substrate protein is unfolded by hydrolases so that it may enter the narrow gate of the 20S particle and then be degraded. The 19S regulatory particle is divided into two subcomplexes called the base and the lid. The base consists of six AAA+ ATPases and three non-ATPase polypeptide chains. The lid includes at least nine non-ATPase polypeptide chains that help remove ubiquitin from the substrates. The lid and base connection is stabilized by the Rpn10 subunit. The base of hexameric ring of 6 ATPases in the 19S regulatory particle facilitates the opening of the 20S gate and is responsible for substrate recognition, deubiquitination, unfolding and translocation into the core particle. However, lack of structural data makes it difficult to understand how the 19S subunits are arranged and how the 19S helps with the opening of the 20S gate. The 20S catalytic core has a narrow gate at the center of the α-subunit ring where substrate proteins enter into this proteolytic degradation chamber. The gate is closed when the N-termini of the α-subunits interact, blocking substrate entry into the chamber. The 19S regulatory particle functions to help open the gate at the center of the α-subunit by interacting with this α ring and facilitate substrate access to the proteolytic chamber. The proteolytic chamber of the 20S core has three types of catalytic activities: chymotrypsin-like, trypsin-like, and caspase-like. These activities are presented by β5, β2, and β1 subunits, respectively. In immune cells the β1, β2, and β5 subunits, which are constitutively expressed, are replaced by β1i, β2i, β5i induced subunits to compose the immunoproteasome. Compared to the normal eukaryotic proteasome, the immunoproteasome has increased chymotrypsin-like and trypsinlike activities which assists in antigen processing. Instead of the 19S regulatory particle, the immunoproteasome utilizes the 11S regulatory particle, in place of 19S, to facilitate the opening of the 20S gate and stimulates substrate unfolding and translocation. Similar to 19S, the 11S binds to the 20S core particle through the

C-terminal tails of its subunits and causes α-ring conformational changes to open the proteolytic gate.

Bortezomib (velcade), is a dipeptide that contains a boronic acid instead of a carboxylic acid at the C-terminus. Bortezomib's boronic acid reversibly binds to the chymotrypsin-like β5 subunit of the catalytic chamber of the 20S particle and inhibits proteasome function [106]. Carfilzomib contains an α,β-epoxyketone moiety that assists in the formation of a morpholino adduct with the N-terminal threonine residue in the proteasome, which inactivates proteasome function irreversibly [107].

One of the earliest explanations for the antimyeloma activity of proteasome inhibition ascribed the cytotoxicity to the accumulation of IkB, the inhibitor of the antiapoptotic factor NFkB, which is implicated in B-cell malignancies. [108-110]. However, more recent data debated this thought because direct inhibitors of NFκB reduce the proliferation of MM cells markedly less effectively than bortezomib [111-112]. Alternative proapoptotic proteins, which are proteasome degraded, were also considered as possible candidates. For instance, the proapoptotic molecule NOXA is induced 20-to-60-folds in certain cancer cells after exposure to proteasome inhibitor [113]. Other groups attributed the antitumoral effects to the inhibition of HIF-1α and repression of HIF-1 transcriptional activity with attenuation of the release of VEGF [114]. However, in the recent years, much of the attention has been directed towards the endoplasmic reticulum (ER) stress response and the accumulation of misfolded proteins destined to be degraded by the proteasome [115-116]. In general, increased misfolded protein levels initiate the unfolded protein response (UPR) signaling, which in turn stimulates splicing of inactive XBP1 [117] whereas spliced XBP1 (XBP1s) modulates genes which are responsible for the ER-associated degradation (ERAD) (e.g., EDEM), ending-up within the proteasome. XBP1s also induces genes which enhance protein folding such as p58IPK and a variety of ER chaperones [118]. Although UPR activation is intended to return protein homeostasis and is normally functions in plasma cell differentiation and survival by induction of various ER chaperones and folding enzymes [119-121], under prolonged and uncompensated ER stress the UPR ends with cellular apoptosis, known as terminal UPR [122-124]. The latter insult is mediated by the proapoptotic transcription factor CHOP (also known as GADD153 and DDIT3), which is induced via PERK and ATF6 pathways. CHOP causes downregulation of BCL2, and thereby leading to caspase-dependent apoptosis [125-126]. In head and neck squamous cell carcinoma cells (HNSCC), bortezomib induces apoptosis through induction of ER stress along with the generation of ROS, which lead to caspase activation whereas inhibition of NFkB alone was not sufficient to induce apoptosis [127]. Additional support to the proapoptotic potential of exaggerated ER stress came from the association between the levels of immunoglobulin chain production and the sensitivity to proteasome inhibition in subclones of the human IgG-secreting myeloma cell line JK-6L and in subclones of the murine myeloma cell line Ag8 transfected with an expression plasmid encoding the μ heavy (H)–chain [128]. Likewise, proapoptotic factors of the ER stress response were induced to a greater extent in subclones producing high levels of μH-chains as compared to subclones producing no μH-chains. Conversely, MM cells became bortezomib resistant through inhibition of unfolded protein accumulation by acquired mutations of the PSMB5 gene which prevented the catastrophic ER stress [129].

In order to find which of the cytotoxic mechanisms mentioned are consistent with the molecular changes appearing in primary tumor cells after treatment with proteasome inhibitors, we compared recently the gene expression profile (GEP) changes, evolving in BM samples from MM patients with bortezomib responsive versus bortezomib resistant myeloma in response to bortezomib treatment in vitro (unpublished data). The MM cases selected had extreme BM infiltration with tumor cells (> 90%), which omitted the need for cell separation procedures, known to modify the expression of numerous genes due to spontaneous switch in their expression in vitro [29]. The microarray data is available in the public Gene Expression Omnibus (GEO), accession number GSE51940. So far, we examined BM samples from an overall group of five MM cases, three of which responded to velcade/dexamethasone (Vel/Dex) combination whereas two failed various velcade regimens; one with newly diagnosed myeloma showing primary resistance to Vel/Dex as reflected by increase in his paraprotein levels and persistence of > 95% plasma cells in repeated BM examination after 6 injections of velcade (days 1, 4, 8, 11, 29, 32, 36, 39); the second refractory case was heavily pre-treated and initially responded to Vel/Dex with VGPR (very good partial response) followed by long term remission after consolidation stem cell transplantation (SCT) with melphalan (200 mg/m2). However, after almost 3-years the patient progressed and received second line treatment with lenalidomide/dexamethasone (Len/Dex) but was refractory to this regimen, then he partially responded to retreatment with Vel/Dex and thereafter received salvage therapy with two cycles of VD-PACE (velcade combined with dexamethasone, platinol, adriamicin and etoposide) followed by second SCT while in VGPR. Once again, after 6 months the patient progressed but now also showing absolute resistance to bortezomib regimens, without any response to Vel/Dex and to VD-PACE treatments, and soon he developed new plasmacytomas, pancytopenia, hypercalcemia, renal failure and rapid increase in his paraprotein levels in the presence of > 95% plasma cells in the marrow. At this stage he entered the study and his BM sample was obtained.

The BM samples from our five MM cases (three bortezomib responsive and two resistant) were cultured and treated in vitro with bortezomib at a concentration of 2 μg/ml, and after 6-8 hours incubation the treated and control cells were released from the bottom wells and fixed with liquid nitrogen. As compared with the control samples, the GEPs analysed from the bortezomib treated samples showed dramatic upregulation of a large subset of genes, mostly encoding for heat shock proteins (HSPs) or related ER stress chaperones, and this observation was common to virtually all five samples examined, irrespective of the clinical response of the patient to bortezomib regimens. A partial list of the upregulated genes includes: HSPA6, HSPA1A, HSPA1B, CHRNA5, HSPB1, HSPH1, DNAJB1, SERPINH1, HSPA7, BAG3, HSP90AA4P, DNAJA4, HSP90AA6P, HSPA4L and HSP90AA2. In contrast, neither NOXA nor HIF-1α, GADD45A, GADD45B, GADD45G, TNFRSF10B, FAS, FASLG, DAP3, CASP8, CASP7 or CASP1, which were all implicated in the apoptosis induced by bortezomib [130-131], were induced markedly in any of the BM samples examined in our series, and no BCL2 repression could be recognized. Furthermore, although the proapoptotic signaling molecule CHOP (DDIT3), which is considered to be induced and activated by ER stress [126-127], was induced to somewhat greater extent in our bortezomib sensitive versus resistant cases, the differences in expression were too small to explain the clinical differences.

Because induction of HSPs is one of the most typical changes induced by proteasome inhibition [132-134], the remarkable in vitro induction of HSPs in our bortezomib resistant cases, and so the lack of in vitro resistance to proteasome inhibition, implies that unlike the resistance acquired in mutant subclones, which is secondary to impaired drug binding [135-140], in the MM cases presented the clinical resistance resulted probably from other mechanisms. One possibility is reduced downstream activation of proapoptotic pathways like p38 and ATF6 [141], Bax and Bak [142], generation of ROS [143-144] or dysregulation of the intracellular calcium [145] following proteasome blockade. Another possibility is that the antitumoral activity is dissociated from the UPR activation, and this option can be tested directly by the response to direct ERAD inhibitors such as Eeyarestatin I [146]. The third possibility is that the clinical resistance results from reduced BM levels of the drug. The last possibility represents also the major limitation of our findings, because the bortezomib concentration used in our cultures was much higher (~20 folds) than the usual peak plasma levels in humans (89-120 ng/ml). However, bortezomib is rapidly and widely distributed in tissues and the mean 24-hour total radioactivity levels (TR) of ^{14}C-bortezomib was found to be 43.5, 30.5 and 27.8 folds higher in the BM versus plasma of Sprague-Dawley rats after the first, third and fourth dose of the drug in a biweekly schedule, respectively [147]. Likewise, the area under the concentration-time curve (AUC; µg-eq. h/g) of TR between 0 and 72 hours post ^{14}C-bortezomib injection ($AUC_{0\text{-}72\ h}$) was 31.7 and 24.1 folds higher in the BM versus plasma after the first and the fourth dose, respectively. Thus, it is still reasonable that the usual bortezomib levels existing in the marrow of treated patients are similar to the concentration used in our cultures, although this issue requires confirmation.

In summary, the mechanism of the antimyeloma activity of proteasome inhibitors is still undefined. The ER stress response seems to be critical, though preserved proteasome inhibition capacity, which elicited potent in vitro induction of HSPs was not predictive for clinical activity of bortezomib in MM patients. On the other hand, the excellent clinical response to bortezomib regimens, despite the remarkable in vitro induction of HSP transcripts in our bortezomib responsive cases, doubts the role attributed to HSP inhibitors in overcoming bortezomib resistance [148-150], though the in vitro observations might be misleading. Another option to overcome resistance to proteasome inhibitors is to combine them with direct ERAD inhibitors [151]. Finally, among all the GEP changes observed after in vitro treatment of primary MM cells with bortezomib, only matrix metalloproteinase-12 (MMP12) was expressed differently in bortezomib responsive versus bortezomib resistant cases. Specifically, MMP12 was induced 6.55, 18.62 and 7.0 folds higher in the BM samples from our bortezomib sensitive cases versus 0.48 and 1.08 folds in the samples from the two bortezomib resistant cases, as compared to the corresponding controls. So far, MMP12 has not been implicated in MM, but is known to participate in tissue remodelling, and is also strongly associated with tumor invasion and pathologies like emphysema and aortic dissection.

Targeted Therapy Using Monoclonal Antibodies

Plasma cells are characterized by the co-expression of CD138 and CD38, which allows their identification in flow cytometry. These terminally differentiated B-cells may lose the expression of surface CD19 and that of CD20 while retaining CD27. When malignant, they can gain a number of other markers such as CD28, CD33, CD56, or CD117 and lose CD27 [152].

The successful assimilation of monoclonal antibodies into the arsenal of treatments for a variety of malignancies, including B cell neoplasms, has encouraged developing similar targeted therapy against myeloma. This effort however has been encountered with difficulties, mainly because of the heterogeneity of the tumor clone, and the obscure phenotype of the cell subset which attains self-renewal capacity. Two terms have been adopted to discriminate specific subset of cells within the malignant plasma cell clone; the first was clonotypic cells, identified by the sharing of the same immunoglobulin heavy chain (IgH) rearrangement as the monoclonal plasma cell population residing in the BM. More recently clonogenic and myelomagenic cell counterparts have been also recognized, likely by an inspiration from the leukemia stem cell research. The existence of clonotypic, non-plasma cells in the blood of MM patients, was firstly described by Leif Bergsagel and Linda Pilarski et al. who showed that in myeloma, certain blood B cells have identical IgH rearrangements as expressed by the BM plasma cells. Specifically, DNA from purified blood B cells and BM plasma cells, taken at the same time, was amplified using Allele-Specific Oligonucleotid (ASO) polymerase chain reaction (PCR) method. In 10/16 patients, a single IgH rearrangement was amplified from the BM plasma cells, and in all the 10 cases the same IgH rearrangement was also amplified from the purified blood B cells [153]. In addition, a significant proportion of the clonotypic CD19+ B cells, aberrantly expressed both CD38 and CD56 [154]. The discovery of a distinct blood B cell population, which is expressing the same IgH rearrangement as the malignant plasma cell clone, readily fueled speculations as to the existence of a malignant B cell compartment with stem-cell like properties, feeding the malignant plasma cell compartment. To quantify the clonotypic B cell subset residing in the circulation, Szczepek and Pilarski et al. analyzed sorted B cells derived from blood of MM patients and healthy donors, using in situ RT-PCR with patient-specific primers. The average proportion of clonotypic B cells in the blood from the patients examined was 66% +/- 4% (range, 9% to 95%), while not detectable among normal blood samples [155]. Whereas the existence of clonotypic B cells was also confirmed by other groups, the proportion of these cells in the blood of MM patients became a subject of debate. Thus, Chen and Epstein from the Arkansas group, estimated the average proportion of CD19+ B lymphocytes in the blood mononuclear cells of nine MM patients as 6% (range, 0.2% to 12.1%), and only a minority of which (range, 0.04% to 0.8%) were clonally related to the MM cell clone [156]. This controversy was later addressed in a phase III clinical trial, conducted by the Eastern Cooperative Oncology Group (ECOG). The study group included 13 newly diagnosed patients with myeloma, and the results excluded any correlation between the number of CD19+ B cells (range, 5% to 51%), and the number of clonal cells in the PB (range, .009% to 3.6%), as estimated by quantitative ASO-PCR. In fact, low CD19+ B cell was associated with clinical stage III disease, while higher levels of CD19+ cells were associated with a longer overall survival. In addition, high CD19+ levels also predicted a better response to treatment and longer event-free survival. There was also a strong and inverse correlation between the level of CD19+ cells at the diagnosis and the incidence of infections within the first 2 months. The number of deaths from infections was also significantly higher in the low versus high CD19+ group. Finally, CD19+ cell quantity was an independent prognostic factor, in addition to plasma cell labeling index, beta2-microglobulin, hemoglobin, and plasmablastic morphology. Taken together, higher CD19+ quantities were associated with a favorable outcome, with no apparent relationship to circulating tumor cells [157]. In line with the ECOG findings, Luque et al. also found that most B lineage cells in the blood of MM patients are polyclonal, and only a minor proportion is clonotypic [158]. However, in contrast to the phenotype described by Pilarski et al., Luque et al. characterized the blood clonotypic cells as expressing CD19- /CD38++/ CD45-/dim CD138++ and monoclonal cytoplasmic immunoglobulin, while being negative for pan-B antigens (CD19, CD20, CD24, DR), surface immunoglobulin and certain adhesion molecules like CD62L, CD18 and CD11a. This phenotype is closely related to the phenotype of malignant plasma cells in the marrow, with the exception of the CD56 antigen. Clinically, clonotypic cells showed a remarkable drug resistance, and could be detected also after treatment albeit in very low proportions (median, 0.004%), and most of which were $CD19^-$ [159]. Clonotypic cells were also detected after high dose therapy and autologous SCT, and the proportion of clonal $CD19^+$ cells ranged between 0.1% and 6.1% (mean, 1.0%) in the cases examined [160].

The idea that the clonotypic cell subset constitutes the main proliferative population in myeloma, was rebutted by their minor proportions as estimated by most groups, as well as by the positive correlation shown by the ECOG between the quantity of blood CD19+ cells and the overall survival, event free survival and lower infection rate. Further skepticism regarding the ability of clonotypic B cells to replenish the BM following treatment, arose from attempts to eradicate this cell reservoir. The first documentation of targeted therapy, directed against residual CD19+/CD20+ clonotypic B cells, which survived HDT was reported by Gemmel et al., who gave B-cell directed consolidation therapy to a patient with plasma cell leukemia in remission after HDT [161]. Prior to antibody therapy, the proportion of clonotypic cells in the PB mononuclear cell fraction, enriched for CD20+ cells, was estimated as 0.093% by PCR assay, based on limiting dilutions. However, despite effective depletion of CD20+ cells from the PB and from the BM following rituximab consolidation (375 mg/m2 on days 1, 8, 15 and 22), the tumor load in boat compartments increased progressively, and by day 120 a relapse was diagnosed clinically and the patient had in the PB 0.65% CD38++/CD138+/CD20- plasma cells, with no detectable CD20+ B cells. This observation excluded, at least for that patient, the possibility that the clonotypic B cell subset represents a major proliferative compartment. More recently, Zojer et al. tested the efficacy of a single course of rituximab monotherapy (375 mg/m2 on days 1, 8, 15 and 22) in patients with relapsed myeloma [162]. The rational for that study was the identification of a population of clonotypic CD20+ B-cells that are believed to be precursors of malignant plasma cells. Before treatment, CD20 was expressed on the cell surface of 10% and 50% of the BM cells from two of the ten patients enrolled. Following rituximab treatment, none of the patients achieved an objective response and no clinical benefit could be recognized, despite the significant reduction in the numbers of circulating B lymphocytes. In another small trial, rituximab given as maintenance therapy to MM patients after autologous SCT, resulted in a shortened time to relapse thereby leading to early termination of the trial [163].

In conclusion, the majority of published studies showed that the clonotypic blood population, detected either before or after treatment, remains consistently minor and relatively static. The clonal diversity seen can be settled with the fact that translocations involving the immunoglobulin locus (14q32), are an early non-transforming event common to MM and MGUS, introduced at the memory B-cell level [164]. Thus, it is not surprising that clonotypic B cells are also detectable in MGUS [165] and therefor might simply represent an earlier stage population, along the ontogenetic course of the tumor clone. On the other hand, in symptomatic MM patients, the persistence of clonotypic cells after treatment or increase in their levels after transplant did correlate with reduced overall survival [166-168]. A possible explanation for the discrepancy mentioned between the "static" behavior of the clonotypic cell population, which shows no expansion even during full blown disease and the unfavorable outcome associated with its persistence, can be that this cell subset is indeed 'innocent' by itself, but its persistence after therapy reflects resistance of the entire clone. An alternative explanation is that the clonotypic blood population does contribute to the tumorigenic actively, but rather than doing so by expansion of the non-plasma cell clonotypic subset, as originally suspected, the expansion is concealed and manifested by gradual replacement of lost plasma cells in the marrow by the non-plasma cell counterparts of the clone, followed by switch in their phenotype after BM engagement, towards the typical mature phenotype. Such scenario may explain the difficulties mentioned to determine the phenotype of the clonotypic cells, being local environment dependent. It may also explain the resistance of the disease to rituximab when given as consolidation or maintenance therapy after HDT, because rituximab can only eliminate the CD20 positive subset of the clone, and not BM engaged or the circulating CD20 negative counterparts identified by Luque et al. [158]. I personally prefer the second explanation, no matter what is the exact phenotype of the clonotypic or clonogenic cells. This is because it is very likely that the relapse initiates from a 'dormant' or hibernated reservoir of clonotypic cells, which are protected from most cytotoxic regimens including HDT, due to their rare biological activities (e.g., replication, metabolism, turnover, recycling, macromolecule repair), and thus reduced dependence on cell resources like ribosomes and proteasome, leading by that to reduced susceptibility to corresponding inhibitors. Indeed, in our experience we were able to maintain primary MM cells for months ex-vivo with minimal supplements to cultures and interestingly, these static cells acquired somewhat different morphology, with less basophilic cytoplasm and less eccentric nuclei (29; and unpublished data).

The phenotype of the clonogenic (or myelomagenic) cells, was firstly reported by Pilarski et al., who identified myeloma initiating cells in granulocyte-colony-stimulating factor (G-CSF) mobilized grafts from symptomatic MM patients. Specifically, after intracardiac injection of the mobilized cells from 3 of 7 patients to mice, the mice developed disease symptoms with a latency of 103 to 157 days, characterized by overall morbidity, hind leg paralysis, and/or boney changes, including easily fractured long bones and macroscopic loss of red marrow. In addition, human B and plasma cells were detected in the BM, spleen, and blood of the mice. Likewise, injection of MM cells directly into the murine sternal BM, led to lytic bone lesions, BM plasma cells, and a high frequency of clonotypic cells in the femoral BM. Finally, the myeloma progenitors underwent self-renewal in murine BM, as demonstrated by the transfer of human myeloma to a secondary recipient mouse [169]. Later, this group showed that injection of CD34-enriched autografts from either fresh or cryopreserved mobilized blood also generates myeloma in NOD/SCID mice. Specifically, the enriched grafts from six of six patients were myelomagenic, as evident by engraftment of clonotypic cells and/or the development of lytic bone lesions. Also the intrasternal route of injection of enriched progenitor fractions led to clonotypic cells in the femoral BM and bone lesions at distant skeletal locations, confirming dissemination of myelomagenic cells. The highly purified CD34+ fractions (separated by immunomagnetic method), contained on the average, 31% clonotypic MM cells and 31% DNA aneuploid cells. Given the lack of morphologically identified plasma cells among enriched progenitors, it was concluded that the xenografting myelomagenic component is unlikely to be plasma cells and appears to be CD34+ CD45 low, similar to normal myeloid progenitors [170]. In line with that conclusion,

Matsui et al. found that CD138- cells from clinical MM samples, were clonogenic both in vitro and in NOD/SCID mice, whereas CD138+ cells were not [171]. Specifically, purified CD138+/CD34− and CD138−/CD34− cells from BM mononuclear cells of 4 MM patients were injected intravenously into NOD/SCID mice. In contrast to CD138+ cells which did not engraft any of the mice, the CD138− cells from one of the patients engrafted 3 of 3 animals, as evident by the presence of human CD138+ cells with light chain restriction, matching the original patient sample within the murine BM and PB. Further analysis of clonotypic CD138- cells from both cell lines and clinical samples, revealed their phenotypic resemblance to post germinal center B cells, suggesting that MM "stem cells" are CD138- B cells, with the ability to replicate and subsequently differentiate into malignant CD138+ plasma cells. In contrast, Hosen et al. showed recently that CD138- cells and CD138+ cells can be both clonogenic [172]. Specifically, CD138- /CD19- /CD38++ plasma cells from 3 out of 9 MM cases propagated in SCID-rab mice model, while CD138+ plasma cells from 4 out of 9 cases propagated too, although more slowly than CD138- cells. In contrast, no engraftment of CD19+ B cells was detected in either SCID-rab mice or in NOD/SCID IL2Rγc(-/-) mice.

As noticed, the controversy encountered in relation to the clonotypic cell phenotype continued with the phenotype of the clonogenic cells. According to Pilarski et al. CD34-enriched grafts are myelomageous while Matsui et al. demonstrated the clonogenic potential of CD138−/CD34− cells and Hosen et al. showed this potential in both CD138- /CD19- /CD38++ and CD138+ cells. These differences could result from the different model used and technical variations. However, another possibility, which was already mentioned, is that the phenotypic variation observed is not necessarily methodological, but represents true clonal diversity, or more intriguingly is the consequence of transition (reversible or not) between two or more 'maturation' states, from the so called 'stem-state' to more proliferative states, possibly depending on timing and local microenvironment. The clonal diversity option is consistent with the cancer stem cell concept and is considered attractive by the potential to eradicate the tumor clone completely by only targeting the minor stem cell counterpart. However, such assumption looks somewhat naïve and elimination of cancer stem cells was never achieved even in core binding AML, where the transforming event can be solitary, the genetic diversity very rare, and the tumor cells "synchronized" in the same maturation arrest stage (due to specific translocation). Also in chronic myeloid leukemia (CML), which is a bona fide single "hit" tumor (t 9;22), there are no evidence for the existence of a minor subset of clonogenic cells, which replenish the tumor clone. Thus, instead of speaking of a distinct subset of cancer stem cells, it is possible that the tumor cells have plasticity up to a certain ontogenetic stage, and can de-differentiate or transit between 'dormant' and more proliferative states (with corresponding phenotypes), leading by that to erroneous conclusions. The existence of a transient 'dormant' state is also predicted from the response to long term maintenance therapy, for example in acute promyelocytic leukemia patients (receiving ATRA + 6-Meraptopurine) or in MM patients (receiving IMiD or proteasome inhibitor maintenance). If this is really the case, then targeted therapy using monoclonal antibodies can be the best option to eliminate the 'dormant' subsets of cells within the malignant clone, provided that their phenotype will be clarified. However, until the exact phenotype of myeloma initiating cells will be determined, the available antibodies will continue to be used empirically.

The available monoclonal antibodies which are currently under clinical assessment, will be now briefly mentioned, starting with the anti CD138 (Syndecan-1) antibody. CD138 is a cell surface receptor for epidermal growth factor ligands, hepatocyte growth factor, Fgf and extracellular molecules such as collagen and fibronectin. It also mediates cell-to-cell adhesion and it was showed to be a differentiation antigen and a co-receptor for MM growth factors. CD138 is expressed on the majority of malignant plasma cells, and at lower level also on normal plasma cells. It is continues to be expressed on MM cells after repeated treatments, thus it can be targeted also in advanced stage disease. In a Phase I/II study, 52% of the patients responded to BT062, an anti CD138-drug conjugated antibody with at least a stable disease, and 4% achieved a PR, when the drug was given weekly for 3 weeks in each 4 week cycle [173]. Two additional surface antigen targets are CS1 (SLAMF7) and CD38. CS1 is a glycoprotein expressed strongly on the surface of normal and malignant plasma cells and elotuzumab is a fully humanized IgG1 anti CS1 monoclonal antibody. As a single agent elotuzumab showed no objective response, although 26% of 34 evaluable patients stayed with a stable disease. Nevertheless, elotuzumab is currently examined in a phase III trial in combination with lenalidomide owing to preclinical evidence for synergism between these agents [174]. CD38 is a type II transmembrane glycoprotein, involved in receptor-mediated adhesion, signaling events and intracellular calcium mobilization. It is relatively highly and uniformly expressed in MM cells, while under normal conditions it is expressed at low levels on lymphoid and myeloid cells. Daratumumab, an anti CD38 antibody showed in dose-escalation study, a marked reduction in paraprotein and BM plasma cells [175]. Such activity was not previously demonstrated with other single-agent monoclonal antibody. Another surface antigen supposedly expressed ubiquitously and preferably on the surface of MM cells was identified recently using comparative GEP [176]. In the above mentioned and in other series GPRC5D expression was extremely higher in primary MM cells than in normal BM cells or non-myeloma tumor cells (e.g., AML, B cell lymphoma cells). This finding justifies further investigation.

Targeting Extracellular Factors

MM cells are strictly dependent on the BM niche for growth and survival. Apart from supplying essential growth factors and nutrient support the BM offers the proper physical conditions required for vital cell-cell interactions among its various inhabitants. Accordingly, targeted therapy which is directed against critical extracellular factors or surface adhesion molecules seems to be an extremely promising approach to threat myeloma. Moreover, unlike the behavior of malignant cells which "escape" therapy due to clonal evolution, soluble and adhesion molecule targets are less likely to "escape" from an antibody. In myeloma, one of the most reasonable targets for such therapy, is soluble factors which drive myeloma bone disease, especially Dkk1 and RANKL. Dkk1 functions as a soluble inhibitor of Wnt/β catenin pathway, and is overexpressed in a subset of MM patients with osteolytic bone lesions. The overexpression of Dkk1 blocks the differentiation of osteoblast precursors and inhibits anabolic bone formation, thus promoting bone resorption. Preclinical studies showed that neutralizing Dkk1 and/or enhancing Wnt/β catenin signaling may be effective in treating bone pathologies [177-178]. BHQ880 is a fully human anti-Dkk1 monoclonal antibody; it increases osteoblast differentiation and bone formation, neutralizes inhibitory effects of MM cells on osteoblastogenesis, reduces IL-6 secretion and inhibits cell adhesion and tumor growth both *in vitro* and in mouse models. These preclinical results provided the rationale for a phase I/II trial evaluating BHQ880 in combination with zolendroic acid and anti-myeloma therapy in patients with relapsed/refractory MM. Preliminary data of phase I trial showed increases in bone mineral density in some patients with a good safety profile [179]. Another ongoing phase II study in patients with previously untreated smoldering MM at risk for progression showed no significant direct anti-myeloma effects but evidence for anabolic bone activity was seen in some patients using novel imaging [180]. RANKL is a type II membrane protein and a member of the tumor necrosis factor (TNF) superfamily. The binding of RANKL to its receptor, RANK increases osteoclastogenesis and activation of osteoclasts. Osteoprotegerin is a natural soluble decoy receptor of RANKL, and it is able to prevent excessive bone resorption by modulating RANKL effects. Denosumab is a fully human monoclonal antibody with high affinity and specificity for RANKL. It was developed to treat patients with skeletal disease mediated by osteoclasts, and it was evaluated in different trials in patients with MM or metastatic bone cancer. None of the documented studies reported any objective response in terms of reduction in serum M protein level. However, the stabilization of disease in some subjects suggested a possible cytostatic effect through alteration of the microenvironment. The available results showed that denosumab was effective in decreasing rapidly bone resorption, measured by changes in serum and urine N-telopeptide X levels. In a recent evaluation of three phase III studies, although similar overall survival and progressive disease were reported, denosumab was significantly more effective than zoledronic acid in preventing or delaying first skeletal-related event (including pathological fracture, radiation to bone, surgery to bone, spinal cord compression), as well as in preventing skeletal complications and hypercalcemia associated with this malignancy [181]. Another MM specific target is the cytokine IL6. IL6 is produced predominantly by the BM stromal cells, and is upregulated by multiple cytokines; it plays a critical role in the proliferation and survival of MM cells. It stimulates at least three different signaling pathways (Ras/MEK/ERK, JAK2/STAT3 and PI3K/Akt cascades). Moreover, IL6 protects against apoptotic cell death induced by several agents, thus conferring resistance to chemotherapeutic agents, including bortezomib and melphalan, and to corticosteroid-induced apoptosis. The combination of the anti IL6 chimeric monoclonal antibody siltuximab (S) directed against IL6 and dexamethasone showed clinical activity, including responses in patients refractory to dexamethasone [182]. Ongoing clinical trials evaluate the addition of S to other agents. The addition of S to the VMP (bortezomib-melphalan-prednisone) regimen was studied in 106 patients who were randomized to receive 9 cycles of VMP or VMP+S (11 mg/kg every 3 weeks) followed by S maintenance. Baseline characteristics were well balanced except for IgA subtype and 17p deletions. With a CR rate of 27% on S+VMP and 22% on VMP, the study did not confirm its hypothesis that the addition of S would increase CR rate by at least 10%. Overall response rate was 88% on S+VMP and 80% on VMP and at least VGPR rates were 71% and 51% (P=0.0382), respectively. Median progression-free survival (17 months) and 1-year overall survival (88%) were identical in the two arms, so it was concluded that the addition of S to VMP did not improve CR rate nor long-term outcomes [183]. Finally, like in any tumor, angiogenesis is also necessary for MM cells. VEGF-A is a pro-angiogenetic factor, overexpressed in MM that also works as growth factor for MM cells, triggers MM cells migration, increases IL6 production and inhibits maturation of dendritic cells. Bevacizumab is a humanized monoclonal antibody directed against VEGF-A. In preclinical studies, bevacizumab inhibited activation of signaling cascades in MM cells, reduced MM and endothelial cells proliferation and inhibited angiogenesis. In a phase II trial on relapsed/refractory patients, only one of 6 patients receiving bevacizumab as a monotherapy responded to treatment while bevacizumab in drug combination led to results similar to single-agent thalidomide, with a substantial lack of efficacy [184].

Acknowledgments

I want to thank Dr. Avraham Kornberg, from Asaf Harofhe Hospital for his endless support and wise advices; to Professor Polliack for teaching me, Professor Dov Zipory for the training in the Weitzmann Institute of Science, Dr. Izhar Hardan for his kind advices, Dr. Osnat Garach-Jehoshua for her great assist in investigation, as well as to Dr Naomy Levine, Dr. Marina Izak, Dr. Katerine Hertzog, Dr. Irena Esterlis, Dr. Odit Gutwein and Alona Meidan for their kind assistance.

References

[1] Jurand, A. Early changes in limb buds of chick embryos after thalidomide treatment. *J Embryol Exp Morphol.*, 1966, 16(2), 289-300.

[2] D'Amato, RJ1; Loughnan, MS; Flynn, E; Folkman, J. Thalidomide is an inhibitor of angiogenesis. *Proc Natl Acad Sci U S A.*, 1994 26, 91(9), 4082-5.

[3] Kruse, FE; Joussen, AM; Rohrschneider, K; Becker, MD; Völcker, HE. Thalidomide inhibits corneal angiogenesis induced by vascular endothelial growth factor. *Graefes Arch Clin Exp Ophthalmol.*, 1998, 236(6), 461-6.

[4] Joussen, AM; Germann, T; Kirchhof, B. Effect of thalidomide and structurally related compounds on corneal angiogenesis is comparable to their teratological potency. *Graefes Arch Clin Exp Ophthalmol.*, 1999, 237(12), 952-61.

[5] Kenyon, BM; Browne, F; D'Amato, RJ. Effects of thalidomide and related metabolites in a mouse corneal model of neovascularization. *Exp Eye Res.*, 1997, 64(6), 971-8.

[6] Or, R; Feferman, R; Shoshan, S. Thalidomide reduces vascular density in granulation tissue of subcutaneously implanted polyvinyl alcohol sponges in guinea pigs. *Exp Hematol.*, 1998, 26(3), 217-21.

[7] Moreira, AL; Friedlander, DR; Shif, B; Kaplan, G; Zagzag, D. Thalidomide and a thalidomide analogue inhibit endothelial cell proliferation in vitro. *J Neurooncol.*, 1999, 43(2), 109-14.

[8] Sauer, H; Günther, J; Hescheler, J; Wartenberg, M. Thalidomide inhibits angiogenesis in embryoid bodies by the generation of hydroxyl radicals. *Am J Pathol.*, 2000, 156(1), 151-8.

[9] Gelati, M; Corsini, E; Frigerio, S; Pollo, B; Broggi, G; Croci, D; Silvani, A; Boiardi, A; Salmaggi, AT. Effects of thalidomide on parameters involved in angiogenesis: an in vitro study. *J Neurooncol.*, 2003, 64(3), 193-201.

[10] Yabu, T; Tomimoto, H; Taguchi, Y; Yamaoka, S; Igarashi, Y; Okazaki, T. Thalidomide-induced antiangiogenic action is mediated by ceramide through depletion

of VEGF receptors, and is antagonized by sphingosine-1-phosphate. *Blood.*, 2005, 106(1), 125-34.

[11] Therapontos, C1; Erskine, L; Gardner, ER; Figg, WD; Vargesson, N., Thalidomide induces limb defects by preventing angiogenic outgrowth during early limb formation. *Proc Natl Acad Sci U S A.*, 2009, 26, 106(21), 8573-8.

[12] Gutman, M; Szold, A; Ravid, A; Lazauskas, T; Merimsky, O; Klausner, JM. Failure of thalidomide to inhibit tumor growth and angiogenesis in vivo. *Anticancer Res.*, 1996, 16(6B), 3673-7.

[13] Fine, HA; Figg, WD; Jaeckle, K; Wen, PY; Kyritsis, AP; Loeffler, JS; Levin VA; Black, PM; Kaplan, R; Pluda, JM; Yung, WK. Phase II trial of the antiangiogenic agent thalidomide in patients with recurrent high-grade gliomas. *J Clin Oncol.*, 2000, 18(4), 708-15.

[14] Short, SC; Traish, D; Dowe, A; Hines, F; Gore, M; Brada, M. Thalidomide as an anti-angiogenic agent in relapsed gliomas. *J Neurooncol.*, 2001, 51(1), 41-5.

[15] Rosiñol, L; Cibeira, MT; Segarra, M; Cid, MC; Filella, X; Aymerich, M; Rozman, M; Arenillas, L; Esteve, J; Bladé, J; Montserrat, E. Response to thalidomide in multiple myeloma: impact of angiogenic factors. *Cytokine.*, 2004, 21, 26(4), 145-8.

[16] Mileshkin, L; Honemann, D; Gambell, P; Trivett, M; Hayakawa, Y; Smyth, M; Beshay, V; Ritchie, D; Simmons, P; Milner, AD; Zeldis, JB; Prince, HM. Patients with multiple myeloma treated with thalidomide: evaluation of clinical parameters, cytokines,angiogenic markers, mast cells and marrow CD57+ cytotoxic T cells as predictors of outcome. *Haematologica.*, 2007, 92(8), 1075-82.

[17] Maïga, S; Gomez-Bougie, P; Bonnaud, S; Gratas, C; Moreau, P; Le, Gouill, S; Pellat-Deceunynck, C; Amiot, M. Paradoxical effect of lenalidomide on cytokine/growth factor profiles in multiple myeloma. *Br J Cancer.*, 2013, 108(9), 1801-6.

[18] Yaccoby, S; Johnson, CL; Mahaffey, SC; Wezeman, MJ; Barlogie, B; Epstein, J. Antimyeloma efficacy of thalidomide in the SCID-hu model. *Blood.*, 2002, 100(12), 4162-8.

[19] Du, W; Hattori, Y; Hashiguchi, A; Kondoh, K; Hozumi, N; Ikeda, Y; Sakamoto, M; Hata, J; Yamada, T. Tumor angiogenesis in the bone marrow of multiple myeloma patients and its alteration by thalidomide treatment. *Pathol Int.*, 2004, 54(5), 285-94.

[20] Cibeira, MT; Rozman, M; Segarra, M; Lozano, E; Rosiñol, L; Cid, MC; Filella, X; Bladé, J. Bone marrow angiogenesis and angiogenic factors in multiple myeloma treated with novel agents. *Cytokine.*, 2008, 41(3), 244-53.

[21] Kuwabara, S; Misawa, S; Kanai, K; Sawai, S; Hattori, T; Nishimura, M; Nakaseko, C. Thalidomide reduces serum VEGF levels and improves peripheral neuropathy in POEMS syndrome. *J Neurol Neurosurg Psychiatry.*, 2008, 79(11), 1255-7.

[22] D'Souza, A1; Hayman, SR; Buadi, F; Mauermann, M; Lacy, MQ; Gertz, MA; Kyle, RA; Kumar, S; Greipp, PR; Lust, JA; Russell, SJ; Zeldenrust, S; Dingli, D; Witzig, TE; Rajkumar, SV; Dispenzieri, A. The utility of plasma vascular endothelial growth factor levels in the diagnosis and follow-up of patients with POEMS syndrome. *Blood.*, 2011, 118(17), 4663-5.

[23] Avecilla, ST1; Hattori, K; Heissig, B; Tejada, R; Liao, F; Shido, K; Jin, DK; Dias, S; Zhang, F; Hartman, TE; Hackett, NR; Crystal, RG; Witte, L; Hicklin, DJ; Bohlen, P; Eaton, D; Lyden, D; de Sauvage, F; Rafii, S. Chemokine-mediated interaction of

hematopoietic progenitors with the bone marrow vascular niche is required for thrombo poiesis. *Nat Med.*, 2004, 10(1), 64-71.

[24] Hoshi, A; Matsumoto, A; Chung, J; Isozumi, Y; Koyama, T. Activation of coagulation by a thalidomide-based regimen. *Blood Coagul Fibrinolysis.*, 2011, 22(6), 532-40.

[25] Lebrin, F; Srun, S; Raymond, K; Martin, S; van den Brink, S; Freitas, C; Bréant, C; Mathivet, T; Larrivée, B; Thomas, JL; Arthur, HM; Westermann, CJ; Disch, F; Mager, JJ; Snijder, RJ; Eichmann, A;
Mummery, CL. Thalidomide stimulates vessel maturation and reduces epistaxis in individuals with hereditary hemorrhagic telangiectasia. *Nat Med.*, 2010, 16(4), 420-8.

[26] Ge, ZZ; Chen, HM; Gao, YJ; Liu, WZ; Xu, CH; Tan, HH; Chen, HY; Wei, W; Fang, JY; Xiao, SD. Efficacy of Thalidomide for Refractory Gastrointestinal Bleeding. *Gastroenterology.*, 2011, 141(5), 1629-37.e1-4.

[27] Feng, Q1; Tan, HH; Ge, ZZ; Gao, YJ; Chen, HM; Xiao, SD. Thalidomide-induced angiopoietin 2, Notch1 and Dll4 downregulation under hypoxic condition in tissues with gastrointestinal vascular malformation and human umbilical vein endothelial cells. *J Dig Dis.*, 2014, 15(2), 85-95.

[28] Kaushal, V; Kaushal, GP; Melkaveri, SN; Mehta, P. Thalidomide protects endothelial cells from doxorubicin-induced apoptosis but alters cell morphology. *J Thromb Haemost.*, 2004, 2(2), 327-34.

[29] Cohen, Y; Garach-Jehoshua, O; Bar-Chaim, A; Kornberg, A. Niche modulated and niche-modulating genes in bone marrow cells. *Blood Cancer J.*, 2012 Dec 14), 2:e97.

[30] Parman, T; Wiley, MJ; Wells, PG. Free radical-mediated oxidative DNA damage in the mechanism of thalidomide teratogenicity. *Nat Med.*, 1999, 5(5), 582-5.

[31] Hansen, JM; Gong, SG; Philbert, M; Harris, C. Misregulation of gene expression in the redox-sensitive NF-kappab-dependent limb outgrowth pathway by thalidomide. *Dev Dyn.*, 2002, 225(2), 186-94.

[32] Hansen, JM; Harris, C. A novel hypothesis for thalidomide-induced limb teratogenesis: redox misregulation of the NF-kappaB pathway. *Antioxid Redox Signal.*, 2004, 6(1), 1-14.

[33] Knobloch, J; Shaughnessy, JD; Jr. Rüther, U. Thalidomide induces limb deformities by perturbing the Bmp/Dkk1/Wnt signaling pathway. *FASEB J.*, 2007, 21(7), 1410-21.

[34] Knobloch, J; Schmitz, I; Götz, K; Schulze-Osthoff, K; Rüther, U. Thalidomide induces limb anomalies by PTEN stabilization, Akt suppression, and stimulation of caspase-dependent cell death. *Mol Cell Biol.*, 2008, 28(2), 529-38.

[35] Knobloch, J; Rüther, U. Shedding light on an old mystery: thalidomide suppresses survival pathways to induce limb defects. *Cell Cycle.*, 2008, 7(9), 1121-7.

[36] Braun, AG; Weinreb, SL. Teratogen metabolism: activation of thalidomide and thalidomide analogues to products that inhibit the attachment of cells to concanavalin A coated plastic surfaces. *Biochem Pharmacol.*, 1984, 33(9), 1471-7.

[37] Nogueira, AC1; Neubert, R; Helge, H; Neubert, D. Thalidomide and the immune system. 3. Simultaneous up- and down-regulation of different integrin receptors on human white blood cells. *Life Sci.*, 1994, 55(2), 77-92.

[38] Neubert, R; Hinz, N; Thiel, R; Neubert, D. Down-regulation of adhesion receptors on cells of primate embryos as a probable mechanism of the teratogenic action of thalidomide. *Life Sci.*, 1996, 58(4), 295-316.

[39] Thiel, R; Kastner, U; Neubert, R. Expression of adhesion receptors on rat limb bud cells and results of treatment with a thalidomide derivative. *Life Sci.*, 2000, 66(2), 133-41.

[40] Thiele, A; Thormann, M; Hofmann, HJ; Naumann, WW; Eger, K; Hauschildt, S. A possible role of N-cadherin in thalidomide teratogenicity. *Life Sci.*, 2000, 16, 67(4), 457-61.

[41] Effects of IMiDs on the interaction between MM cells and BM stromal cells. Chang, X; Zhu, Y; Shi, C; Stewart, AK. Mechanism of immunomodulatory drugs' action in the treatment of multiple myeloma. *Acta Biochim Biophys Sin (Shanghai).*, 2014, 46(3), 240-53.

[42] Chang, X; Zhu, Y; Shi, C; Stewart, AK. Mechanism of immunomodulatory drugs' action in the treatment of multiple myeloma. *Acta Biochim Biophys Sin (Shanghai).*, 2014, 46(3), 240-53.

[43] Görgün, G; Calabrese, E; Soydan, E; Hideshima, T; Perrone, G; Bandi, M; Cirstea, D; Santo, L; Hu, Y; Tai, YT; Nahar, S; Mimura, N; Fabre, C; Raje, N; Munshi, N; Richardson, P; Anderson, KC. Immunomodulatory effects of lenalidomide and pomalidomide on interaction of tumor and bone marrow accessory cells in multiple myeloma. *Blood.*, 2010, 116(17), 3227-37.

[44] Gordon, G. The mechanism of thalidomide deformities correlated with the pathogenic effects of prolonged dosage in adults. *Dev Med Child Neurol.*, 1966, 8(6), 761-7.

[45] Fullerton, PM; O'Sullivan, DJ. Thalidomide neuropathy: a clinical, electrophysiological, and histological follow-up study. *J Neurol Neurosurg Psychiatry.*, 1968, 31(6), 543-51.

[46] McCredie, J; McBride, WG. Some congenital abnormalities: possibly due to embryonic peripheral neuropathy. *Clin Radiol.*, 1973, 24(2), 204-11.

[47] McBride, WG. Studies of the etiology of thalidomide dysmorphogenesis. *Teratology.*, 1976), 14(1), 71-87.

[48] Stokes, PA; Lykke, WJ; McBride, WG. Ultrastructural changes in the dorsal root ganglia evoked by thalidomide in rabbits. *Experientia.*, 1976, 15, 32(5), 597-9.

[49] McCredie, J; North, K; de Iongh, R. Thalidomide deformities and their nerve supply. *J Anat.*, 1984, 139 (Pt 3), 397-410.

[50] McCredie, J; Willert, HG. Longitudinal limb deficiencies and the sclerotomes. An analysis of 378 dysmelic malformations induced by thalidomide. *J Bone Joint Surg Br.*, 1999, 81(1), 9-23.

[51] Stephens, TD; McNulty, TR. Evidence for a metameric pattern in the development of the chick humerus. *J Embryol Exp Morphol.*, 1981, 61, 191-205. The segmental pattern of limb development was consistent with the segmental pattern of limb deformities.

[52] Egar, M; Wallace, H; Singer, M. Partial denervation effects on limb cartilage regeneration. *Anat Embryol (Berl).*, 1982, 164(2), 221-8.

[53] Strecker, TR; Stephens, TD. Peripheral nerves do not play a trophic role in limb skeletal morphogenesis. *Teratology.*, 1983, 27(2), 159-67.

[54] Somers, GF. Pharmacological properties of thalidomide (alpha-phthalimido glutarimide), a new sedative hypnotic drug. *Br J Pharmacol Chemother.*, 1960, 111-6.

[55] Kanbayashi, T; Nishino, S; Tafti, M; Hishikawa, Y; Dement, WC; Mignot, E. Thalidomide, a hypnotic with immune modulating properties, increases cataplexy in canine narcolepsy. *Neuroreport.*, 1996, 7(12), 1881-6.

[56] Kanbayashi, T; Nishino, S; Tafti, M; Hishikawa, Y; Dement, WC; Mignot, E. Thalidomide, immune modulation and narcolepsy. *Sleep.*, 1996, 19(2), 116.

[57] Kanbayashi, T; Shimizu, T; Takahashi, Y; Kitajima, T; Takahashi, K; Saito, Y; Hishikawa, Y. Thalidomide increases both REM and stage 3-4 sleep in human adults: a preliminary study. *Sleep.*, 1999, 22(1), 113-5.

[58] Etori, K; Saito, YC; Tsujino, N; Sakurai, T. Effects of a newly developed potent orexin-2 receptor-selective antagonist, compound 1 m, on sleep/wakefulness states in mice. *Front Neurosci.*, 2014, 8, 8.

[59] Dugovic, C; Shelton, JE; Yun, S; Bonaventure, P; Shireman, BT; Lovenberg, TW. Orexin-1 receptor blockade dysregulates REM sleep in the presence of orexin-2 receptor antagonism. *Front Neurosci.*, 2014, 8:28.

[60] Lu, J; Sherman, D; Devor, M; Saper, CB. A putative flip-flop switch for control of REM sleep. *Nature.*, 2006, 441(7093), 589-94.

[61] Boissard, E; Fort, P; Gervasoni, D; Barbagli, B; Luppi, P. Localization of the GABAergic and non-GABAergic neurons projecting to the sublaterodorsal nucleus and potentially gating paradoxical sleep onset. *Eur J Neurosci*, 2003, 18, 1627-39.

[62] Boeve, BF; Silber, MH; Saper, CB; Ferman, TJ; Dickson, DW; Parisi, JE; Benarroch, EE; Ahlskog, JE; Smith, GE; Caselli, RC; Tippman-Peikert, M; Olson, EJ; Lin, SC; Young, T; Wszolek, Z; Schenck, CH; Mahowald, MW; Castillo, PR; Del Tredici, K; Braak, H. Pathophysiology of REM sleep behaviour disorder and relevance to neurodegenerative disease. *Brain.*, 2007, 130(Pt 11), 2770-88.

[63] Neubert, D. Never-ending tales of the mode of the teratogenic action of thalidomide. *Teratog Carcinog Mutagen.*, 1997, 17(1), i-ii.

[64] Hansen, JM; Harris, KK; Philbert, MA; Harris, C. Thalidomide modulates nuclear redox status and preferentially depletes glutathione in rabbit limb versus rat limb. *J Pharmacol Exp Ther.*, 2002, 300(3), 768-76.

[65] Hendrickx, AG; Sawyer, RH. Developmental staging and thalidomide teratogenicity in the green monkey (Cercopithecus aethiops). *Teratology.*, 1978, 18(3), 393-404.

[66] Hendrickx, AG. The sensitive period and malformation syndrome produced by thalidomide in crab-eating monkey (Macaca fascicularis). *J Med Primatol.*, 1973, 2(5), 267-76.

[67] Hendrickx, AG; Peterson, PE. Perspectives on the use of the baboon in embryology and teratology research. *Hum Reprod Update.*, 1997, 3(6), 575-92.

[68] Hendrickx, AG; Helm, FC. Non teratogenicity of a structural analog of thalidomide in pregnant baboons. *Teratology.*, 1980, 22(2), 179-82. (Papio cynocephalus).

[69] Scott, WJ; Wilson, JG; Helm, FC. A metabolite of a structural analog of thalidomide lacks teratogenic effect in pregnant rhesus monkeys. *Teratology.*, 1980, 22(2), 183-5.

[70] Günzler, V. Thalidomide in human immunodeficiency virus (HIV) patients. A review of safety considerations. *Drug Saf.*, 1992, 7(2), 116-34.

[71] Bai, N; Cui, XY; Wang, J; Sun, CG; Mei, HK; Liang, BB; Cai, Y; Song, XJ; Gu, JK; Wang, R. Determination of thalidomide concentration in human plasma by liquid chromatography-tandem mass spectrometry. *Exp Ther Med.*, 2013, 5(2), 626-630.

[72] Teo, SK; Colburn, WA, Thomas, SD. Single-dose oral pharmacokinetics of three formulations of thalidomide in healthy male volunteers. *J Clin Pharmacol, 39,* 1162-1168, 1999.

[73] Lyons, K; Ezaki, M. Molecular Regulation of Limb Growth. Lyons. K Ezaki M. *J Bone Joint Surg Am.*, 2009, 91 Suppl 4, 47-52.
[74] Tabin, CG. A developmental model for thalidomide defects. *Nature.*, 1998, 26, 396(6709), 322-3
[75] Neubert, R; Merker, HJ; Neubert, D. Developmental model for thalidomide action. *Nature.*, 1999, 29, 400(6743), 419-20.
[76] Galloway, JL; Delgado, I; Ros, MA; Tabin, CJ. A reevaluation of X-irradiation-induced phocomelia and proximodistal limb patterning. *Nature.*, 2009, 460(7253), 400-4.
[77] Henkel, L; Willert, HG. Dysmelia. A classification and a pattern of malformation in a group of congenital defects of the limbs. *J Bone Joint Surg Br.*, 1969, 51(3), 399-414.
[78] Smithells, RW; Newman, CG. Recognition of thalidomide defects. *J Med Genet.*, 1992, 29(10), 716-23.
[79] Al-Qattan, MM. WNT pathways and upper limb anomalies. *J Hand Surg Eur Vol.*, 2011, 36(1), 9-22.
[80] Koyama, E; Leatherman, JL; Noji, S; Pacifici, M. Early Chick Limb Cartilaginous Elements Possess Polarizing Activity and Express Hedgehog-Related Morphogenetic Factors. *Dev Dyn.*, 1996, 207(3), 344-54.
[81] Litingtung, Y; Dahn, RD; Li, Y; Fallon, JF; Chiang, C. Shh and Gli3 are dispensable for limb skeleton formation but regulate digit number and identity. *Nature.*, 2002, 418(6901), 979-83.
[82] Adolphe, C; Hetherington, R; Ellis, T; Wainwright, B. Patched1 functions as a gatekeeper by promoting *cell cycle* progression. *Cancer Res.*, 2006, 66(4), 2081-8.
[83] Goodrich, LV; Milenkovic, L; Higgins, KM; Scott, MP. Altered neural cell fates and medulloblastoma in mouse patched mutants. *Science*, 1997, 277, 1109–13.
[84] Ruiz, I; Altaba, A. Gli proteins encode context-dependent positive and negative functions: implications for development and disease. *Development*, 1999, 126 (14), 3205–16.
[85] Pi-Roig, A; Martin-Blanco, E; Minguillon, C. Distinct tissue-specific requirements for the zebrafish tbx5 genes during heart, retina and pectoral fin development. *Open Biol.*, 2014, 4(4), 140014.
[86] Robert, B. Bone morphogenetic protein signaling in limb outgrowth and patterning. *Dev Growth Differ.*, 2007, 49(6), 455-68.
[87] Topol, L; Jiang, X; Choi, H; Garrett-Beal, L; Carolan, PJ; Yang, Y. Wnt-5a inhibits the canonical Wnt pathway by promoting GSK-3- independent b catenin degradation. *J Cell Biol.*, 2003, 162, 899–908.
[88] St-Jacques, B; Hammerschmidt, M; McMahon, AP. Indian hedgehog signaling regulates proliferation and differentiation of chondrocytes and is essential for bone formation. *Genes Dev.*, 1999, 13(16), 2072-86.
[89] Hagen, EO. Congenital malformations in a thalidomide baby: a postmortem anatomical study. *Can Med Assoc J.*, 1965, 92, 283-6.
[90] Zakany, J; Duboule, D. The role of Hox genes during vertebrate limb development. *Curr Opin Genet Dev.*, 2007, 17(4), 359-66.
[91] Tian, E; Zhan, F; Walker, R; Rasmussen, E; Ma, Y; Barlogie, B; Shaughnessy, JD, Jr. The role of the Wnt-signaling antagonist DKK1 in the development of osteolytic lesions in multiple myeloma. *N Engl J Med.*, 2003, 349(26), 2483-94.

[92] Dela, Cruz, F; Terry, M; Matushansky, I. A transgenic, mesodermal specific, Dkk1 mouse model recapitulates a spectrum of human congenital limb reduction defects. *Differentiation.*, 2012, 83(4), 220-30.

[93] Ma, G; Yu, J; Xiao, Y; Chan, D; Gao, B; Hu, J; He, Y; Guo, S; Zhou, J; Zhang, L; Gao, L; Zhang, W; Kang, Y; Cheah, KS; Feng, G; Guo, X; Wang, Y; Zhou, CZ; He, L. Indian hedgehog mutations causing brachydactyly type A1 impair Hedgehog signal transduction at multiple levels. *Cell Res.*, 2011, 21(9), 1343-57

[94] Ema, M; Ise, R; Kato, H; Oneda, S; Hirose, A; Hirata-Koizumi, M; Singh, AV; Knudsen, TB; Ihara, T. Fetal malformations and early embryonic gene expression response in cynomolgus monkeys maternally exposed to thalidomide. *Reprod Toxicol.*, 2010, 29(1), 49-56.

[95] Yaccoby, S; Wezeman, MJ; Henderson, A; Cottler-Fox, M; Yi, Q; Barlogie, B; Epstein, J. Myeloma interacts with the bone marrow microenvironment to induce osteoclastogenesis and is dependent on osteoclast activity. *Br J Haematol.*, 2002, 116(2), 278-90.

[96] Dezorella, N; Pevsner-Fischer, M; Deutsch, V; Kay, S; Baron, S; Stern, R; Tavor, S; Nagler, A; Naparstek, E; Zipori, D; Katz, BZ. Mesenchymal stromal cells revert multiple myeloma cells to less differentiated phenotype by the combined activities of adhesive interactions and interleukin-6. *Exp Cell Res.*, 2009, 315(11), 1904-13.

[97] Ito, T; Ando, H; Suzuki, T; Ogura, T; Hotta, K; Imamura, Y; Yamaguchi, Y; Handa, H. Identification of a primary target of thalidomide teratogenicity. *Science.*, 2010, 327(5971), 1345-50.

[98] Zhu, YX; Braggio, E; Shi, CX; Bruins, LA; Schmidt, JE; Van, Wier, S; Chang, XB; Bjorklund, CC; Fonseca, R; Bergsagel, PL; Orlowski, RZ; Stewart, AK. Cereblon expression is required for the antimyeloma activity of lenalidomide and pomalidomide. *Blood.*, 2011, 118(18), 4771-9.

[99] Broyl, A; Kuiper, R; van, Duin, M; van der Holt, B; el Jarari, L; Bertsch, U; Zweegman, S; Buijs, A; Hose, D; Lokhorst, HM; Goldschmidt, H; Sonneveld, P; Dutch-Belgian HOVON group; German GMMG Group. High cereblon expression is associated with better survival in patients with newly diagnosed multiple myeloma treated with thalidomide maintenance. *Blood.*, 2013, 121(4), 624-7.

[100] Heintel, D; Rocci, A; Ludwig, H; Bolomsky, A; Caltagirone, S; Schreder, M; Pfeifer, S; Gisslinger, H; Zojer, N; Jäger, U; Palumbo, A. High expression of cereblon (CRBN) is associated with improved clinical response in patients with multiple myeloma treated with lenalidomide and dexamethasone. *Br J Haematol.*, 2013, 161(5), 695-700.

[101] Gandhi, AK; Kang, J; Havens, CG; Conklin, T; Ning, Y; Wu, L; Ito, T; Ando, H; Waldman, MF; Thakurta, A; Klippel, A; Handa, H; Daniel, TO; Schafer, PH; Chopra, R. Immunomodulatory agents lenalidomide and pomalidomide co-stimulate T cells by inducing degradation of T cell repressors Ikaros and Aiolos via modulation of the E3 ubiquitin ligase complex CRL4(CRBN.). *Br J Haematol.*, 2014, 164(6), 811-21.

[102] Spoorendonk, KM; Peterson-Maduro, J; Renn, J; Trowe, T; Kranenbarg, S; Winkler, C; Schulte-Merker, S. Retinoic acid and Cyp26b1 are critical regulators of osteogenesis in the axial skeleton. *Development.*, 2008, 135(22), 3765-74.

[103] Chevy, F; Illien, F; Wolf, C; Roux, C. Limb malformations of rat fetuses exposed to a distal inhibitor of cholesterol biosynthesis. *J Lipid Res.*, 2002, 43(8), 1192-200.

[104] Aguilar, A; Wu, S; De Luca, F. P450 oxidoreductase expressed in rat chondrocytes modulates chondrogenesis via cholesterol- and Indian Hedgehog-dependent mechanisms. *Endocrinology.*, 2009, 150(6), 2732-9

[105] Ardecky, R; Magnuson, GK; Zou, J; Ganji, SR; Brown, B; Ngo, T; Lee, J; Zeng, FY; Sun, Q; Stonich, D; Salaniwal, S; Sakata, T; Rack, PG; Casabar, JKT; Mangravita-Novo, A; Smith, LH; Sergienko, E; Chung, TDY; Pinkerton, AB; Pass, I; Chen, JK. Small-molecule antagonists of Gli function. Probe Reports from the NIH Molecular Libraries Program [Internet]. Bethesda (MD): National Center for Biotechnology Information (US)): 2010-2012 Dec 17 [updated 2013 Mar 22].

[106] Ruschak, AM; Slassi, M; Kay, LE; Schimmer, AD. Novel proteasome inhibitors to overcome bortezomib resistance. *J Natl Cancer Inst*, 2011, 103(13), 1007-1017.

[107] Tsukamoto, S; Yokosawa, H. Inhibition of the ubiquitin-proteasome system by natural products for cancer therapy. *Planta Med.*, 2010, 76(11), 1064-74.

[108] Alkalay, I; Yaron, A; Hatzubai, A; Jung, S; Avraham, A; Gerlitz, O; Pashut-Lavon, I; Ben-Neriah, Y. In vivo stimulation of I kappa B phosphorylation is not sufficient to activate NF-kappa B. *Mol Cell Biol.*, 1995, 15(3), 1294-301.

[109] Alkalay, I; Yaron, A; Hatzubai, A; Orian, A; Ciechanover, A; Ben-Neriah, Y. Stimulation-dependent I kappa B alpha phosphorylation marks the NF-kappa B inhibitor for degradation via the ubiquitin-proteasome pathway. *Proc Natl Acad Sci U S A.*, 1995, 92(23), 10599-603.

[110] Kanarek, N; London, N; Schueler-Furman, O; Ben-Neriah, Y. Ubiquitination and degradation of the inhibitors of NF-kappaB. Cold Spring *Harb Perspect Biol.*, 2010, 2(2), a000166.

[111] Mitsiades, N; Mitsiades, CS; Poulaki, V; Chauhan, D; Richardson, PG; Hideshima, T; Munshi, N; Treon, SP; Anderson, KC. Biologic sequelae of nuclear factor-kappaB blockade in multiple myeloma: therapeutic applications. *Blood*, 2002, 99(11), 4079-86.

[112] Hideshima, T; Chauhan, D; Richardson, P; Mitsiades, C; Mitsiades, N; Hayashi, T; Munshi, N; Dang, L; Castro, A; Palombella, V; Adams, J; Anderson, KC. NF-kappa B as a therapeutic target in multiple myeloma. *J Biol Chem.*, 2002, 277(19), 16639-47.

[113] Fernández, Y; Verhaegen, M; Miller, TP; Rush, JL; Steiner, P; Opipari, AW, Jr; Lowe, SW; Soengas, MS. Differential regulation of noxa in normal melanocytes and melanoma cells by proteasome inhibition: therapeutic implications. *Cancer Res.*, 2005, 65(14), 6294-304.

[114] Befani, CD; Vlachostergios, PJ; Hatzidaki, E; Patrikidou, A; Bonanou, S; Simos, G; Papandreou, CN; Liakos, P. Bortezomib represses HIF-1α protein expression and nuclear accumulation by inhibiting both PI3K/Akt/TOR and MAPK pathways in prostate cancer cells. *J Mol Med (Berl).*, 2012, 90(1), 45-54.

[115] Nawrocki, ST; Carew, JS; Pino, MS; Highshaw, RA; Dunner, K, Jr; Huang, P; Abbruzzese, JL; McConkey, DJ. Bortezomib sensitizes pancreatic cancer cells to endoplasmic reticulum stress-mediated apoptosis. *Cancer Res.*, 2005, 65(24), 11658–66.

[116] Nawrocki, ST; Carew, JS; Dunner, K; Jr. Boise, LH; Chiao, PJ; Huang, P; Abbruzzese, JL; McConkey, DJ. Bortezomib inhibits PKR-like endoplasmic reticulum (ER) kinase and induces apoptosis via ER stress in human pancreatic cancer cells. *Cancer Res.*, 2005, 65(24), 11510–19.

[117] Yoshida, H; Matsui, T; Yamamoto, A; Okada, T; Mori, K. XBP1 mRNA is induced by ATF6 and spliced by IRE1 in response to ER stress to produce a highly active transcription factor. *Cell*, 2001, 107(7), 881-91.

[118] Lee, AH; Iwakoshi, NN; Glimcher, LH. XBP-1 regulates a subset of endoplasmic reticulum resident chaperone genes in the unfolded protein response. *Mol Cell Biol.*, 2003, 23(21), 7448-59.

[119] Iwakoshi, NN; Lee, AH; Glimcher, LH. The X-box binding protein-1 transcription factor is required for plasma cell differentiation and the unfolded protein response. *Immunol Rev.*, 2003, 194, 29-38.

[120] Reimold, AM; Iwakoshi, NN; Manis, J; Vallabhajosyula, P; Szomolanyi-Tsuda, E; Gravallese, EM; Friend, D; Grusby, MJ; Alt, F; Glimcher, LH. Plasma cell differentiation requires the transcription factor XBP-1. *Nature*, 2001, 412(6844), 300-7.

[121] Iwakoshi, NN; Lee, AH; Vallabhajosyula, P; Otipoby, KL; Rajewsky, K; Glimcher, LH. Plasma cell differentiation and the unfolded protein response intersect at the transcription factor XBP-1. *Nat Immunol.*, 2003, 4(4), 321-29.

[122] Gass, JN; Gifford, NM; Brewer, JW. Activation of an unfolded protein response during differentiation of antibody-secreting B cells. *J Biol Chem.*, 2002, 277(5), 49047–54.

[123] Kim, R; Emi, M; Tanabe, K; Murakami, S. Role of the unfolded protein response in cell death. *Apoptosis*, 2006, 11(1), 5–13.

[124] Sano, R; Reed, JC. ER stress-induced cell death mechanisms. *Biochim Biophys Acta*, 2013, 1833(12), 3460-70.

[125] McCullough, KD; Martindale, JL; Klotz, LO; Aw, TY; Holbrook, NJ. Gadd153 sensitizes cells to endoplasmic reticulum stress by down-regulating Bcl2 and perturbing the cellular redox state. *Mol Cell Biol.*, 2001, 21(4), 1249-59.

[126] Harding, HP; Zhang, Y; Bertolotti, A; Zeng, H; Ron, D. Perk is essential for translational regulation and cell survival during the unfolded protein response. *Mol Cell*, 2000, 5(5): 897-904.

[127] Fribley, A; Zeng, Q; Wang, CY. Proteasome inhibitor PS-341 induces apoptosis through induction of endoplasmic reticulum stress-reactive oxygen species in head and neck squamous cell carcinoma cells. *Mol Cell Biol.*, 2004, 24(22), 9695–704.

[128] Meister, S; Schubert, U; Neubert, K; Herrmann, K; Burger, R; Gramatzki, M; et al. Extensive immunoglobulin production sensitizes myeloma cells for proteasome inhibition. *Cancer Res.*, 2007, 67(4), 1783-92.

[129] Ri, M; Iida, S; Nakashima, T; Miyazaki, H; Mori, F; Ito, A; Inagaki, A; Kusumoto, S; Ishida, T; Komatsu, H; Shiotsu, Y; Ueda, R. Bortezomib-resistant myeloma cell lines: a role for mutated PSMB5 in preventing the accumulation of unfolded proteins and fatal ER stress. *Leukemia*, 2010, 24(8), 1506-12.

[130] Mujtaba, T; Dou, QP. Advances in the understanding of mechanisms and therapeutic use of bortezomib. *Discov Med*, 2011, 12(67), 471-480.

[131] Mitsiades, N; Mitsiades, CS; Poulaki, V; Chauhan, D; Fanourakis, G; Gu, X; Bailey, C; Joseph, M; Libermann, TA; Treon, SP; Munshi, NC; Richardson, PG; Hideshima, T; Anderson, KC. Molecular sequelae of proteasome inhibition in human multiple myeloma cells. *Proc Natl Acad Sci U S A.*, 2002, 99(22), 14374-379.

[132] Obeng, EA; Carlson, LM; Gutman, DM; Harrington, WJ Jr; Lee, KP; Boise, LH. Proteasome inhibitors induce a terminal unfolded protein response in multiple myeloma cells. *Blood*, 2006, 107(12), 4907–16.

[133] Mancini, R; Fagioli, C; Fra, AM; Maggioni, C; Sitia, R. Degradation of unassembled soluble Ig subunits by cytosolic proteasomes: evidence that retrotranslocation and degradation are coupled events. *FASEB J.*, 2000, 14(5), 769-78.

[134] Werner, ED; Brodsky, JL; McCracken, AA. Proteasome-dependent endoplasmic reticulum-associated protein degradation: an unconventional route to a familiar fate. *Proc Natl Acad Sci U S A.*, 1996, 93(24), 13797-801.

[135] O'Hare, T; Wiens, GD; Whitcomb, EA; Enns, CA; Rittenberg, MB. Cutting edge: proteasome involvement in the degradation of unassembled Ig light chains. *J Immunol.*, 1999, 163(1), 11-14.

[136] Wacker, SA; Houghtaling, BR; Elemento, O; Kapoor, TM. Using transcriptome sequencing to identify mechanisms of drug action and resistance. *Nat Chem Biol.*, 2012, 8(3), 235-37.

[137] Stessman, HA; Baughn, LB; Sarver, A; Xia, T; Deshpande, R; Mansoor, A; Walsh, SA; Sunderland, JJ; Dolloff, NG; Linden, MA; Zhan, F; Janz, S; Myers, CL; Van Ness, BG. Profiling bortezomib resistance identifies secondary therapies in a mouse myeloma model. *Cancer Ther.*, 2013, 12(6), 1140-50.

[138] Shuqing, Lü; Jianmin, Wang. The resistance mechanisms of proteasome inhibitor bortezomib. *Biomarker Research.*, 2013, 1(1), 13.

[139] Suzuki, E; Demo, S; Deu, E; Keats, J; Arastu-Kapur, S; Bergsagel, PL; Bennett, MK; Kirk, CJ. Molecular mechanisms of bortezomib resistant adenocarcinoma cells. *PLoS One*, 2011, 6(12), e27996.

[140] Franke, NE; Niewerth, D; Assaraf, YG; van, Meerloo, J; Vojtekova, K; van, Zantwijk, CH; Zweegman, S; Chan, ET; Kirk, CJ; Geerke, DP; Schimmer, AD; Kaspers, GJ; Jansen, G; Cloos, J. Impaired bortezomib binding to mutant β5 subunit of the proteasome is the underlying basis for bortezomib resistance in leukemia cells. *Leukemia*, 2012, 26(4), 757-68.

[141] Leung-Hagesteijn, C; Erdmann, N; Cheung, G; Keats, JJ; Stewart, AK; Reece, DE; Chung, KC; Tiedemann, RE. Xbp1s-negative tumor B cells and pre-plasmablasts mediate therapeutic proteasome inhibitor resistance in multiple myeloma. *Cancer Cell*, 2013, 24(3), 289-304.

[142] Zong, WX; Li, C; Hatzivassiliou, G; Lindsten, T; Yu, QC; Yuan, J; Thompson, CB. Bax and Bak can localize to the endoplasmic reticulum to initiate apoptosis. *J Cell Biol.*, 2003, 162(1), 59–69.

[143] Selimovic, D; Porzig, BB; El-Khattouti, A; Badura, HE; Ahmad, M; Ghanjati, F; Santourlidis, S; Haikel, Y; Hassan, M. Bortezomib/proteasome inhibitor triggers both apoptosis and autophagy-dependent pathways in melanoma cells. *Cell Signal.*, 2013, 25(1), 308-18.

[144] Yu, C; Rahmani, M; Dent, P; Grant, S. The hierarchical relationship between MAPK signaling and ROS generation in human leukemia cells undergoing apoptosis in response to the proteasome inhibitor Bortezomib. *Exp Cell Res.*, 2004, 295(2), 555-66.

[145] Landowski, TH; Megli, CJ; Nullmeyer, KD; Lynch, RM; Dorr, RT. Mitochondrial-mediated disregulation of Ca2+ is a critical determinant of Velcade (PS-341/bortezomib) cytotoxicity in myeloma cell lines. *Cancer Res.*, 2005, 65(9), 3828–36.

[146] Wang, Q; Shinkre, BA; Lee, JG; Weniger, MA; Liu, Y; Chen, W; Wiestner, A; Trenkle, WC; Ye, Y. The ERAD inhibitor Eeyarestatin I is a bifunctional compound

with a membrane-binding domain and a p97/VCP inhibitory group. *PLoS One*, 2010, 12, 5(11), e15479.

[147] Hemeryck, A; Geerts, R; Monbaliu, J; Hassler, S; Verhaeghe, T; Diels, L; Verluyten, W; van Beijsterveldt, L; Mamidi, RN; Janssen, C; De Coster, R. Tissue distribution and depletion kinetics of bortezomib and bortezomib-related radioactivity in male rats after single and repeated intravenous injection of 14 C-bortezomib. *Cancer Chemother Pharmacol.*, 2007, 60(6), 777-87.

[148] Davenport, EL; Moore, HE; Dunlop, AS; Sharp, SY; Workman, P; Morgan, GJ; Davies, FE. Heat shock protein inhibition is associated with activation of the unfolded protein response pathway in myeloma plasma cells. *Blood*, 2007, 110(7), 2641-49.

[149] Khong, T; Spencer, A. Targeting HSP 90 induces apoptosis and inhibits critical survival and proliferation pathways in multiple myeloma. *Mol Cancer Ther.*, 2011, 10(10), 1909-17.

[150] Roué, G; Pérez-Galán, P; Mozos, A; López-Guerra, M; Xargay-Torrent, S; Rosich, L; Saborit-Villarroya, I; Normant, E; Campo, E; Colomer, D. The Hsp90 inhibitor IPI-504 overcomes bortezomib resistance in mantle cell lymphoma in vitro and in vivo by down-regulation of the prosurvival ER chaperone BiP/Grp78. *Blood*, 2011, 117(4), 1270-79.

[151] Auner, HW1; Moody, AM; Ward, TH; Kraus, M; Milan, E; May, P; Chaidos, A; Driessen, C; Cenci, S; Dazzi, F; Rahemtulla, A; Apperley, JF; Karadimitris, A; Dillon, N. Combined inhibition of p97 and the proteasome causes lethal disruption of the secretory apparatus in multiple myeloma cells. *PLoS One*, 2013, 17, 8(9), e74415.

[152] Robillard, N; Wuillème, S1; Moreau, P2; Béné, MC1. Immunophenotype of normal and myelomatous plasma-cell subsets. *Front Immunol.*, 2014, 5, 137.

[153] Bergsagel, PL; Masellis, Smith, A; Belch, AR; Pilarski, LM. The *blood* B-cells and bone marrow plasma cells in patients with multiple myeloma share identical IgH rearrangements. *Curr Top Microbiol Immunol.*, 1995, 194, 17-24.

[154] Bergsagel, PL; Smith, AM; Szczepek, A; Mant, MJ; Belch, AR; Pilarski, LM. In multiple myeloma, clonotypic B lymphocytes are detectable among CD19+ peripheral blood cells expressing CD38, CD56, and monotypic Ig light chain. *Blood.*, 1995, 85(2), 436-47.

[155] Szczepek, AJ; Seeberger, K; Wizniak, J; Mant, MJ; Belch, AR; Pilarski, LM. A high frequency of circulating B cells share clonotypic Ig heavy-chain VDJ rearrangements with autologous bone marrow plasma cells in multiple myeloma, as measured by single-cell and in situ reverse transcriptase-polymerase chain reaction. *Blood.*, 1998, 92(8), 2844-55.

[156] Chen, BJ; Epstein, J. Circulating clonal lymphocytes in myeloma constitute a minor subpopulation of B cells. *Blood.*, 1996, 87(5), 1972-6.

[157] Kay, NE; Leong, T; Kyle, RA; Greipp, P; Billadeau, D; Van Ness, B; Bone, N; Oken, MM. Circulating blood B cells in multiple myeloma: analysis and relationship to circulating clonal cells and clinical parameters in a cohort of patients entered on the Eastern Cooperative Oncology Group phase III E9486 clinical trial. *Blood.*, 1997, 90(1), 340-

[158] Luque, R; Brieva, JA; Moreno, A; Manzanal, A; Escribano, L; Villarrubia, J; Velasco, JL; López-Jiménez, J; Cerveró, C; Otero, MJ; Martínez, J; Bellas, C; Roldán, E. Normal and clonal B lineage cells can be distinguished by their differential expression

of B cell antigens and adhesion molecules in peripheral blood from multiple myeloma (MM) patients--diagnostic and clinical implications. *Clin Exp Immunol.*, 1998, 112(3), 410-8.

[159] Cremer, FW; Ehrbrecht, E; Kiel, K; Benner, A; Hegenbart, U; Ho, AD; Goldschmidt, H; Moos, M. Evaluation of the kinetics of bone marrow tumor load in the course of sequential high-dose therapy assessed by quantitative PCR as predictive factor in patients with multiple myeloma. *Bone Marrow Transplant.*, 2000, 26(8), 851-8.

[160] Cremer, FW; Ehrbrecht, E; Kiel, K; Benner, A; Hegenbart, U; Ho, AD; Goldschmidt, H; Moos, M. Evaluation of the kinetics of bone marrow tumor load in the course of sequential high-dose therapy assessed by quantitative PCR as predictive factor in patients with multiple myeloma. *Bone Marrow Transplant.*, 2000, 26(8), 851-8.

[161] Gemmel, C; Cremer, FW; Weis, M; Witzens, M; Moldenhauer, G; Koniczek, KH; Imbach, U; Ho, AD; Moos, M; Goldschmidt, H. Anti-CD20 antibody as consolidation therapy in a patient with primary plasma cell leukemia after high-dose therapy and autologous stem cell transplantation. *Ann Hematol.*, 2002, 81(2), 119-23.

[162] Zojer, N; Kirchbacher, K; Vesely, M; Hübl, W; Ludwig, H. Rituximab treatment provides no clinical benefit in patients with pretreated advanced multiple myeloma. *Leuk Lymphoma.*, 2006, 47(6), 1103-9.

[163] Musto, P; Carella, AM, Jr; Greco, MM; Falcone, A; Sanpaolo, G; Bodenizza, C; Cascavilla, N; Melillo, L; Carella, AM. Short progression-free survival in myeloma patients receiving rituximab as maintenance therapy after autologous. *Br J Haematol.*, 2003, 123(4), 746-7.

[164] Rasmussen, T. The presence of circulating clonal CD19+ cells in multiple myeloma. *Leuk Lymphoma.*, 2001, 42(6), 1359-66.

[165] Zojer, N; Schuster-Kolbe, J; Assmann, I; Ackermann, J; Strasser, K; Hübl, W; Drach, J; Ludwig, H. Chromosomal aberrations are shared by malignant plasma cells and a small fraction of circulating CD19+ cells in patients with myeloma and monoclonal gammopathy of undetermined significance. *Br J Haematol.*, 2002, 117(4), 852-9.

[166] Rottenburger, C; Kiel, K; Bösing, T; Cremer, FW; Moldenhauer, G; Ho, AD; Goldschmidt, H; Moos, M. Clonotypic CD20+ and CD19+ B cells in peripheral blood of patients with multiple myeloma post high-dose therapy and peripheral blood stem cell transplantation. *Br J Haematol.*, 1999, 106(2), 545-52.

[167] Fenk, R; Ak, M; Kobbe, G; Steidl, U; Arnold, C; Korthals, M; Hünerlitürkoglu, A; Rohr, UP; Kliszewski, S; Bernhardt, A; Haas, R; Kronenwett, R. Levels of minimal residual disease detected by quantitative molecular monitoring herald relapse in patients with multiple myeloma. *Haematologica.*, 2004, 89(5), 557-66.

[168] Korthals, M; Sehnke, N; Kronenwett, R; Schroeder, T; Strapatsas, T; Kobbe, G; Haas, R; Fenk, R. Molecular monitoring of minimal residual disease in the peripheral blood of patients with multiple myeloma. *Biol Blood Marrow Transplant.*, 2013, 19(7), 1109-15.

[169] Pilarski, LM; Hipperson, G; Seeberger, K; Pruski, E; Coupland, RW; Belch, AR. Myeloma progenitors in the blood of patients with aggressive or minimal disease: engraftment and self-renewal of primary human myeloma in the bone marrow of NOD SCID mice. *Blood.*, 2000, 95(3), 1056-65..

[170] Pilarski, LM; Belch, AR. Clonotypic myeloma cells able to xenograft myeloma to nonobese diabetic severe combined immunodeficient mice copurify with CD34 (+) hematopoietic progenitors. *Clin Cancer Res.*, 2002, 8(10), 3198-204.

[171] Matsui, W; Huff, CA; Wang, Q; Malehorn, MT; Barber, J; Tanhehco, Y; Smith, BD; Civin, CI; Jones, RJ. Characterization of clonogenic multiple myeloma cells. *Blood.*, 2004, 103(6), 2332-6.

[172] Hosen, N; Matsuoka, Y; Kishida, S; Nakata, J; Mizutani, Y; Hasegawa, K; Mugitani, A; Ichihara, H; Aoyama, Y; Nishida, S; Tsuboi, A; Fujiki, F; Tatsumi, N; Nakajima, H; Hino, M; Kimura, T; Yata, K; Abe, M; Oka, Y; Oji, Y; Kumanogoh, A; Sugiyama, H. CD138-negative clonogenic cells are plasma cells but not B cells in some multiple myeloma patients. *Leukemia.*, 2012, 26(9), 2135-41.

[173] Heffner, LT; Jagannath, S; Zimmerman, TM; et al. BT062, an antibody-drug conjugate directed against CD138, given weekly for 3 weeks in each 4 week cycle: safety and further evidence of clinical activity. *Blood* (ASH Annual Meeting Abstract), 2012, 120, Abstract # 4042.

[174] Zonder, JA; Mohrbacher, AF; Singhal, S; et al. A phase 1, multicenter, open-label, dose escalation study of elotuzumab in patients with advanced multiple myeloma. *Blood*, 2012, 120, 552-9.

[175] Lokhorst, H; Plesner, T; Gimsing, P; et al. A CD38 monoclonal antibody study in advanced multiple myeloma - an open label, dose-escalation followed by open label extension in a single arm phase I/II study (abstract S576). *EHA Abstract*, 2013, 98(Suppl 1), 241.

[176] Cohen, Y; Gutwein, O; Garach-Jehoshua, O; Bar-Haim, A; Kornberg, A. GPRC5D is a promising marker for monitoring the tumor load and to target multiple myeloma cells. *Hematology.*, 2013, 18(6), 348-51.

[177] Pinzone, JJ; Hall, BM; Thudi, NK; Vonau, M; Qiang, YW; Rosol, TJ; Shaughnessy, JD, Jr. The role of Dickkopf-1 in bone development, homeostasis, and disease. *Blood.*, 2009, 113(3), 517-25.

[178] Pozzi, S; Fulciniti, M; Yan, H; Vallet, S; Eda, H; Patel, K; Santo, L; Cirstea, D; Hideshima, T; Schirtzinge, L; Kuhstoss, S; Anderson, KC; Munshi, N; Scadden, D; Kronenberg, HM; Raje, N. In vivo and in vitro effects of a novel anti-Dkk1 neutralizing antibody in multiple myeloma. *Bone.*, 2013, 53(2), 487-96.

[179] Padmanabhan, S; Beck, JT; Kelly, KR; Munshi, NC; Dzik-Jurasz, A; Gangolli, E; Ettenberg, S; Miner, K; Bilic, S; Whyte, W; Mehdi, F; Chiang, LM; Rae, PL; Spencer, A; Shah, J; Anderson, KC; Giles, FJ; Stewart, AK. A phase I/II sttudy of BHQ880, a novel osteoblast activating, anti-DKK1 human monoclonal antibody, in relapsed and refractory multiple myeloma (MM) patients treated with zoledronic acid (Zol) and anti-myeloma therapy (MM Tx). *Blood* (ASH Annual Meeting Abstracts), 2009, 114, Abstract 750.

[180] Munshi, NC; Abonour, R; Beck, JT; Bensinger, W; Facon, T; Stockerl-Goldstein, K; Baz, R; Siegel, DS; Neben, K; Lonial, S; Suvannasankha, A; Bilic, S; Chica, S; Mukhopadhyay, S; Isaacs, R; Jagannath, S. Early evidence of anabolic bone activity of BHQ880, a fully human anti-DKK1 neutralizing antibody: results of a phase 2 study in previously untreated patients with smoldering multiple myeloma at risk for progression. *Blood* (ASH Annual Meeting Abstracts), 2012, 120, Abstract 331.

[181] Lipton, A; Fizazi, K; Stopeck, AT; Henry, DH; Brown, JE; Yardley, DA; Richardson, GE; Siena, S; Maroto, P; Clemens, M; Bilynskyy, B; Charu, V; Beuzeboc, P; Rader, M; Viniegra, M; Saad, F; Ke, C; Braun, A; Jun, S. Superiority of denosumab to zoledronic

acid for prevention of skeletal-related events: a combined analysis of 3 pivotal, randomised, phase 3 trials. *Eur J Cancer.*, 2012, 48(16), 3082-92.

[182] Voorhees, PM1; Manges, RF; Sonneveld, P; Jagannath, S; Somlo, G; Krishnan, A; Lentzsch, S; Frank, RC; Zweegman, S; Wijermans, PW; Orlowski, RZ; Kranenburg, B; Hall, B; Casneuf, T; Qin, X; van, de, Velde, H; Xie, H; Thomas, SK. A phase 2 multicentre study of siltuximab, an anti-interleukin-6 monoclonal antibody, in patients with relapsed or refractory multiple myeloma. *Br J Haematol.*, 2013, 161(3), 357-66.

[183] San, Miguel, J; Bladé, J; Shpilberg, O; Grosicki, S; Maloisel, F; Min, CK; Polo, Zarzuela, M; Robak, T; Prasad, SV; Goh, YT; Laubach, J; Spencer, A; Mateos, MV; Palumbo, A; Puchalski, T; Reddy, M; Uhlar, C; Qin, X; van de Velde, H; Xie, H; Orlowski, RZ. Randomized, open label, phase 2 study of siltuximab (an anti IL 6 mAb) and bortezomib melphalan prednisone versus bortezomib-melphalan-prednisone in patients with newly diagnosed multiple myeloma. *Blood.*, 2014. pii: blood-2013-12-546374.

[184] Somlo, G; Lashkari, A; Bellamy, W; Zimmerman, TM; Tuscano, JM; O'Donnell, MR; Mohrbacher, AF; Forman, SJ; Frankel, P; Chen, HX; Doroshow, JH; Gandara, DR. Phase II randomized trial of bevacizumab versus bevacizumab and thalidomide for relapsed/refractory multiple myeloma: a California Cancer Consortium trial. *Br J Haematol*, 2011, 154(4), 533-5.

Index

A

B

C

D

E

J

K

L

M

N

O

P

Q

R

S

T

U

V

W

X

Z